MASTERING
Documentation

MASTERING
Documentation

Springhouse Corporation
Springhouse, Pennsylvania

Staff

Executive Director, Editorial
Stanley Loeb

Senior Publisher
Matthew Cahill

Clinical Manager
Cindy Tryniszewski, RN, MSN

Art Director
John Hubbard

Senior Editor
June Norris

Clinical Project Director
Patricia Dwyer Schull, RN, MSN

Clinical Editors
Beverly Tscheschlog, RN; Carol Calianno, RN, BSN; Tina R. Dietrich, RN, BSN; Mary Jane McDevitt, RN, BS

Editors
Edith McMahon (book editor), Crystal Norris, Marylou Ambrose, Neal Fandek, Beth Mauro, Gale Sloan, Elizabeth Weinstein

Copy Editors
Cynthia C. Breuninger (manager), Lynette High, Doris Weinstock, Lewis Adams, Priscilla DeWitt, Jennifer George Mintzer, Nancy Papsin

Designers
Stephanie Peters (associate art director), Lorraine Lostracco Carbo (book designer), Kaaren Mitchel, Susan Hopkins Rodzewich

Typographers
Diane Paluba (manager), Elizabeth Bergman, Joyce Rossi Biletz, Phyllis Marron, Robin Mayer, Valerie Rosenberger

Manufacturing
Deborah Meiris (director), T.A. Landis, Anna Brindisi

Editorial Assistants
Maree DeRosa, Beverly Lane, Mary Madden, Dianne Tolbert

Indexer
Robin Hipple

Printed in the United States of America.

MD-051097

℞ A member of the Reed Elsevier plc group

Library of Congress Cataloging-in-Publication Data

Mastering documentation.
    p.   cm.
Includes bibliographical references and index.
1. Nursing records.   I. Springhouse Corporation.
[DNLM: 1. Nursing Records.   2. Medical Records—nurses' instruction.   3. Documentation—nurses' instruction.   WY 100.5 M423 1994]
RT50.M38   1994
610.73—dc20
DNLM/DLC   94-29557
ISBN 0-87434-749-1   CIP

Contents

Contributors

Dorothy T. Arnold, RN, BSN
Education Coordinator
Neshaminy Manor Home
Doylestown, Pa.

Bonita Largent Cloyd, RN, MSN
Certified Enterostomal Therapist Nurse
Western Baptist Hospital
Paducah, Ky.

Mary C. Crellin, RN, CPHQ
Director of Quality Assurance
Asco Healthcare, Inc.
Columbia, Md.

Marion B. Dolan, RN
President
Heritage Home Health and
Heritage Hospice
Meredith, N.H.

Georgette Fedor, RN, BSN, CCRN
Critical Care Staff Nurse
Doylestown (Pa.) Hospital

Janine Fiesta, BSN, JD
Vice-President, Legal Services and Risk
Management
Lehigh Valley Hospital
Allentown, Pa.

Pamela A. Henderson, RN
Director of Health and Nursing Services
St. Mary's Manor
Lansdale, Pa.

Kathy Malloch, RN, MBA, CNA
Vice-President, Patient Care Services
Del E. Webb Memorial Hospital
Sun City West, Ariz.

Roseanne M. Matricciani, RN, JD
Chief Operating Officer
Medical and Chirurgical Faculty
of Maryland
Baltimore

Edwinna A. McConnell, RN, MSN, PhD
Independent Nurse Consultant
Madison, Wis.

Karen E. Michael, RN, MSN
Case Manager
Greater Atlantic Health Service
Philadelphia

Mary A. Mishler, RN, MSN, CNN, CS
Medical-Surgical Clinical Nurse Specialist
Our Lady of Lourdes Medical Center
Camden, N.J.

Paula L. Rich, RN, MSN
President
Professional Nursing Development
Mountaintop, Pa.

Linda F. Roy, RN, MSN, CCRN
Clinical Education Coordinator
Doylestown (Pa.) Hospital

Carol L. Schaffer, RN, MSN, JD
President and Chief Executive Officer
CCF Health Care Ventures, Inc.
Valley View, Ohio

Frances U. Warwick, RN,C, BSN
Patient Care Director
Doylestown (Pa.) Hospital

Acknowledgments

The publisher and editors thank the following institutions for their help in preparing this book:

Doylestown Hospital
Doylestown, Pa.

Heritage Home Health
Meredith, N.H.

Medical College Hospitals
Bucks County Campus
Warminster, Pa.

Our Lady of Lourdes Medical Center
Camden, N.J.

St. Mary's Manor
Lansdale, Pa.

Foreword

The importance of documentation is unparalleled in health care today. Compiled in various records, documentation is the foremost source of reference and communication among health care professionals. To meet the challenge of delivering ever more specialized care, you must provide and interpret others' detailed information about your patients' condition. And like all members of the health care team, you must record your assessment, interventions, and evaluations in the patient's medical record. This information then spurs health care decisions and subsequent interventions by doctors, nurses, physical therapists, social workers, and others—all charged with ensuring the quality and continuity of patient care.

Several other factors contribute to the current emphasis on documentation. Among the most significant are health care economics (rising costs force providers to streamline services for maximum efficiency), increasingly stringent professional standards, and consumer demand for improved health care.

In nursing alone, documentation requirements multiply daily. Your carefully constructed plan of care must fulfill its objectives and must withstand the scrutiny of third-party reimbursers (insurance companies, Medicare, and Medicaid), the Joint Commission on Accreditation of Healthcare Organizations (JCAHO) and other accrediting bodies and regulatory agencies, and the legal community's malpractice attorneys. In short, accurate documentation is as crucial to the health care industry's well-being as it is to the patient's.

To help you meet these ever-increasing documentation demands, *Mastering Documentation* takes a comprehensive view. This reference provides detailed instructions on charting all aspects of care, employing various methods and charting systems—for patients in various health care settings. Using this text and the more than 100 completely filled-in documentation samples, you'll soon chart confidently at each stage of the nursing process—from assessment through evaluation. You'll streamline your technique for charting any situation requiring written or computerized notations—without sacrificing the detail and accuracy necessary to minimize the risk of malpractice.

Chapter 1, Nursing Documentation and the Medical Record, provides an overview of documentation, discusses the medical record and its components, and reviews the latest trends and social factors that influence your responsibilities in documentation.

Chapter 2, Legal and Ethical Implications of Documentation, addresses the legal relevance of the medical record, the elements of malpractice, risk management, and ethical concerns, with special emphasis on the patient's rights.

Chapter 3, Quality Improvement and Reimbursement, demonstrates documentation as the bridge between the quality of your nursing care and prompt reimbursement by third-party payers.

Chapter 4, Documentation Systems, describes the advantages and disadvantages of virtually all types of documentation systems—traditional narrative, POMR, PIE, Focus, CBE, FACT, Core, Outcome, and computerized charting.

Chapter 5, Documentation Methods, does the same for the many forms and methods used to document care not only in acute care but also in long-term and home care settings.

Chapter 6, Documentation of the Nursing Process, shows you how to precisely record your assessments, nursing diagnoses and expected outcomes, plans of care, interventions, and evaluations.

Chapter 7, Documentation of Everyday Events, presents common clinical situations and samples of accurate charting for the patient's medical record. Situations include medication administration, I.V. therapy, patient noncompliance, codes, and others.

Chapter 8, Legally Perilous Charting Practices, outlines the basics of defensive charting in potentially hazardous, legally threatening situations. Two examples include cautious countersigning of the medical record and chronicling the behavior of problematic patients.

The final chapter, Malpractice Lawsuits, outlines the steps of a malpractice suit, your role in the eyes of the law, and tips for defending yourself on the witness stand.

Throughout *Mastering Documentation,* you'll see examples of correct charting with completed forms and actual phrases and sentences you can use to chart specific situations. Other features for your convenience are logos — graphic symbols that direct your attention to key points. The *Charting guidelines* logo suggests ways to improve your nursing documentation and build a defense against malpractice lawsuits. *Charting timesavers* points out shortcuts to reduce charting time by minutes — even hours — while maintaining accuracy, standards of care, and legal safety. *Better charting* signals a completed form — with handwritten notations — showing you precisely how to document every observation and action during patient care. The *On trial* symbol highlights accounts of actual court cases and legal scenarios that discuss actual or alleged documentation errors by nurses.

Mastering Documentation concludes with a series of appendices spotlighting the abbreviations and symbols commonly used in the medical record, the American Nurses' Association's standards of nursing practice, the North American Nursing Diagnosis Association's taxonomy of nursing diagnoses, the JCAHO's documentation standards, and more.

Even the most experienced nurse will benefit from using *Mastering Documentation.* If you regularly practice the documentation solutions presented here, you can expect to increase your charting skills, accuracy, speed, and confidence and, most important, enhance the quality of your nursing care.

Audrey Stephan, RN, EdD
Assistant Professor of Nursing
Bergen Community College
Paramus, N.J.

CHAPTER ONE

Nursing Documentation and the Medical Record

Broadly speaking, documentation refers to the preparation and maintenance of records that describe a patient's care. If you document with attention to detail, you'll clearly show the quality of care your patient received, the outcome of that care, and the treatment he still needs.

The detailed information you assemble will be scrutinized by many reviewers, including other health care team members; accrediting, certifying, and licensing organizations; quality improvement monitors; peer reviewers; and Medicare and insurance company reviewers. Your documentation may also be examined by attorneys and judges. And researchers and educators may use it to improve patient care and to provide continuing education.

This chapter spells out what you need to document satisfactorily for these reviewers. After summarizing the history of documentation, it describes the development of the medical record and covers the two basic types—source-oriented and problem-oriented. Next, the chapter reviews the principles of sound documentation, including using computers to promote efficiency. It goes on to discuss current nursing documentation requirements and new documentation systems.

Overview of documentation

Traditionally, nurses recorded their *observations* of patients, creating documents only under the direction of doctors. The chief purposes of these documents were to ensure that the doctors' orders had been followed and to demonstrate to the facility that its policies had been observed and all requisite care had been provided.

Charting began as a checklist of cursory observations, noting such details as whether the patient "ate well" or "slept well." Beyond such simple notations, nurses were reluctant to record their own ideas and observations.

Florence Nightingale, the 19th-century British nurse, is customarily regarded as the founder of nursing documentation. In *Notes on Nursing,* she stressed the importance of gathering patient information in a clear, concise, organized manner. As her theories gained acceptance, nurses began to be trained in her concept of lucid, formal nursing documentation. Gradually, nurses' perceptions and observations about patient care gained credence and respect.

Much later, in the 1970s, nurses began creating their own vocabulary for documentation based on nursing diagnoses. However, nursing diagnoses have thus far failed to be the basis for independent reimbursement, and insurance companies and Medicare do not reimburse for nursing services rendered under a nursing diagnosis.

The current reimbursement trend is to compensate nurses, especially nurse practitioners and home health care nurses, for skilled care that meets eligibility requirements. This care includes assessing a patient's condition, creating a plan of care, and following a strict treatment regimen.

More than ever before, nursing documentation plays a vital role in ensuring reimbursement by verifying—and justifying—a nurse's actions.

Understanding the medical record

Typically, a patient's medical record contains many forms, including the initial assessment form, daily assessment flow sheets, problem or nursing diagnosis lists, and other flow sheets. Forms vary with the policies, procedures, and organizational and patient needs in individual health care facilities.

Because of the medical record's complexity, many nurses organize the data by category, placing undue focus on format over content. But a medical record is more than a summary of a patient's illness and recovery. It's an incremental record of a patient's care in a health care facility and a road map of potential patient care problems. The record should be well organized, easy to read, and accessible to all reviewers.

Many nurses approach the medical record with trepidation—needlessly. Think of the medical record as an ally, not an enemy. It serves as a central site for organizing your thoughts about patient care and recording your actions. Used properly, it can help you identify problem areas and plan better patient care.

Nursing documentation makes up one critical part of the complete medical record, which contains contributions from all health care team members. Your contribution has many purposes, including verifying the quality of your care, helping all caregivers to coordinate treatment, ensuring reimbursement, and providing legal protection for you and your employer. (See *Guarding against liability*.)

Guarding against liability

Good documentation should offer legal protection to you, the patient's other caregivers, and the health care facility.

Admissible in court as a legal document, the medical record provides proof of the care received by the patient and the standards by which the care was provided. Medical records typically serve as evidence in disability, personal injury, and mental competency cases. They're also used in malpractice cases. And how and what you document—or don't document—can mean the difference between winning and losing a case, not only for you but also for your employer.

For the best legal protection, make sure that your documentation shows that you not only adhere to professional standards of nursing care but also follow your employer's policies and procedures—especially in high-risk situations.

Purpose of the medical record

The medical record provides evidence of the quality of patient care. The record is used by various groups to help evaluate patient care.

Evidence of the quality of care

To verify the quality of your care, you must describe what you've done for your patient and provide evidence that it was necessary. You also should describe your patient's response to the care and any changes made in his plan of care. And you must be sure to document this information in accordance with professional practice standards—those published by the American Nurses' Association (ANA) and the Joint Commission on Accreditation of Healthcare Organizations (JCAHO), for instance.

Accreditation, certification, and licensure

Organizations, most notably the JCAHO, accredit health care facilities that meet their standards. (Some states also require all health care facilities—including home health care facilities—to become licensed.) Health care facilities need JCAHO accreditation not only to demonstrate that they provide quality care, but also to ensure their eligibility for government funds. The federal government also contracts with state organizations that certify health care facilities as being eligible to receive Medicare reimbursement.

In deciding whether a facility should receive accreditation, an accrediting organization looks at the structure and function of the facility. It also reviews the medical record to ensure that the facility meets the required standards. Then, at regular intervals, the organization checks the facility for compliance. The accrediting organization conducts surveys to assess the standard and quality of care and audits the facility to ensure that it's complying with those standards.

Most accrediting organizations have some common standards for documentation. For example, most require that each patient's medical record contains an assessment, a plan of care, medical orders, progress notes, and a discharge summary. Several organizations even spell out what these components must contain. Then, the nurse-manager must establish and implement documentation guidelines that meet the accrediting organization's requirements. These guidelines should specify the format that must be used as well as the topics that must be covered in the documentation.

Quality assurance and improvement

Mandated by state and JCAHO regulations, quality improvement activities are designed, conducted, and analyzed by designated employees of the health care facility. These employees—including doctors, nurses, pharmacists and administrative personnel—report their findings to their board of trustees.

Quality assurance committees monitor, evaluate, and seek ways to improve the quality of patient care. Committee members develop standards, or indicators, of care. They must choose well-defined, objective, readily measurable indicators that allow them to assess the structure, process, and outcome of patient care. They can then use these indicators to monitor and evaluate the contents of the medical record.

Peer review

Peer review organizations (PROs) are mandated by federal law to evaluate the quality of care in health care facilities. These organizations consist of employees who are paid by the federal government. They evaluate a sample of a health care facility's medical records and compare their findings with established generic standards or *screens*—a list of basic conditions that a group of similar health care facilities should meet. The reviewers use these screens to determine whether the health care facility or particular caregivers provided appropriate care. (See *How PROs evaluate performance*.)

How PROs evaluate performance

Your nursing documentation is vitally important to peer review organizations (PROs), which can fine or sanction a health care facility that fails to provide quality care. Using established screens, the PROs scrutinize medical records to determine whether a health care facility or particular caregivers have provided appropriate patient care. The screens identify the following problem areas.

Necessary admission
Reviewers look at the medical record to determine whether a health care facility justifiably admitted a particular patient and whether the patient received appropriate treatment.

Nosocomial infection
If the reviewers find that a health care facility has an excessive rate of nosocomial infection, for example, they must examine the medical records to determine the causes.

Medical stability
If the record shows that a patient has a pattern of elevated temperature after insertion of an indwelling catheter, reviewers may question whether health care personnel have maintained the patient's medical stability.

Unscheduled returns to surgery
Reviewers are alert for unscheduled surgery—repeat surgery for infection, for example.

Discharge planning
Reviewers check whether the health care facility provides a formal discharge planning process as evidenced by the forms used by that facility.

Avoidable trauma and death
When a patient dies unexpectedly during or after surgery or after a return to the critical care unit within 24 hours of being transferred out of the unit, the PROs must determine if the health care facility could have prevented the death.

If they find that the facility or specific caregivers were negligent, they can discipline those at fault and suggest steps to minimize the recurrence of such incidents.

Medicare complaints
PROs review complaints made by Medicare patients about care received at health care facilities. If they find problems with the quality of care a patient received, they can invoke fines or sanctions or deny reimbursement for care provided.

Reimbursement requirements
Documentation helps determine the amount of reimbursement a health care facility receives. The federal government, for instance, uses a prospective payment system based on diagnosis-related groups (DRGs) to determine its Medicare reimbursements, paying a fixed amount for a particular diagnosis.

For the health care facility to receive payment, the patient's medical record at discharge must contain the correct DRG codes and show that the patient received the proper care. Your documentation should support your nursing diagnoses and indicate that appropriate patient teaching and discharge planning were provided.

Faulty documentation can have a direct impact on the amount of reimbursement a facility receives. For example, a home health care agency can be denied payment retroactively for home care visits deemed unreasonable and unnecessary—a determination strongly influenced by documentation.

Numerous patients have been discharged from home health care plans because the payer would no longer agree to pay for improperly documented care. This has the added negative effect of denying patients the care they need. (For more information, see Chapter 3, Quality Improvement and Reimbursement.)

Organization of the medical record

The basic methods of organizing the medical record include the traditional source-oriented narrative record and the more innovative problem-oriented medical record. Each health care facility selects the method—or a variation of it—that best suits its needs.

Source-oriented narrative record

This method requires members of each discipline—the sources—to record information in a separate section of the medical record, which is its main drawback. Segregating entries according to discipline discourages communication among personnel. The reader must consult various parts of the record to gain a complete picture of the patient's care.

Another problem of this type of documentation is its lack of coordination. Information is disjointed, topics are seldom clearly identified, and data are difficult to retrieve.

To allow you to determine a patient's progress more easily, progress notes can be grouped together with a different color page for each discipline. To retrieve information more readily, nursing documentation can be organized with Focus charting and PIE (*Problem-Intervention-Evaluation*) charting, both explained in Chapter 4, Documentation Systems.

Problem-oriented medical record

This type of record consists of baseline data, a problem list, a plan of care for each problem, and progress notes. Baseline data, which are obtained from all departments involved in patient care, focus on the patient's present complaints and illness.

The information gathered relates to the patient's social and emotional status, medical status, health history, initial assessment findings, and diagnostic test results. A problem list is then distilled from this baseline to construct a plan of care. The plan of care addresses each of the patient's problems, which are routinely updated both in the plan of care and in the part of the medical record known as progress notes. (See *What makes up the medical record?*)

Other formats

Some health care facilities may adapt the source-oriented or problem-oriented organization to better meet their documentation needs. This places you in the position

What makes up the medical record?

Each health care facility has its own medical record-keeping system, typically composed of the documents named below. Depending on the patient's needs, the medical record may include some or all of these items.

Face sheet
The first page of the medical record, this form includes information identifying the patient by name, birth date, social security number, address, and marital status. It also lists his closest relative or guardian, food or drug allergies, admitting diagnosis, assigned diagnosis-related group, and the attending doctor.

Medical history and physical examination
Completed by the doctor, this form contains the patient's initial medical examination and evaluation data.

Initial nursing assessment form
This document contains nursing data including the health history and physical assessment findings.

Doctor's order sheet
This is the record of the doctor's medical orders.

Problem or nursing diagnosis list
Known as a problem list or a nursing diagnosis list in health care facilities that follow the problem-oriented medical record system, this record lists the patient's problems. Some health care facilities list nursing diagnoses on a separate form.

Nursing plan of care
This is a statement of the nurse's plan of patient care. Usually included with the basic medical record forms, it's sometimes kept in a separate folder at the nurses' station until the patient's discharge.

Graphic sheet
Known by various titles assigned by the health care facility, this graph is a type of flow sheet that tracks the patient's temperature, pulse rate, respiratory rate, blood pressure and, possibly, daily weight. Additional graphic sheets may be designed for recording such information as skin care, blood glucose levels, urinalysis results, neurologic assessment data, and patient intake and output. These forms usually allow you to show that you've completed a certain task or assessment by simply dating, initialing, or checking off the appropriate column.

Medication administration record
This document contains a record of each medication a patient receives, including the dosage and the administration route, site, date, and time.

Nurses' progress notes
This record details patient care information, nursing interventions, and the patient's responses.

Doctors' progress notes
Like the nurses' progress notes, this record contains the doctor's observations and notes on the patient's progress. It includes treatment data as well.

(continued)

What makes up the medical record? *(continued)*

Diagnostic findings
These forms contain diagnostic and laboratory data—for example, hematology, pathology, radiology, and X-ray test results.

Health care team records
This part of the medical record includes information from such professional personnel as the physical therapist, respiratory therapist, and social worker.

Consultation sheets
These forms include evaluations made by doctors, clinical specialists, and others consulted for diagnostic and treatment recommendations.

Discharge plan and summary
This document presents a brief account of the patient's time in the health care facility and plans for care after discharge. Pertinent data may include dietary and medication instructions and follow-up medical appointments or referrals.

to influence the type and style of documentation you'll provide for the medical record. Keep in mind that your documentation should clearly reflect the essential quality of the nursing care you deliver every day.

In home health care settings, for example, nurses have created many documentation forms—including the initial assessment form, problem list, day-visit sheet, and discharge summary to better reflect the services and essential quality of care provided. These forms were designed to meet the nurse's documentation needs while at the same time complying with state and federal laws and other regulations.

Elements of sound documentation

Sound documentation demonstrates a logical approach to problem solving. Nursing documentation typically begins with assessment data, which provide a baseline definition of the patient's health care needs or problems currently and throughout hospitalization. Next, nursing documentation provides evidence that patient care has been planned, and it continues by reflecting nursing interventions and the patient's response and progress.

Essentially, effective documentation is a systematic, accurate, well-written account of nursing practice. To produce sound documentation, you'll need to set aside time for completing charts and other forms. Try to schedule a regular time for charting so that your records are current and up-dated. And you'll need to use proper forms to ensure accuracy and consistency.

Legible and clearly written charts that demonstrate professionalism and diligence will withstand litigation, ensure reimbursement, and satisfy reviewer requirements of the medical record.

Besides learning and applying documentation fundamentals, mastering documentation skills may involve improving existing documentation habits, using more efficient methods, adopting new systems, and applying new technology to documentation.

Of course, your documentation requirements will differ depending on where you work—in a hospital, nursing home, home health care agency, or other community facility. For instance, perioperative, critical, and emergency care areas have specialized criteria and forms for documenting nursing care. And requirements may change depending on the patient population—for example, requirements in obstetric settings differ from those in geriatric settings.

Three C's

Documentation is both demanding and complex, a professional challenge for novice and expert alike. When documenting, remember the three C's of good charting—*c*larity, *c*onciseness, and *c*onsistency. Be sure to use correct spelling and approved abbreviations and symbols, avoid altering notations, and make legible and neat entries. Include your signature along with the date and time of posting.

Documentation should demonstrate the nursing process—from assessment, nursing diagnosis, and planning care to nursing interventions and evaluation. Your documentation should also demonstrate pre-charting plans (such as the nursing plan of care, Kardex, or activity sheets). What's more, it must comply with standards established by accrediting and licensing organizations, state and federal agencies, insurance companies, and your health care facility.

Efficient methods

To ensure thoroughness and accuracy, adopt efficient documentation methods. Such methods may include tape-recorded dictation and transcription services; computerized documentation; and special charting forms, such as standardized flow sheets, checklists, admission forms, initial care plans, and progress notes. These methods support data about the intensity of nursing care and the patient's condition, provide formats that help you make precise entries, and supply information that can be retrieved at a glance.

New systems

Several effective documentation systems currently in use were developed to respond to the expanded purposes and functions of the medical record—a result of the changes within the health care delivery system and the technologic advances in health care.

Each record-keeping system has advantages, disadvantages, and distinguishing features that may make it more or less suitable for a given situation. A documentation system known as charting-by-exception (CBE), for example, is most appropriate for summarizing patient care, whereas a system known as Focus charting is better suited for reporting a patient's rapidly changing condition.

Charting by computer

Today, computers play an increasing role in completing the medical record from admission through discharge. The benefits of computerized charting include greater legibility, fewer errors, decreased recording time and costs, improved communication among health care team members, and greater access to medical data for education, research, and quality improvement.

Nursing plans of care, progress notes, medication records, vital signs records, intake and output sheets, and patient classifications may be filed on computers. Some hospitals have installed bedside workstations to allow quick entry of information and access to it.

Additional developments may be forthcoming as nurses are being consulted by software companies. In all likelihood, more hospitals will adopt automated charting as computer equipment becomes less expensive and more accessible.

An effective automated documentation system must feature the capacity to:
• record and send data to the appropriate department
• adapt easily to the health care facility's needs
• display highly selective information on command
• provide easy access and retrieval for all trained personnel.

Nursing informatics

In acknowledging the importance of computers in nursing, the ANA has recognized a field known as nursing informatics as an area of specialization.

Nursing informatics aims to standardize documentation; improve communication; support decision making; develop and share new knowledge; enhance the quality, effectiveness, and efficiency of health care; and advance the science of nursing through the use of data, information, and knowledge.

Requirements of nursing documentation

State and professional organizations mandate certain documentation requirements. Some requirements are incorporated into laws, such as nurse practice acts, which vary from state to state. Other requirements—for example, accountability or a health care facility's documentation policies—are not mandated by law but are accepted under the general scope of nursing as practiced today.

Adherence to nurse practice acts

Nurse practice acts are state laws designating the activities that each nurse can perform in that state. Cumulative changes in the regulations that govern nursing have resulted in redefinitions or revisions of the acts in many states. Trends point to substantial revisions of existing documentation requirements in nurse practice acts. Today, state regulations consider nurses to be managers of care as well as practitioners.

These and other revisions in state laws and regulations require that complete descriptions of nursing judgment and provision of care be documented in nurses' records as evidence of compliance with standards.

Accountability

Proper nursing documentation provides evidence that you have acted as required or ordered. You must demonstrate your accountability by complying with the documenting requirements established by your health care facility, professional organizations, and state law.

Policies affecting documentation

Usually, health care facilities establish documentation policies that meet the requirements of insurance agencies and accrediting bodies. A facility's board of trustees typically appoints a committee to investigate various documentation systems and to make recommendations—for example, on adopting a particular format and style of documentation.

The health care facility may then move to adopt or modify a system to support its goals and preserve its accreditation and licenses.

Meeting requirements in special settings

In certain health care environments—acute or critical care, long-term care, intermediate care, or home care, for example—documentation requirements may be considerably more demanding. In such environments, take extra care to review your facility's documentation policies and follow them accurately.

Acute or critical care

Generally, documentation policies in acute or critical care settings require you to record nursing interventions, patient responses, and patient outcomes. Much of critical care unit documentation is entered on flow sheets accompanied by brief commentary or critical data, such as an electrocardiogram.

Long-term and intermediate care

These settings offer more time to document but less flexibility. State laws and Medicare's conditions of participation determine a great deal of what you must record. Some institutions choose the CBE documentation system for these settings.

Home care

Again, Medicare's conditions of participation strongly influence the documentation required. To increase efficiency and avoid licensing, accreditation, and reimbursement difficulties, most health care facilities have abandoned narrative notes in favor of individualized visit sheets and physical discomfort forms. (See *Charting home care in the electronic era,* page 12.)

Understanding length of stay and patient awareness

As the average patient's length of hospitalization declines, documentation must include all exceptional problems and interventions. This becomes particularly important when reimbursing agents and insurance companies insist on evidence to support a patient's extended stay in the health care facility.

Charting home care in the electronic era

Some home care agencies have embraced computer charting in a "small" way. Growing in popularity are computer notebooks—portable devices combining hardware and software—that generate and complete standardized documentation forms at the press of a finger or a probe.

Speeding reimbursement
Such equipment can handle the more routine aspects of charting and offers uniformity and thoroughness to ensure timely updates and speedy reimbursement.

Cutting down on paperwork
This technology also speeds and streamlines paperwork for the home care agency. In the past, completing certain charts and other paperwork were the sole responsibility of the office nurse-manager. She would review the field nurse's written information, apply it to accepted reimbursement tables and the health care agency's internal forms, and send the data to the appropriate office for processing.

Today, the properly equipped field nurse can obtain the appropriate data and complete the necessary forms during her health care visit by using a hand-held computer.

Patient awareness also influences documentation. Patients today are increasingly aware of the nurse's role in documenting and the patient's right to view the medical record. More and more patients may ask you for a copy of the medical record. Though the patient is entitled to this information, of course, you should always consult your legal department or attorney for advice. Keep in mind that the request for these documents may be preliminary to a lawsuit.

Understanding utilization review

Reimbursing agents maintain control over health care providers through utilization review programs that focus on length of hospital stay, treatment regimen, validation of diagnostic tests and procedures, and verification that medical supplies and equipment were used. To determine if utilization is proper, they commonly rely on nursing documentation.

Among specific data you may need to document (to comply with utilization review policy) are the type and quantity of I.V. needles, infusion pumps, drains, tubes, and other equipment that you've used. Usually, doctors don't record their use of supplies. Utilization review policies can also affect where treatment occurs—in the hospital, doctor's office, or patient's home, for example.

Documentation formats and trends

Because narrative charting takes considerable time but rarely provides a quantifiable measure of a patient's condition, some health care facilities have implemented more efficient documentation systems. Among them are SOAP charting, the CBE method, Focus charting, computerized record keeping, and others. (For detailed information, see Chapter 4, Documentation Systems.)

Choosing formats

Briefly, specific documentation systems offer specific advantages in specific situations. For example, SOAP charting, a vital component of the problem-oriented medical record, organizes record keeping by *S*ubjective, *O*bjective, *A*ssessment, and *P*lanning data. A variation, SOAPIE charting, adds two more categories: *I*ntervention and *E*valuation. CBE documentation saves you time by requiring you to enter notes in the patient's chart only to record exceptional circumstances, and Focus charting provides a specific structure for progress notes.

Recognizing trends

By the early 1990s, handwritten plans of care came to be regarded as a thing of the past. The JCAHO no longer requires a formal plan of care, concluding that it doesn't necessarily affect patient outcomes. As a result, new documentation tools have arisen, including standardized plans of care, critical pathways, and patient-out-come time lines. What's more, the increased use of computers, fax machines, and other technologies are changing the way you'll document the plan of care.

Standardized plans of care

Today, standardized plans of care or case maps that correspond with a DRG or other guidelines are growing in use. Specifically, the emphasis is on concise plans of care that reflect the patient's needs. Here, home health care nurses are on the cutting edge because Medicare's conditions of participation require that plans of care be tailored to specific patient needs.

Critical pathways

A merger of medical and nursing plans of care, critical pathways outline such key elements as expected patient outcomes, essential medical and nursing interventions, and other patient variables for each DRG. Doctors and nurses are each responsible for establishing a care track, or case map, for each DRG. The care track defines a patient's daily care requirements and desired outcomes, consistent with the average length of stay for the specified DRG.

Patient-outcome time lines

Another valuable documentation tool, the patient-outcome time line allows all practitioners to note essential diagnostic tests, interventions, patient outcomes, and other parameters to attain the average length of stay for each DRG.

For example, the patient-outcome time line for a patient who's had abdominal surgery might recommend that he be out of bed and into a chair the day after surgery and walking in the hallway 4 days after surgery. This plan will also list key interventions needed to achieve the expected outcomes and will be used to monitor the patient's progress during each shift.

Technologic advances

In the near future, charting by discipline will probably be replaced by a computerized medical record reflecting a collaborative overview of a patient's care. Because the data will be recorded on computerized flow sheets, information will be more accessible, with much of the vital data displayed on graphs for easy interpretation.

One handy channel of information is already in widespread use—the fax machine. Home health care agencies communicate with their nurses mainly by fax, and this efficient mode of communicating information will likely carry over into most areas of nursing.

Charting will continue to change rapidly—which makes it all the more essential for you to understand and explore new approaches as documentation systems become more efficient and improve communication among health care personnel.

New technology—and new ways of organizing your observations—should help you save time, eliminate confusion and, most of all, improve patient care.

Selected references

Joint Commission on Accreditation of Healthcare Organizations. *1994 Accreditation Manual for Hospitals.* Oakbrook Terrace, Ill.: Joint Commission on Accreditation of Healthcare Organizations, 1993.

Atkinson, L.D., and Murray, M.E. *Understanding the Nursing Process: Fundamentals of Care Planning,* 4th ed. New York: Pergamon Press, 1990.

Fiesta, J. *Twenty Legal Pitfalls for Nurses to Avoid.* Albany, N.Y.: Delmar Publishers, Inc., 1994.

Iyer, P.W. "New Trends in Charting," *Nursing91* 21(1):48-50, January 1991.

Sinioris, M.E. "TQM: The New Frontier for Quality and Productivity Improvement in Health Care," *Journal of Quality Assurance, 12*(4), 14-17, 1990.

Legal and Ethical Implications of Documentation

As your professional responsibility grows, so does your accountability. And with increased accountability comes awareness. In today's health care environment, you know that keeping accurate records is more important than ever before. Your documentation demonstrates that the patient care you provide meets not only the needs and expressed wishes of your patient, but also the accepted standards of nursing care that are mandated by law, your profession, and the health care facility in which you practice.

While your records protect you, they're also one of the best instruments for communicating important clinical information to caregivers. Failure to document appropriately is a key factor in clinical mishaps and a pivotal issue in many malpractice cases as well.

Knowing what your legal and ethical obligations are and careful documenting to show that the care you provide meets these obligations are the keys to conveying information and protecting yourself legally.

This chapter discusses the important issues involved when documenting your patient's condition and your nursing care. These include the legal relevance of the medical record; malpractice litigation; how policies and procedures affect legal decisions; the nature of support programs, such as risk management and quality improvement programs; and important ethical considerations in patient care.

Legal relevance of medical records

Accurately and completely documenting the nature and quality of your nursing care helps the other members of the health care team confirm their impressions of the patient's condition and progress—or points out the need for adjustments in the therapeutic regimen. This clinical account of a patient's condition, treatment, and responses is also used as evidence in the courtroom—for example, in malpractice suits, workers' compensation litigation, and personal injury cases.

Intent of documentation

To be sure, the number of medical records that appear in court are miniscule compared with the number you deal with daily. If you think of the medical record first and foremost as a clinical communication that you documented carefully, you needn't panic if the court subpoenas it. However, if you think only of legal implications or document to protect yourself, your part of the medical record will sound self-serving and defensive. Such documentation tends to have a negative impact on a judge and jury.

Standards of documentation

Ideally, what nursing information appears in a medical record isn't dictated by standards set by the courts. It is governed by standards developed over the years by the nursing profession.

Documentation that meets these standards communicates the patient's status, medical treatment, and nursing care. Professional organizations such as the American Nurses' Association (ANA) have established that documentation must be systematic, continuous, accessible, communicated, recorded, and readily available to all members of the health care team. The ANA sets specific standards for most of the nursing specialties.

Although documentation goals have changed little since their inception, documentation methods have changed greatly. For example, most nurses no longer need to spend valuable time writing long narrative notes. Instead, today's nurses have devised flow sheets, graphic records, and checklists to ease and speed the flow of significant clinical information. In malpractice cases, the courts recognize several different documentation systems as long as the system provides comprehensive, factual information relevant to the patient's care.

Malpractice litigation

Though you document first to convey information, never lose sight of documentation's legal import. Depending on how well you administer care and record your activities and observations, the records may or may not support a plaintiff's accusation of nursing malpractice. Legally, malpractice focuses on these four elements: duty, breach of duty, damage, and causation.

Duty and breach of duty

The terms duty and breach of duty refer to your obligation to provide patient care and to follow appropriate standards. The courts have ruled that a nurse has a *duty* to provide care once a nurse-patient relationship is established. The relationship may be established in person—at admission, for example—or at a distance—during a telephone conversation, for example. (Therefore, even telephone calls need careful documentation, especially with outpatient care on the rise.)

Breach of duty can be difficult to prove because nursing responsibilities typically overlap those of doctors and other health care providers. A key question to ask when investigating a breach of duty is this: "How would a reasonable, prudent nurse with comparable training and experience have acted in the same or similar circumstances?" In judging a nurse guilty of breach of duty, the courts must prove that she failed to provide the appropriate care, as they did in the following case.

In *Collins v. Westlake Community Hospital*, 312 N.E. 2d 614 (Ill. 1974), a 6-year-old boy was hospitalized for a fractured leg, which was put in a cast and placed in traction. Although the doctor ordered the nurse on duty to monitor the condition of the boy's toes, the medical record didn't contain evidence that she did so. In fact, 7 hours elapsed between documented nursing entries in the medical record. The boy's leg was later amputated, and the parents sued.

Because a nurse is responsible for continually assessing patients and because documentation of these assessments didn't appear in the record, the nurse was found guilty of breach of duty.

On the other hand, no breach of duty was found in *Stone v. Sisters of Charity of House of Providence*, 469 P. 2d 229 (Washington 1970), in which the court ruled that constant patient monitoring by nurses is unreasonable. In this case, a nurse decided to change the abdominal binder of a postoperative patient. After the nurse removed the binder and left the room to get a clean one, the patient felt an urge to cough and tried to call the nurse back, but she didn't hear him.

When the nurse returned 5 minutes later, the patient had coughed, causing a dehiscence that required additional surgery. The court ruled that no breach of duty occurred. It was not convinced that the binder would have contained the patient's wound (whether or not he coughed) or that the nurse's presence would have prevented either the coughing or the dehiscence.

Damage and causation

Once the plaintiff establishes a breach of duty, he must then prove that the breach caused his injury. (See *Failing to monitor and review the record.*) Of the four malpractice factors, causation is the most difficult to prove, as the case below illustrates.

Lenger v. Physicians' General Hospital, Inc., 455 S.W. 2d 730 (Texas 1970), involved a patient who mistakenly received trays of solid food for three meals after a colon resection. Although the patient questioned the type of diet and asked the nurse to call the doctor, the nurse refused, saying that she didn't want to bother him. She assured the patient that the food wouldn't have been sent if it wasn't appropriate for him to eat. Although the patient did require a second operation, he couldn't prove that the solid food had caused the complication.

Policies, procedures, and the law

While most discussions about documentation center on writing in the patient's chart, other types of documentation also affect nurses. One example is the documentation of policies and procedures contained in health care facility employee and nursing manuals. Deviation from these rules suggests that an employee failed to meet the facility's standards of care.

Whether such policies establish a standard of care has been debated in some malpractice cases. But in *every* nursing malpractice case, the actions of the nurse are compared with the appropriate nursing standard of care. The jury measures the nurse's actions or omissions against the performance of a reasonable, prudent nurse with comparable training and experience, using regularly updated, national minimum standards as guidelines.

Keep in mind, however, that the defense can always challenge the presumption of the standard—by introducing expert testimony among other strategies.

Cases involving health care facility policy

A classic example of a policy setting the standard of care occurred in *Utter v. United Hospital Center, Inc.*, 236 S.E. 2d 313 (West Virginia 1977). The hospital's nursing manual stated that a nurse who

Failing to monitor and review the record

The following case shows how failing to monitor and review the record can cause the patient harm, lead to litigation, and result in a ruling of nursing negligence. In *Sanchez v. Bay General Hospital,* 172 Cal. Rptr. 342 (California Ct. App 1981), a patient's family proved several areas of damage because of nursing negligence. In 1975, Mrs. Sanchez entered Bay General Hospital for an elective laminectomy. Before the surgery, the doctor implanted an atrial catheter to minimize the chance that an air embolism would form in the patient's heart.

Nursing errors
After Mrs. Sanchez was transferred to the postanesthesia unit, the nurses made several errors. According to the medical record, they:
• failed to take vital signs
• neglected to perform neurologic examinations
• failed to review the chart and therefore assumed that the atrial catheter was a peripheral I.V. line.

Later, when the patient began vomiting and complaining of pain, the nurses didn't call the doctor.

When the patient was transferred to her room, the neglect continued. Finally, the patient went into cardiac arrest. The emergency department doctor who responded didn't recognize the atrial catheter for what it was and injected medication through it. The medication was delivered directly to Mrs. Sanchez's heart. Mrs. Sanchez then experienced brain death.

Her actual death occurred after the cuff of a tracheostomy tube eroded through the back of her trachea and damaged an artery, causing her to bleed to death.

The Sanchez children sued the hospital for the wrongful death of their mother, and the jury awarded them $400,000. The court held the nurses negligent for failing to monitor the patient, for failing to notify the doctor of significant signs and symptoms, and for failing to review the patient's record to learn that an atrial catheter was in place. The nurses also failed in their responsibility to identify the atrial line for the doctor responding to the emergency. Later, they failed to provide standard care required for a tracheostomy tube.

In this claim, the plaintiffs proved duty, breach of duty, damages, and causation.

has any doubts or questions about a patient's care should contact the attending doctor. If the question isn't resolved, then the nurse should call the department chairperson. In this case, a patient's arm, which was in a cast, became progressively swollen, black, and edematous; it also emitted a foul-smelling drainage. The patient had a high fever, was delirious at

times, and couldn't retain oral antibiotics. Although the patient's nurse called the doctor and reported these signs and symptoms, the doctor didn't visit the patient or prescribe treatment. The nurse took no further action. The patient's arm had to be amputated at the shoulder.

The doctor testified that the nurse notified him that the patient's condition had worsened, but he didn't recall her reporting either the foul-smelling drainage or the delirium. He said that had he known about these conditions, he would have taken action immediately. The court ruled in favor of the patient and against the nurse, saying that the nurse's duty was to observe her patient's condition and to take a positive course of action if it worsened. The nurse failed to provide the standard care required by hospital policy.

In another case related to a health care facility's policies, the court was pressed to distinguish between a hospital's policies and goals.

In *H.C.A. Health Services v. National Bank,* 1745 S.W. 2d 120 (Ark. 1988), three nurses were working in a nursery comprising three connecting rooms. After report, one nurse cared for a baby in the first (admissions) room. The other two nurses went into the second room, which housed 11 babies (two of whom were premature and one of whom was jaundiced). For 1½ hours, none of the nurses went into the third room, which had six babies. When the first nurse finally entered the third room, she found that one of the infants had stopped breathing and had no heartbeat.

Both the hospital's executive director and the nurse who found the baby testified that, according to the hospital's manual, no infant is ever to be left alone without a member of the nursery staff present. However, they also testified that this was a goal—not a policy. Another doctor testified that the baby's problem would have been avoided if a nurse had been present. The court disagreed with the distinction between policies and goals and ruled against the hospital and nurses and in favor of the plaintiff.

A policy doesn't even have to be in writing to be considered a policy. In *Hartman v. Riverside Methodist Hospital,* 577 N.E. 2d 112 (Ohio 1989), a patient needed emergency surgery, even though she had a full stomach. After transferring the patient to the postanesthesia unit, the anesthetist informed the patient's nurse about the patient's full stomach so that she could take precautions to prevent aspiration, such as not administering a sedative. During the patient's stay in the postanesthesia unit, the patient's nurse did administer pain medication without obtaining the doctor's approval and, unfortunately, the patient did aspirate and die. Although the doctor's policy on medication wasn't written, the court held that it was a valid policy.

Risk management: Outgrowth of documentation

Sometimes documentation reveals potential problems within a health care facility. For example, perhaps a particular procedure repeatedly leads to patient injury or another type of accident. To reduce preventable injuries and accidents and minimize financial loss, health care facilities have instituted risk management programs. In the past, these programs concentrated on maintaining and improving facilities and equipment and ensuring employee, visitor, and patient safety.

Today, however, risk management (and quality improvement) efforts focus on identifying, evaluating, and reducing the risk of patient injury in specialty units, such as general surgery and obstetrics, because these areas represent the greatest malpractice risks.

Preventing adverse events

The primary objectives of a risk management program are:
• to reduce the frequency of preventable injuries and accidents leading to liability claims by maintaining or improving quality of care
• to decrease the chance of a claim being filed by promptly identifying and following up on adverse events (incidents)
• to help control costs related to claims by identifying trouble spots early and intervening with the patient and his family.

Early warning systems

A key part of a risk management program involves developing a system for identifying adverse events that are an abnormal consequence of a patient's condition or treatment and that precede a potential lawsuit. These events may or may not be caused by a health care provider's breach of duty or the standard of care.

Such warning systems are crucial. They permit early investigation and intervention, which help minimize additional adverse consequences and legal action. They also provide valuable data bases for building strategies to prevent repeated incidents.

The most common early warning systems are known as occurrence reporting and occurrence screening.

Occurrence reporting

In *occurrence reporting,* certain criteria are used to define events that must be reported by doctors, nurses, or other hospi-

tal staff either when they're observed or shortly after. Examples of such events include the unplanned return of a patient to the operating room or a medication error requiring intervention.

Occurrence screening

In contrast, *occurrence screening* techniques flag adverse events through a review of all or some of the medical charts. These reviews use generic criteria (such as a nosocomial infection or medication error). More specific reviews may focus on specialty- or service-specific criteria, such as an incorrect sponge count during surgery.

Over the years, generic and focused criteria have been developed for reporting and screening systems, and a growing body of literature exists to compare the effectiveness of various approaches.

Although these early warning systems pinpoint much useful information, they aren't effective without a strong organizational structure; the commitment of key staff (such as doctors, nurses, administrators, and chiefs of high-risk services, such as perinatal care) to analyze the information; and cooperation between risk management and quality improvement departments.

Of great importance is bringing adverse events to the attention of the appropriate clinical chairperson, who may then talk with the staff member involved or study the medical records more closely. If a particularly serious event or pattern of events occurs, he may recommend remedial education, required proctoring, or restricted privileges.

Legal & Ethical Implications

Coordinated risk management and quality improvement

Rather than support two separate programs, many health care facilities now coordinate their risk management and quality improvement programs to ensure that they fulfill their legal duty to provide reasonable care. In so doing, the facility may also coordinate the programs' educational efforts—for example, in reaching out to a specific employee, such as a nurse or doctor, who's been identified as having a particular problem or to a larger population, such as new residents and nurses.

The health care facility places high priority on teaching new residents and nurses about risk management and quality improvement. Required teaching topics for new employees are malpractice claims, staff members' particular reporting obligations, proper informational and reporting channels, and principles of risk management and quality improvement.

Keep in mind, however, that a coordinated system usually continues its dual focus on different aspects of health care delivery. Risk management focuses on the patients' and families' perception of the care provided, and quality improvement focuses on the role of the health care provider.

A hospital's reputation for safe, reliable, effective service is its primary defense against liability claims. Systematic, well-coordinated risk management and quality improvement demonstrate to the public that the hospital is being managed in a legally responsible manner. When complaints do arise, risk managers handle them promptly to contain the damage and minimize liability claims.

Documenting adverse events

Despite risk management and other programs, adverse events, such as incidents, do occur.

Sources of information

In investigating an adverse event, incident reports (sometimes called occurrence reports) have been a primary source of information for identifying health care dangers or trends and for attorneys involved in potential lawsuits. Other sources of information are equally important.

Nurses

Nurses are typically the first to recognize potential problems because they spend so much time with patients and their families. They can identify patients who are dissatisfied with their care and particularly those with complications that may result in injuries.

Patient representatives

Another information source is the patient representative's office, which keeps a file of patient complaints. The representatives are trained to identify litigious patients; they also maintain communications with the patient and his family after an incident has occurred.

Business and related offices

Additional sources of information are the business office and the medical records department. Sometimes, a patient may decide to sue after he receives his bill. Or, the first clue of an impending lawsuit may be a patient's or attorney's request for a copy of the medical record. Highly dissatisfied patients may also be known to social workers, hospital clergy, volunteers, and patient escorts.

Reports from the engineering department about the safety of the hospital environment and from purchasing, biomedical engineering, and the pharmacy on the safety and adequacy of products and equipment are also informative.

Of course, reports from all sources should be documented thoroughly. For nurses, this means charting on the patient's medical record and filling out an incident report.

Managing adverse events

Once the risk manager learns of a potential or actual lawsuit, he notifies the medical records department and the hospital's insurance carrier. The medical records department makes copies of the patient's chart and files the original in a secure place to prevent tampering.

A claim notice should also trigger a quality improvement–peer review of the medical record. This review may be conducted by the chairperson of the department involved, the risk management or quality improvement department, or an external reviewer to measure the health care provider's conduct against the professional standards of conduct for the particular situation.

The reasonable professional standard required for a successful defense isn't necessarily the same as the hospital's optimal, high-quality standard. This review helps the risk manager investigate the claim's merit and also helps to define the hospital's responsibility for care in particular situations.

Filing an incident report

Incident reports are continually being revised, and some may be computerized. If these newer incident reports don't allow enough space to fully describe an incident, nurses can usually attach an additional page of comments. (See *Tips for writing an incident report*, page 24, and *Completing an incident report*, pages 25 to 27.) Note that computer processing permits classifying and counting of incidents to indicate trends.

Completing progress notes

When documenting the incident in the patient's medical record, keep the following in mind:

• Write a factual account of the incident, including the treatment and follow-up care provided and the patient's response. If you don't document the incident, the plaintiff's lawyer might think that you're hiding something. This documentation shows that the patient was closely monitored after the incident. If the case goes to court, the jury may be asked to determine if the patient received appropriate care after the incident.

• Don't write "incident report completed" after discussing the event. This destroys the confidential nature of the report and may result in a lawsuit. If a doctor writes an order for an incident report to be completed, ask him not to do this for the same reason.

• Include in the progress notes and in the incident report anything the patient or his family says about their role in the incident. For example, you might write: "Patient stated, 'The nurse told me to ask for help before I went to the bathroom, but I decided to go on my own.'"

This kind of statement helps the defense attorney prove that the patient was guilty of contributory or comparative neg-

Tips for writing an incident report

If a malpractice suit reached the courtroom in years past, the plaintiff's attorney wasn't allowed to see incident reports (administrative records of adverse events affecting a patient of the health care facility). Today, however, the plaintiff in many states is legally entitled to a record of the incident if he requests it through proper channels.

When writing an incident report, keep in mind the people who may read it and follow these guidelines.

Write objectively
Record the details of the incident in objective terms, describing exactly what you saw and heard. For example, unless you actually saw a patient fall, write: "Found patient lying on the floor." Then describe only the actions you took to provide care at the scene, such as helping the patient get back into bed or assessing him for injuries.

Include only essential information
Document the exact time and place of the incident and the name of the doctor who was notified.

Avoid opinions
Don't commit your opinions to writing in the incident report. Rather, verbally share your suggestions or opinions on how an incident may be avoided with your supervisor and risk manager.

Assign no blame
Don't admit to liability or blame or point your finger at colleagues or administrators. Steer clear of such statements as "Better staffing would have prevented this incident." Only state what happened.

Avoid hearsay and assumptions
Each staff member who knows about the incident should write a separate report. If one of your patients is injured in another department, the staff in that department is responsible for documenting the details of the incident.

File the report properly
Don't file the incident report with the medical record. Send the report to the person designated to review it according to your hospital's policy.

---

ligence. Contributory negligence is conduct that contributed to the patient's injuries. Comparative negligence involves determining the percentage of each party's fault. For example, the nurse might be found 25% negligent and the patient, 75% negligent.

The law and you

Claims data support the perception that lawsuits naming the nurse as a specific defendant continue to increase. The expanding role of nurses and the breakdown of the nurse-patient relationship are major

(Text continues on page 28.)

BETTER CHARTING

Completing an incident report

When you witness a reportable event, you must fill out an incident report. Forms vary, but most include the following information.

INCIDENT REPORT

Name of person

Raymond Thomas

Address

18 N. Central, Chicago, Ill. 60612

Date of report	Date of incident	Time of incident	If ED patient, give unit number.
1/10/95	*1/10/95*	*1800*	

LOCATION OF INCIDENT
- ☑ patient room
- ☐ patient bathroom
- ☐ OR
- ☐ ED
- ☐ hospital grounds
- ☐ nurses' station
- ☐ other _____

IDENTIFICATION
- ☑ inpatient
- ☐ ED patient
- ☐ outpatient
- ☐ employee

- ☐ volunteer
- ☐ visitor
- ☐ other _____

Admitting diagnosis of patient
CHF

CONDITION BEFORE INCIDENT

Level of consciousness (previous 4 hours)
- ☑ alert
- ☐ confused, disoriented
- ☐ uncooperative
- ☐ sedated (drug: ____)
- ☐ unconscious

Ambulation
- ☐ OOB
- ☑ OOB with assistance
- ☐ bed rest with BRP
- ☐ complete bed rest
- ☐ not specified
- ☐ other (specify) _____

Side rails
- ☐ up
- ☑ partially up
- ☐ down

Restraints
present ☐ yes ☑ no
ordered ☐ yes ☑ no

Call button within reach
- ☑ yes
- ☐ no

Bed height
- ☐ high
- ☑ low

NATURE OF INCIDENT

Fall
- ☐ while ambulatory
- ☑ while sitting
  - ☐ chair
  - ☑ commode
- ☐ from bed
- ☐ off table, stretcher, or equipment
- ☐ found on floor
- ☐ other _____

Medication
- ☐ error in patient identification
- ☐ incorrect drug
- ☐ incorrect dosage
- ☐ incorrect route
- ☐ timing
- ☐ duplication
- ☐ omission
- ☐ incorrect I.V. solution hung
- ☐ incorrect I.V. rate
- ☐ other _____

Surgical
- ☐ consent problem
- ☐ incorrect sponge and instrument count
- ☐ foreign object left in patient
- ☐ other _____

Burn
- ☐ chemical
- ☐ cigarette
- ☐ treatment
- ☐ hot liquid
- ☐ other _____

(continued)

Completing an incident report *(continued)*

NATURE OF INCIDENT *(continued)*

Equipment
- ☐ Type _____
- ☐ Control and serial number
- ☐ malfunction
- ☐ shock
- ☐ burn
- ☐ other _____
- ☐ date of last maintenance
- ☐ BioMed notified
   ☐ yes ☐ no
- ☐ Risk Management notified
   ☐ yes ☐ no

Miscellaneous
- ☐ patient refuses treatment
- ☐ needle stick
- ☐ injuries in treatment
- ☐ infection
- ☐ discharge against medical advice
- ☐ struck by door
- ☐ other _____

Personal property
- ☐ damaged
- ☐ lost
- ☐ other _____

Describe the items.
_____
_____
_____
_____

Describe the incident.
Pt. found sprawled on floor in front of commode chair. Chair next to foot of bed. Stated he fell from chair while trying to get up.

Witnesses: ☐ yes ☑ no

If yes, note names, addresses, and phone numbers, and indicate if they're employees, visitors, etc.

1. _____
2. _____

DISPOSITION

Seen by
- ☑ attending doctor
- ☐ ED doctor
Name: *James P. Spencer, M.D.*

Examination findings:
Pain in L knee

Doctor's signature:
James P. Spencer MD

Treatment
- ☐ not indicated
- ☐ treatment given
- ☐ reatment refused
- ☑ X-ray ordered
- ☐ admitted to hospital
- ☐ follow-up care indicated

Notification

(include your name, the date, and the time)

Attending doctor notified ☑ yes ☐ no
Nora Martin, RN 1/10/95 1815

Supervisor notified ☑ yes ☐ no
Nora Martin, RN 1/10/95 1815

Noted in chart ☑ yes ☐ no
Nora Martin, RN 1/10/95 1815

Sick call request completed ☐ yes ☐ no
_____

Patient or family notified ☐ yes ☑ no
_____

Documented in progress notes ☑ yes ☐ no

BETTER CHARTING

Completing an incident report *(continued)*

GENERAL DATA

Attending doctor: _James P. Spencer, MD_

Patient's room number: _511_   **Bed number:** _2_   **Shift:** ☐ 1 ☑ 2 ☐ 3

Additional details of incident

Pt. states he attempted to get off the commode, became dizzy, and fell to the floor, banging his Ⓛknee as he fell. Pt. assisted back to bed. Pt. complaining of pain in Ⓛ knee. BP, 134/76; P, 100. Dr. Spencer notified at 1815.

Signature: _Nora Martin_   **Title:** _RN_   **Date:** _1/10/95_

Director's summary (detail follow-up to above incident and action taken)

Signature: **Title:**   **Date:**

factors in this increase. You have less time to establish relationships with patients than you once did because they now move out of the acute care system very quickly or they're transferred to other units. All of this leads to unfamiliarity, which leads to errors. Try to develop a rapport with your patients, even on a short-term basis.

Although the chance of actually being sued is small, the fear of a malpractice suit is pervasive and stress-producing among nurses.

Preliminary steps in a lawsuit

When a patient (the plaintiff) takes legal action against a health care provider, an out-of-court settlement can usually be made. A plaintiff who was injured because the health care provider was negligent deserves compensation without going through the stress and expense of litigation. All parties named as defendants (usually the doctor, hospital, and nurse), as well as the insurance companies and attorneys, try to work toward a fair settlement.

Preparations for adjudication

If the parties can't agree or if the plaintiff isn't satisfied with the settlement offer, he may take his claim to court for adjudication.

With the patient's written authorization, the attorney will request a copy of the medical records. The attorney will scour the records for evidence to support the plaintiff's claim. Typically he looks for poorly documented information—especially in the nurses' notes—and evidence that other errors, incidents, or adverse

events occurred that may strengthen or expand the patient's claim.

That's what happened in one case. A patient visited an attorney to discuss an adverse reaction to a blood transfusion he received during surgery. In reviewing the medical record, the attorney realized that the blood was the correct type, that all policies and procedures had been properly followed, and that the policy itself had set a reasonable standard. He could find no evidence of negligence—the patient had simply had an unexpected reaction to the blood transfusion.

However, the lawyer noted two important documentation errors: a signed surgical consent form was missing from the chart, and a nurse had charted "incident report filed" because she'd forgotten to give a dose of medication. One omission and one inappropriate notation led to one full-blown lawsuit.

Many attorneys immediately forward a medical record to a qualified doctor or nurse for review to determine whether a basis for a lawsuit exists. The expert reviewer evaluates whether a reasonable standard of care was met and whether the record indicates damage and causation.

If the attorney fails to do this, he runs the risk of being sued for malpractice for not initiating a valid claim. Some large law firms employ nurses to perform this first evaluation.

Activity on the defendant's side begins when the medical records department receives an attorney's request for a medical record and notifies the risk management department, which also reviews the situation. An in-house investigation usually takes place immediately, and the health care facility's insurance carrier is alerted. The doctor involved in the lawsuit will also be notified and given a chance to review the record.

Remember: No one should make changes in the medical record after a lawsuit is initiated. If the record is incomplete or inaccurate, this should be clarified in an addendum with the correct date documented. The jury will think that you were covering up something if you try to explain changes made to the medical record after it was requested by a lawyer.

Complaint

Once the attorney reviews the record and determines that the claim is appropriate and timely, he'll file a *complaint* — a summary of what the injured party aims to prove. This legal document is filed in the courthouse, and copies are presented to each defendant personally, along with a *summons*. A summons notifies the defendant of the plaintiff's charges and gives the latest date an *answer* to the complaint can be filed.

In most jurisdictions, the complaint goes to a lower court judge. In jurisdictions with an arbitration system, an arbitration panel receives the complaint and initially hears the case. The case may then be appealed to the designated court.

Discovery

Once the attorney files the complaint, the discovery period begins. Discovery has two purposes: to give each party time to gather evidence and learn all the facts and allegations involved in the case, and to encourage an out-of-court settlement when appropriate.

The most important type of discovery for the nurse-defendant is the deposition, or testimony under oath.

Deposition

During a deposition, attorneys question the defendants, plaintiffs, and witnesses one by one, while a court stenographer records the interactions.

During her deposition, a nurse will be asked questions by the plaintiff's lawyer and sometimes by other lawyers representing additional parties. The nurse's own attorney will be present to protect her rights and help her with the answers but he probably won't ask her questions. If the case goes to trial, transcripts from the deposition may be introduced as evidence and compared with courtroom testimony for any discrepancies or contradictions.

The deposition process may sound innocuous but it isn't. Lawyers spend considerable time preparing defendants for it. The same goes for nurses subpoenaed (served with a written notice to appear in court) to testify at depositions as fact witnesses (as opposed to named defendants).

Although nurses will be discussing their care of the patient but not offering their opinion as an expert witness would, they should still be represented by an attorney. No one should ever go to a deposition unprepared.

Interrogatories

During the deposition, some attorneys use interrogatories (lists of written questions) to determine what evidence is available. The plaintiff's attorney may ask the health care facility for all records, policies, procedures, and committee minutes pertaining to the plaintiff. These documents may be protected from discovery under peer review acts, but each jurisdiction has different statutes governing what may be made available to opposing counsel.

Nurse's response

After being named in a malpractice suit, the nurse-defendant will need to devote considerable time to preparing her case. She will spend most of her time preparing for and responding to discovery requests from the plaintiff's attorney. In addition, the nurse's own attorney will rely on her to provide accurate information on the plaintiff's nursing care and other treatment issues. (For more information, see Chapter 9, Malpractice Lawsuits.)

The attorney may also ask for the nurse's help in selecting the right type of expert witnesses for the defense and in developing questions to ask the plaintiff's expert witnesses.

In many complex malpractice suits, the discovery period lasts 1 or 2 years or even longer. When this period is over, both sides are ready to testify in court.

Courtroom hearings

Witnesses will include people with knowledge of the actual incident, expert witnesses offering opinions about the case, and family members who may attest to the plaintiff's pain and suffering.

In cases heard in a court, rather than by an arbitration panel, a jury weighs the credibility of the people testifying, listens to all the evidence, and then decides whose testimony it believes.

In malpractice cases, the parties involved almost always make contradictory statements. For example, the plaintiff may testify that she fell and fractured her hip

on the way to the bathroom because the nurse never answered her call light. However, the nurse may testify that she did answer the patient's call and that she told her she'd be there in a minute and not to get out of bed alone.

The differences in testimonies may not always be a question of who's telling the truth and who's lying—it may be that the parties involved simply don't quite remember what happened after months or years have elapsed.

Role of documentation

Good documentation can save a nurse in a credibility dispute. In one case, a house doctor didn't respond to a nurse's calls about a patient's deteriorating neurologic condition for more than an hour. After repeated calls, the nurse finally notified the neurosurgeon directly. The patient had an epidural hematoma and left-sided hemiparesis. The house doctor claimed that he never received the calls, but the nurse had documented each one. The jury decided against the house doctor.

Lack of documentation doesn't always imply negligence—but juries often believe it does. You've probably heard the expression, "If it wasn't charted, it wasn't done." Juries may think that this statement applies to all situations, when in reality, you can't possibly document every word and action. Fair or not, this misconception can lead to a negative outcome in a malpractice case when no negligence occurred. (See *Not charted, not done.*)

Role of the judge

In a malpractice case, the judge's role is to monitor the testimony, to decide legal questions about how the evidence is presented, and to determine questions of law.

ON TRIAL

Not charted, not done

Even though you provide appropriate care, you risk a lawsuit if you fail to document. Consider the case of *Jarvis v. St. Charles Medical Center,* 713 P.2d 620 (Oregon 1986).

Concerned that his patient with a fractured leg was developing compartment syndrome, the patient's doctor spread the cast and instructed the nurses on duty to perform hourly tests (assessments and observations) and to notify him if problems developed.

Two days later, at 2030 hours, the doctor noticed that the patient's foot was white and pulseless. A nurse's entry at 1600 hours on the progress notes indicated no change in circulation, movement, or sensation.

Although emergency surgery was performed, the patient was left with restricted use of her leg.

Court's decision

In the malpractice suit that followed, the hospital argued that muscle death was gradual and that the doctor didn't manage the patient appropriately. The doctor claimed that a sudden change had occurred and that the nurses didn't notify him.

The court ruled that the doctor was negligent and added that because the progress notes indicated only sporadic testing, the nurses had contributed to the doctor's negligence by failing to conduct regular examinations.

In this case, it didn't matter whether the nurses assessed the patient hourly and provided care as ordered. What mattered was that the records didn't demonstrate that the ordered care was provided. The result: a judgment of negligence.

After all the testimony has been presented, the judge discusses with the jury how the law should be applied.

Role of the jury

The jury decides whether negligence has occurred and, if so, what conpensation should be awarded. At any point before the jury's decision, the opposing parties can decide to settle the case out of court. These settlements rarely receive as much publicity as jury verdicts. In fact, one stipulation of an out-of-court settlement may be that the amount of the award be kept confidential.

Ethical relevance of medical records

Since the 1960s, ethical problems in health care have increased in quantity and complexity. As a nurse, you routinely take part in decisions about removing life-support systems, guarding patient confidentiality, and obtaining informed consent. Often, you deal with ethical dilemmas long before the courts even contemplate them.

Ethical problems are complex enough, but several factors further complicate them: fear of death and dying, technologic advances that prolong life, the legal right of a competent adult to refuse care, increased consumer sophistication, and hospital problems, such as limited financial resources, reimbursement issues, and computerized health care systems.

As ethical problems increase, your challenge is to respond in compassionate, legally sound, and morally justifiable ways. You need to listen to your patients' requests about their care, communicate their wishes to doctors and family members, and then document these conversations carefully.

Meticulous documentation can prove that proper ethical and clinical decisions were made. When ethical issues are at stake, you're especially vulnerable to being sued. Patient care situations with ethical overtones require special types of documentation. Among the most commonly encountered ethical situations are those related to informed consent, living wills, confidentiality, and refusal of treatment.

Informed consent

Required before most treatments and procedures, informed consent means that the patient understands the proposed therapy and its risks and agrees to undergo it by signing a consent form. Legally, the doctor performing the procedure is responsible for obtaining the patient's informed consent. Depending on your hospital's policy, you may be asked to witness the patient's signature. (See *Witnessing informed consent*.)

Legal requirements

For informed consent to be legally binding, the patient must be mentally competent and the doctor must:
• explain the patient's diagnosis and the nature and purpose of the treatment or procedure to him, identifying any aspect that's considered experimental
• describe any risks associated with the treatment or procedure
• explain the possible consequences of not undergoing the treatment or procedure
• describe alternative treatments and procedures as appropriate
• inform the patient that he has the right to refuse the treatment or the procedure without having other care or support withdrawn; this includes withdrawing his consent after giving it
• obtain consent without coercing the patient; performing a procedure without voluntary consent may be considered battery.

The requirements for informed consent can be waived in only two situations: if the patient himself waives them by saying that he doesn't want to know the details about a treatment or procedure or if an urgent medical or surgical situation occurs. Many hospitals have policies specifying how you should document such an emergency. Make sure that you're familiar with your hospital's policy.

Questions about informed consent

Most hospitals use a standard consent form that also includes the legal requirements for a consent. If the patient doesn't understand the doctor's explanation or asks for more information, answer any questions that fall within the scope of your practice. Then be sure to document your interaction with the patient.

Witnessing informed consent

After the doctor informs the patient about a medical procedure, you may be asked to obtain the patient's signature on the consent form and sign as a witness. To ensure that you're a competent witness to a legally binding consent form, use this checklist:

• Always make sure the patient's record contains a signed consent form before he undergoes any scheduled treatment or procedure for which the hospital requires written consent.

• If you need to obtain the patient's signature, make sure he's competent, awake, alert, and aware of what he's doing. Also make sure he's not under the influence of alcohol, illicit drugs, or any medications that impair his understanding or judgment.

• Ask the patient if the doctor explained the diagnosis, proposed treatment, and expected outcome to his satisfaction.

• Ask the patient if he's been told about risks associated with a specific treatment or procedure, the possible consequences of refusing it, and any alternative treatments or procedures available.

• Ask if the patient has any concerns or questions about his condition or the information he's received.

• Help the patient get any additional information he needs from his doctor or other appropriate sources.

• Inform the patient that he has the right to refuse the treatment without having other care or support withdrawn and that he may withdraw his consent after giving it.

• Notify your nurse-manager and the doctor immediately if you suspect the patient is concerned about the information he's received, has doubts about his condition or the procedure, or hasn't been properly informed.

• Using objective language, document your assessment of the patient's understanding in the chart, noting the situation, his responses, and any actions taken.

• When (and *only* when) you're satisfied that the patient is well informed, have him sign the consent form (including the date and time); then sign your name as witness.

• Remember that you're responsible for obtaining *oral* informed consent for any procedures that you'll be performing, such as inserting an I.V. line or a urinary catheter.

Living wills

In a living will, a legally competent person declares what medical care he wants or doesn't want in a terminal illness. Living wills may apply only to treatment decisions made after a terminally ill patient becomes comatose and has no reasonable chance of recovery. Typically, a will authorizes the doctor to withhold or discontinue lifesaving measures.

Statutory requirements

All states recognize living wills as valid legal documents. Although the legal requirements vary, generally the laws:

• define the circumstances under which a living will applies

• indicate the people authorized to make a living will (usually only competent adults)
• cover any limitations or restrictions in the care that can be refused (for example, some statutes don't acknowledge the refusal of food and water)
• describe the elements the will must contain to be considered a legal document, including witnessing requirements
• identify who's immune from liability for following a living will's directions
• address the procedure for rescinding a living will.

Health care facility requirements
When a patient presents you with a living will, consult your facility's policy manual for information on how to proceed. Carefully document the circumstances surrounding the presentation of the will and your handling of the situation. (See *Filing a living will*.)

Confidentiality
One of your documentation responsibilities includes protecting the confidentiality of the patient's medical record. Usually, you can't reveal confidential information without the patient's permission. Besides your legal responsibilities, you also have professional and ethical responsibilities (as specified by the ANA, the Joint Commission on Accreditation of Healthcare Organizations, and other professional bodies in their codes and standards) to protect your patient's privacy.

The ANA Code of Ethics states that the nurse safeguards the patient's right to privacy by judiciously protecting confidential information. In most states, all health care records, including clinical data obtained from examinations, treatments, observa-tions, and conversations, are considered confidential. Specific state statutes may restrict disclosure of this information. (See *Ethical codes for nurses*, pages 36 to 38.)

Nurse's role
You assume a primary role in maintaining confidentiality and in safeguarding the privacy of medical records. Breaches in confidentiality can result from unintentional release of information, unauthorized entry into a patient's record, or even a casual conversation that's overheard by others. Avoid discussing patient concerns in areas where you can be overheard.

While the patient is hospitalized, you are the primary custodian of the record and you control access to it. This is especially true in settings where the record is kept at the bedside.

Never release patient records to unauthorized parties—this includes family members and police officers. If some person or agency requests information, consult your policy manual for guidance, and report the request to your nurse-manager. Also notify her if you're in doubt about the validity of a request. She may want to notify the hospital administrator. Refer all requests from insurance investigators or representatives to the appropriate administrator.

Keep in mind that the law requires you to disclose confidential information in certain situations—for example, in instances of alleged child abuse cases, matters of public health and safety, and criminal cases. Certain government agencies—such as state and local tax bureaus, the Internal Revenue Service, and public health departments—also can order you to reveal confidential information.

(*Text continues on page 38.*)

Filing a living will

If your patient has filled out a living will, it may resemble this one. However, its specific wording may differ to reflect both his wishes and the appropriate state statute. Consult your health care facility's policy on filing the patient's living will. Some facilities keep a photocopy of the will in the patient's medical record.

LIVING WILL DECLARATION

Declaration made this ___*17th*___ day of ___*January*___, 199___*5*___.I, ___*Bryan McCarthy*___, being of sound mind, willfully and voluntarily make known my desires that my dying shall not be artificially prolonged under the circumstances set forth below, and do declare:

If at any time I should have an incurable injury, disease, or illness certified to be a terminal condition by two (2) doctors who have personally examined me, one of whom shall be my attending doctor, and the doctors have determined that my death will occur whether or not life-sustaining procedures are used and where the application of life-sustaining procedures would serve only to artificially prolong the dying process, I direct that such procedures be withheld or withdrawn and that I be permitted to die naturally with only the administration of medication or the performance of any medical procedure deemed necessary to provide me with comfort or care or to alleviate pain.

In the absence of my ability to give directions regarding the use of such life-sustaining procedures, I want this declaration to be honored by my family and doctor(s) as the final expression of my legal right to refuse medical or surgical treatment and accept the consequences from such refusal.

I understand the full import of this declaration, and I am emotionally and mentally competent to make this declaration.

Signed ___*Bryan McCarthy*___   Address ___*19 Sawmill Rd, Sellersville, Pa.*___

I believe the declarant to be of sound mind. I did not sign the declarant's signature above for or at the direction of the declarant. I am at least 18 years of age and am not related to the declarant by blood or marriage, entitled to any portion of the estate of the declarant according to the laws of intestate succession of the ___*State of Pennsylvania*___ or under any will of the declarant or codicil thereto, or directly financially responsible for declarant's medical care. I am not the declarant's attending doctor, an employee of the attending doctor, or an employee of the health care facility in which the declarant is a patient.

Witness ___*James Cook*___   Witness ___*Mary Campbell*___

Address ___*20 Deerwood Lane, Perkasie, Pa*___   Address ___*1941 2nd St., Warrington, PA*___

Before me, the undersigned authority, on this ___*18th*___ day of ___*January*___, 199___*5*___, personally appeared ___*Bryan McCarthy*___ and ___*James Cook and Mary Campbell*___, known to me to be the Declarant and the witnesses, respectively, whose names are signed to the foregoing instrument, and who, in the presence of each other, did subscribe their names to the attached declaration (Living Will) on this date, and that said declarant at the time of execution of said declaration was over the age of eighteen (18) years and of sound mind.

(SEAL) My commission expires: ___*March 1, 1996*___   Notary Public ___*Susan Reinhart*___

Ethical codes for nurses

Two of the most important ethical codes for registered nurses are the American Nurses' Association (ANA) code and the Canadian Nurses' Association (CNA) code. Licensed practical and vocational nurses (LPNs and LVNs) also have an ethical code. The International Council of Nurses, an organization based in Geneva, Switzerland, that seeks to improve the standards of and status of nursing worldwide, has also published a code of ethics.

ANA code of ethics
The ANA views both nurses and patients as individuals who possess basic rights and responsibilities and who should command respect for their values and circumstances at all times. The ANA code provides guidance for carrying out nursing responsibilities consistent with the ethical obligations of the profession.

According to the ANA code, the nurse:
• provides services with respect for human dignity and the uniqueness of the patient unrestricted by considerations of social or economic status, personal attributes, or the nature of health problems
• safeguards the patient's right to privacy by judiciously protecting information of a confidential nature
• acts to safeguard the patient and the public when health care and safety are affected by the incompetent, unethical, or illegal practice of any person
• assumes responsibility and accountability for individual nursing judgments and actions
• maintains competence in nursing
• exercises informed judgment and uses individual competence and qualifications as criteria in seeking consultation, accepting responsibilities, and delegating nursing activities to others
• cooperates in activities that contribute to the ongoing development of the profession's body of knowledge
• participates in the profession's efforts to implement and improve standards of nursing
• takes part in the profession's efforts to establish and maintain conditions of employment conducive to high-quality nursing care
• shares in the profession's efforts to protect the public from misinformation and misrepresentation and to maintain the integrity of nursing
• collaborates with members of the health care professions and other citizens in promoting community and national efforts to meet the health needs of the public.

CNA code of ethics
The CNA code consists of four sources of nursing obligations.

Patients
• A nurse is obligated to treat patients with respect for their individual needs and values.
• Based on respect for patients and regard for their rights to control their own care, nursing care should reflect respect for patients' right of choice.
• The nurse is obligated to hold confidential all information about patients learned in the health care setting.
• The nurse is obligated to be guided by consideration for the dignity of patients.
• The nurse is obligated to provide competent care to patients.
• The nurse is obligated to represent the ethics of nursing before colleagues and others.

Ethical codes for nurses *(continued)*

• The nurse is obligated to advocate patients' interests.

• In all professional settings, including education, research, and administration, the nurse retains a commitment to the patient's welfare. The nurse has an obligation to act in a fashion that will maintain trust in nurses and nursing.

Health care team

• Patient care should represent a cooperative effort, drawing on the expertise of nursing and other health care professions. By acknowledging personal or professional limitations, the nurse recognizes the perspective and expertise of colleagues from other disciplines.

• The nurse, as a member of the health care team, is obligated to take steps to ensure that patients receive competent and ethical care.

Social context of nursing

• Conditions of employment should contribute to patient care and to the professional satisfaction of nurses. Nurses are obligated to work toward securing and maintaining conditions of employment that satisfy these goals.

Responsibilities of the profession

• Professional nurses' organizations recognize a responsibility to clarify, secure, and sustain ethical nursing conduct. The fulfillment of these tasks requires professional organizations to remain responsive to the rights, needs, and interests of patients and nurses.

Code for LPNs and LVNs

The code for LPNs and LVNs seeks to provide a motivation for establishing, maintaining, and elevating professional standards. It includes the following imperatives:

• Know the scope of maximum utilization of the LPN and LVN as specified by the nurse practice act, and function within this scope.

• Safeguard the confidential information acquired from any source about the patient.

• Provide health care to all patients regardless of race, creed, cultural background, disease, or lifestyle.

• Refuse to give endorsement to the sale and promotion of commercial products or services.

• Uphold the highest standards in personal appearance, language, dress, and demeanor.

• Stay informed about issues affecting the practice of nursing and delivery of health care and, where appropriate, participate in government and policy decisions.

• Accept the responsibility for safe nursing by keeping oneself mentally and physically fit and educationally prepared to practice.

• Accept responsibility for membership in the National Federation of Licensed Practical Nurses, and participate in its efforts to maintain the established standards of nursing practice and employment policies that lead to quality patient care.

International Council of Nurses code of ethics

According to the International Council of Nurses, the fundamental responsibility of the nurse is fourfold: to promote health, to prevent illness, to restore health, and to alleviate suffering.

The International Council of Nurses further states that the need for nursing is universal. Inherent in nursing is respect for life, dignity, and the rights of man. It is unrestricted by

(continued)

Ethical codes for nurses   (continued)

considerations of nationality, race, creed, color, age, sex, politics, or social status.

Nurses and people
• The nurse's primary responsibility is to those who require nursing care.
• The nurse, in providing care, respects the beliefs, values, and customs of the individual.
• The nurse holds in confidence personal information and uses judgment in sharing this information.

Nurses and practice
• The nurse carries personal responsibility for nursing practice and for maintaining competence by continual learning.
• The nurse maintains the highest standards of nursing care possible within the reality of a specific situation.
• The nurse uses judgment in relation to individual competence when accepting and delegating responsibilities.
• The nurse, when acting in a professional capacity, should at all times maintain standards of personal conduct that would reflect credit upon the profession.

Nurses and society
• The nurse shares with other citizens the responsibility for initiating and supporting action to meet the health and social needs of the public.

Nurses and coworkers
• The nurse sustains a cooperative relationship with coworkers in nursing and other fields.
• The nurse takes appropriate action to safeguard the individual when his care is endangered by a coworker or any other person.

Nurses and the profession
• The nurse plays the major role in determining and implementing desirable standards of nursing practice and nursing education.
• The nurse is active in developing a core of professional knowledge.
• The nurse, acting through the professional organization, participates in establishing and maintaining equitable social and economic working conditions in nursing.

But even when circumstances call for disclosure, be sure to uphold your patient's right to privacy as much as possible. Obtain a written consent from your patient before disclosing any confidential information to anyone, and consult your nurse-manager if you're in doubt.

What do you do if the patient wants to see his own record? Although he has this right, first ask if he has any questions about his treatment. A patient may ask for his records because he's confused about the care he's receiving. Talking to him can help clear up such confusion.

Safeguards for computer records
A computerized system of clinical records dramatically increases the risk of unauthorized access to confidential information. To combat this, some safeguards have

been added to protect patients' privacy. The main safeguard is the signature code, which permits access only to signature code holders.

Never tell anyone your signature code, and promptly notify your nurse-manager if you suspect that someone is using it.

Refusing and withholding treatment

Any mentally competent adult can legally refuse treatment if he's been fully informed about his medical condition and the likely consequences of his refusal. Thus any mentally competent adult can legally refuse mechanical ventilation, tube feedings, antibiotics, fluids, and other treatments that will clearly result in the patient's death if they're withheld.

Besides asking a patient if he has a living will, more and more health care facilities (both acute and long-term care) are informing patients soon after admission about their future treatment options. Discuss the patient's wishes and document the discussion for use later in case the patient becomes unable to participate in decision making.

Release forms

When a competent patient refuses treatment, the doctor should inform him of the risks involved and have him sign a refusal-of-treatment release form. (See *Witnessing refusal of treatment,* page 40.) This form legally protects the nurse, doctor, and hospital by indicating that the appropriate treatment would have been given with the patient's consent. If the patient refuses to sign the release form, document his refusal in the progress notes.

Treatment withheld

The ethical and legal implications of withholding treatment center on documenting the patient's wishes. To prevent problems, be sure to take these steps:
• Confirm and record the patient's condition and prognosis in the medical record.
• Check that the doctor has documented that the patient understands the consequences of his refusal of treatment, such as the pain he might have and the possibility of a decreased life expectancy and quality of life.
• Review the patient's medical record for a copy of a living will, a health care proxy statement, or even letters from people who heard the patient express his wishes. Documentation should include dates of conversations, full names of people involved, the circumstances, and exactly which treatments and medical conditions were discussed.
• Scrutinize the medical record for a complete and accurate summary of all conversations between the patient and health care providers. The record should also document the conversation concerning the patient's final decision about withholding treatment.
• Exercise extreme caution when taking do-not-resuscitate (DNR) orders over the phone or verbally. If you can't avoid taking such an order, have another nurse listen to the conversation, and make sure that the doctor signs the order within the time set by your hospital's policy.
• Refuse orders for a "slow code"—they're unethical and illegal. A slow code may specify calling the doctor before resuscitating a patient, doing cardiopulmonary resuscitation (CPR) but withholding drugs, giving oxygen but withholding CPR, or not putting a patient on a ventilator. Such

BETTER CHARTING

Witnessing refusal of treatment

To prevent possible misunderstandings and potential lawsuits if a patient refuses treatment, the doctor must first explain the risks involved in making this choice. Then, if the patient still refuses treatment, the doctor will ask him to sign a refusal-of-treatment release form, such as the one below, which you also may need to sign as a witness.

REFUSAL-OF-TREATMENT RELEASE FORM

I, _Brenda Lyndstrom_, refuse to allow anyone to _administer blood or blood products_.
   (patient's name)   (insert treatment)

The risks attendant to my refusal have been fully explained to me, and I fully understand the benefits of this treatment. I also understand that my refusal of treatment seriously reduces my chances for regaining normal health and may endanger my life.

I hereby release _____ _Mercy General_ _____, its nurses and employees, together with all doctors in any way
                       (name of hospital)
connected with me as a patient, from liability for respecting and following my express wishes and direction.

Susan Reynolds, R.N.   _Brenda Lyndstrom_
(Witness's signature)   (Patient's or legal guardian's signature)

_11/29/94_   _54_
(Date)   (Patient's age)

---

orders indicate that the doctor either doesn't know the correct procedure for writing a DNR order or has a problem accepting the patient's death or discussing DNR orders with the family.

• Suggest that the hospital set up an ethics committee to resolve problems about terminating treatment. This committee may include nurses, doctors, social workers, clergy, and risk management or legal counsel.

DNR policies

Health care facilities need to develop policies and procedures for DNR orders, which are implemented if a patient has a sudden cardiac arrest. If no policies exist, a DNR order may be written by the attending doctor if it is medically appropriate and:

• the patient understands the impact of the DNR order

• the patient is incompetent and an appropriate surrogate gives consent. A DNR order may be appropriate if the patient has a terminal illness, is permanently unconscious, won't respond to resuscitation, or would be extraordinarily burdened by CPR.

DNR orders should be reviewed periodically or whenever a significant change occurs in the patient's clinical status.

Selected references

"A Question of Timing," *Nursing91* 21(11):88, November 1991.

Bennett, B. "Quality Care Through Risk Management," *Orthopedic Nursing* 12(3):54-55, May-June 1993.

Buchanan-Chell, M., et al. "Use of Generic Quality Improvement Chart Review to Recognize Nosocomial Infection," *American Journal of Infection Control* 20(6):310-14, December 1992.

Freedland, B. "Moving Toward Continuous Quality Improvement," *Journal of Intravenous Nursing* 15(5):278-82, September-October 1992.

Grange, N. "Witnessing Informed Consent," *Nursing94* 24(5):17, May 1994.

Hayden, L.S. "Risk Management Strategies," *Journal of Intravenous Nursing* 15(5):288-90, September-October 1992.

Hogue, E.E. "Be Aware of Increased Liability When RNs Switch Work Sites," *Hospital and Home Health* 10(6):82-83, June 1993.

Hudson, T. "Medical Record Analysis Can Show Legal Risks," *Hospitals* 66(22):46, 48, November 20, 1992.

Joint Commission on Accreditation of Healthcare Organizations. *1994 Accreditation Manual for Hospitals.* Oakbrook Terrace, Ill.: Joint Commission on Accreditation of Healthcare Organizations, 1993.

Lesparre, M. "Evolution in Progress: From Quality Assurance to Continuous Quality Improvement," *The Quality Letter for Healthcare Leaders* 1(2):1-7, February 1989.

MacDonald, J. "Elements of a Hospital Risk Management Program," *Canadian Journal of Infection Control* 6(4):94, Winter 1991.

Mamaril, M. "Standard of Care: Legal Implications in the Postanesthesia Care Unit," *Journal of Postanesthesia Nursing* 8(1):13-20, February 1993.

Mandell, M. "What You Don't Say Can Hurt You," *American Journal of Nursing* 93(8):15-16, August 1993.

Moniz, D.M. "The Legal Danger of Written Protocols and Standards of Practice," *Nurse Practitioner* 17(9):58-60, September 1992.

Nurse's Handbook of Law and Ethics. Springhouse, Pa.: Springhouse Corp., 1992.

"Nursing and Risk: The Politics of Responsibility," *American Nurse* 25(7):44, July-August 1993.

Patterson, C.H. "Joint Commission Nursing Care Standards: The Framework for a Comprehensive Program to Assess and Improve Quality," *Journal of Nursing Care Quality* 7(2):1-14, January 1993.

Quigley, F.M. "Applying Standards of Care in Legal Proceedings," *Focus on Critical Care* 18(6):474-75, March 1992.

Schiala, T., et al. "Communication: The Key to Avoiding Query and Reporting Standards Violations," *Journal of Health-care Quality* 15(3):15-21, May-June 1993.

Stodart, K. "Incident Forms: The Right Way to Use Them," *New Zealand Nursing Journal* 85(2):14, March 1992.

"Understanding Incident Reporting Systems," *Minimally Invasive Surgical Nursing* 7(1):5, Spring 1993.

White, L. "Quality Improvement Consumer Influence on Perioperative Services," *Association of Operating Room Nurses Journal* 58(1):96, 98-101, July 1993.

Zuffoletto, J.M. "The Doctrine of *res ipsa loquitur* Places Burden on Perioperative Personnel...The Thing Speaks for Itself," *Association of Operating Room Nurses Journal* 56(2)J:342-43, August 1992.

Quality Improvement and Reimbursement

The impact of nursing documentation on the quality of patient care and the reimbursement for patient care extends throughout—and beyond—the patient's stay in a health care facility. What makes this documentation so important? In most cases, nursing documentation constitutes a major part of the medical record. It helps prove or disprove that a health care facility provides acceptable care and qualifies for reimbursement. This means that the various parties interested in quality health care, reimbursement standards, and legal practices will study a great deal of nursing documentation.

Quality watchdogs

Who are these parties? Typically, they include representatives of the Joint Commission on Accreditation of Healthcare Organizations (JCAHO), Medicare and Medicaid auditors, peer review organizations (PROs), quality improvement teams, and others, such as those involved in assigning patients to appropriate diagnostic groups and meeting legal requirements. These parties are directly charged with improving quality and justifying government and insurance company disbursements for health care.

To accomplish their mission, they scrutinize medical records to evaluate care that they can't observe firsthand. Because what you document or don't document either supports or challenges the quality standards and appropriateness of care, your notes directly affect your health care facility's accreditation, financial reimbursement, and legal security.

Documentation and quality improvement

The JCAHO, PROs, quality improvement teams, and case managers are just a few of the groups who will periodically validate your facility's quality of care and overall nursing competency.

JCAHO quality standards

The JCAHO routinely surveys health care facilities in the United States to make sure that they meet its standards as accredited health care providers. A health care facility submits to these surveys mainly to demonstrate that it provides high-quality, safe health care. It also seeks JCAHO accreditation to qualify for reimbursement and other funding from governmental and private insurance agencies. These agencies require health care facilities to hold JCAHO accreditation before they're eligible to receive Medicare, Medicaid, or private funds. (For information on Medicare and Medicaid reimbursement benefits, see *Comparing Medicare and Medicaid.*)

Besides being concerned with documentation that demonstrates measurable overall quality care, the JCAHO requires that nursing documentation meets certain quality standards. Specifically, reviewers examine medical records containing patient assessments, plans of care, and personnel records, such as clinical nurse evaluations, nursing licenses and credentials, and nursing assignments.

Because the JCAHO depends on nursing documentation to evaluate patient care, what and how you document plays a crucial role in the accreditation process.

Comparing Medicare and Medicaid

Both Medicare and Medicaid were established in 1966 under the Social Security Act. As the following chart shows, the two organizations differ in their reimbursement policies, regulations, and documentation guidelines.

MEDICARE	MEDICAID
Federal health insurance benefits program for persons over age 65. Part A covers skilled nursing home and hospital care; Part B covers care by doctors, hospital equipment, and supplies.	Combined state and federal insurance and medical assistance plan for qualified needy individuals of any age. Encourages home care as an alternative to institutional care.
Benefits are uniform for eligible recipients nationwide.	Benefits differ from state to state.
Pays for skilled medical and nursing care only.	Pays for home nursing care (not necessarily skilled care).
Patients must be confined to home to receive reimbursement for part-time or intermittent skilled nursing care.	Patients aren't required to be confined to home.
Documentation is required to support the need for skilled medical and nursing care and its delivery.	Documentation is required to ensure payment but varies according to setting.
Doesn't pay for custodial care.	Pays for custodial care in specified care settings.
A doctor's order initiates service.	The patient's qualifying need initiates service.

To be accredited by the JCAHO, a health care facility must have an organized, systematic, and ongoing method for documenting quality (see *Documenting to reflect standards,* page 46). The JCAHO recommends a monitoring and evaluation process based on a 10-step model.

Step 1: Assigning responsibility for quality care

Ultimately, the responsibility for quality lies with a hospital's governing body—its board of directors. In general, the board charges the health care facility administrator to appoint someone to oversee monitoring and evaluation activities throughout the facility. In turn, this person assigns hands-on, quality improvement responsibilities to the group responsible for each service. For example, the responsibility for monitoring and evaluating nursing care may pass through a long chain of command from the board to the administrator, to the quality improvement director, to the vice president of nursing, and to the nurse-manager.

Specifically, the medical staff monitors doctors, the nursing department evaluates

Documenting to reflect standards

When representatives of the Joint Commission on Accreditation of Healthcare Organizations (JCAHO) review medical records, they look for indications that the health care facility provides quality care.

Of particular interest to the JCAHO is evidence that the health care facility has an organized and systematic method for monitoring and evaluating patient care. And, of course, your documentation should reflect this method.

As you chart care, keep in mind that your documentation can prove detrimental or beneficial to your facility during JCAHO reviews. Ideally, it would show that your facility:
• monitors and evaluates health care activities and caregivers
• defines the scope of care provided
• recognizes the most important aspects of care provided

• identifies indicators (a sign or set of signs) and appropriate clinical criteria for monitoring the important aspects of care
• establishes thresholds (or limits) for the indicators to trigger evaluation of care
• collects and organizes data for each indicator to analyze and monitor the important aspects of care
• evaluates health care when thresholds are reached to identify problems or opportunities to improve care
• acts to correct identified problems or to improve care
• assesses the effectiveness of corrective actions and documents improvements in care
• communicates the results of the monitoring and evaluation to relevant individuals, departments or services, quality improvement administrators and, in general, the entire health care staff.

nursing care, and pharmacists review pharmacy service. The director of each group then appoints a committee or quality improvement team to identify indicators of key elements of patient care, collect data, evaluate care, and take corrective actions or initiate improvements.

Step 2: Defining the scope of care
As a basis for future monitoring, the team members of each service must clearly define their group's function. To do so, they consider the types and numbers of patients treated, the patients' diagnoses, the treatments performed, the staff members

providing the service, and the locations and times of care.

Step 3: Defining key aspects of care
To pinpoint where quality improvement activities will begin, team members identify their group's most important functions by considering the type of care their service provides and determining which kinds of care:
• occur most frequently
• affect the greatest number of patients
• carry the greatest current risk or have posed the most problems for patients or staff in the past.

Step 4: Identifying indicators

The team members evaluate the latest information presented by researchers, journals, and professional organizations in relation to local, state, and national standards of care. They undertake these studies to identify indicators for each key aspect of care. Basically, indicators measure the structures, processes, and outcomes of care (see *Understanding JCAHO indicators,* page 48).

Step 5: Establishing thresholds

Before data collection, team members must establish a threshold: a boundary that alerts the team to the need for an intensive review. For example, a mental health unit may establish a threshold for individual treatment plans (ITPs), requiring the staff to complete 95% of ITPs within 24 hours of admission. If the actual compliance rate is 92%, then the threshold would remain unmet, which would trigger an investigation. Depending on the threshold at issue, the staff may need to review resources, staff education, or even a doctor's response time.

Occasionally, failing to meet a threshold may be justifiable. However, a pattern of noncompliance points to a problem requiring correction.

Not all thresholds are, or should be, set at 100%. Such a target would be unrealistic and, possibly, counterproductive. However, certain crucial aspects of care, such as the requirement to type all blood before a transfusion, should always have a threshold of 100%. Failing to meet this threshold—or any threshold that would jeopardize a patient's survival—should trigger an immediate, extensive review.

Step 6: Collecting data

Once the team members establish thresholds, they can begin collecting and organizing data for each one. (See *Collecting and organizing data,* page 49.)

Step 7: Analyzing data

The team members study the data, looking for trends or patterns to determine whether a problem exists or whether they need to investigate further. If no problem exists, or if the team members find acceptable care, they take no further action. If the team members find unacceptable care or if they identify a problem, they proceed with appropriate action.

Step 8: Taking action

If possible, the team members recommend and initiate corrective action themselves. However, if the required action is beyond their authority, they make their recommendations to the person or department that does have the authority to act. A corrective action plan should identify:
• who or what needs to change
• who is responsible for implementing the action
• the specific action required in view of the problem's cause and severity
• when the change should occur.

Step 9: Evaluating the outcome

After suggesting or taking action, the team members continue to monitor and evaluate the problem area to assess whether the action resulted in a measurable improvement in patient care.

Step 10: Communicating findings

Whatever the findings, the quality improvement team members must report their findings to the health care facility's

Understanding JCAHO indicators

The Joint Commission on Accreditation of Healthcare Organizations (JCAHO) expects accredited health care facilities to establish indicators of quality health care. A measurable sign of standard patient care, an indicator may reflect a patient's care structure, process, or outcome.

In constructing or identifying indicators, the quality improvement team asks such questions as "What is required for care?" and "What does care involve?" and "What is the outcome of care?"

Structure indicator

This indicator identifies key elements required for care. It describes the patient care environment, including required equipment and qualifications of caregivers. A structure indicator also helps the quality improvement team assess how well a particular department functions. For example, structure indicators for a telemetry unit might include the following:
• The unit has a nurse-to-patient ratio of 1:4.
• All registered nurses (RNs) on the unit have completed the hospital's coronary care continuing education program.

Process indicator

In determining what care involves, the quality improvement team focuses on nursing procedures (or actions), such as assessment, plans of care, and complication management. A process indicator may demonstrate that the nursing staff routinely takes and documents a patient's pulse rate before administering certain medications (as required by the JCAHO). For patients with diabetes mellitus, process indicators might include the following:

• RNs assess the patient's blood glucose level every 8 hours or more frequently if his condition warrants.
• They assess the patient's peripheral pulses every 8 hours or more frequently if his condition warrants.
• They assess the patient's skin integrity daily or more frequently if his condition warrants.
• They weigh the patient daily.
• They teach the patient and his caregiver about insulin preparation, administration, storage, and disposal of used syringes.
• They teach the patient and his caregiver how to test blood glucose levels and how to recognize and respond to hypoglycemia and hyperglycemia.

Outcome indicator

When studying the results of patient care, the quality improvement team members focus on complications or adverse events as well as the long-term effects of care measures on the patient's health. Then they try to construct indicators that are well-defined, objective, and measurable.

General outcome indicators may measure the incidence of nosocomial infections or record unplanned transfers to the critical care unit. Specific outcome indicators—for Crohn's disease, for instance—might include the following:
• The patient reports no episodes of bloody diarrhea within 72 hours of discharge.
• Diet and medication regimens effectively control abdominal pain.
• The patient's blood test results show no evidence of a continued drop in hemoglobin level and hematocrit.

Collecting and organizing data

To make sure that the data collected for evaluation accurately represent the patient care provided, a health care facility's evaluators must establish a procedure for collecting and tabulating information.

Searching resources

First, the evaluators must decide exactly which areas of care they need to know more about. Then they'll choose relevant resources for scrutiny. For example, they may collect data from parts of the medical record, such as the nurses' progress notes and laboratory reports, and medication administration records or other documents, such as occurrence reports and logs.

Choosing a method

The evaluators must decide how to collect the information needed to review the quality of patient care. The methods used are retrospective, concurrent, or prospective.

Deciding on the sample size

Next, the evaluators must determine how many instances of care — procedures, treatments, or patients with the same diagnosis, for example — they'll need to study.

Typically they'll base their decision on frequency. For example, for an aspect of care that produces a rare complication, the evaluators may need a sample from only one source or a set of sources; on the other hand, for an aspect of care that produces problems consistently, they may need to collect much more data from many more sources.

Determining frequency

When deciding on the frequency of data collection, the evaluators must review such factors as the number of patients involved, the anticipated risk of the procedure or treatment being studied, the regularity of the care being studied, the extent to which the care measures have been problem-free, and so forth. However, they must collect data frequently enough for comparison with threshold data.

Evaluating results

Ideally, cumulative data for each indicator should be available for periodic comparison with corresponding thresholds. Evaluating indicators and thresholds in this way helps determine early on whether intensive reviews and corrective actions (or improvements) are needed.

quality improvement program director and to relevant staff members, departments, and services. This allows the quality improvement personnel to trace trends and issues between medical staff services and other health care facility departments.

Besides being used when the JCAHO reviews the health care facility for accreditation, data collected by the quality improvement team also helps justify third-party insurance reimbursement and assignment of medical staff privileges.

PRO emphasis

The PROs rely heavily on documentation in the medical record. Developed to assist in utilization review processes, PROs consist of groups of doctors and nurses required by the federal government to monitor and evaluate the quality and appropriateness of care given.

PROs evaluate a sample of a health care facility's medical records. They compare the data with specific screening criteria to assess the need for and appropriateness of medical services. Their screening criteria lists basic standards or conditions that a comparable group of health care facilities can reasonably be expected to meet. In studying a sample of the medical records, the PROs focus on the intensity of services and the severity of illnesses. (For more information on PROs, see Chapter 1, Nursing Documentation and the Medical Record.)

Because a PRO's primary focus is quality patient care carried out within cost-containment guidelines, the reviewers also scrutinize documented care as a means for determining reimbursements.

Just as it confirms quality care, nursing documentation may also supply the justification needed for approving full reimbursement. Familiarity with the PRO's criteria usually helps target nursing documentation. (See *How peer reviewers screen specialized care.*)

Case management focus

A case management system provides an additional way for health care facilities to improve quality and contain costs. Case managers help to coordinate a patient's long-term care by using resources throughout a community. One of their primary goals is to control costs. In the process, they influence both the type of health care services a patient receives and where he receives them.

Case management began as an offshoot of the Medicare and Medicaid waiver-demonstration projects, which made exceptions to usual federal Medicare and Medicaid eligibility requirements. The exceptions (or waivers) extended health care coverage to certain patients who could use community and nursing services at home. The intent was to prevent unnecessary nursing home admissions; the result is an expanded role for many nurses.

Nurses as case managers

Case managers direct patient care to the most cost-effective health care setting while still meeting quality health care standards. Today's case manager must ensure that the patient's care and reimbursement for care is appropriate for his diagnosis—or diagnosis-related group (DRG).

The case management system forces health care facilities to deliver care economically without compromising quality. If you become a case manager, your role will change from giving hands-on nursing care to coordinating cost-effective health care settings. You'll manage a closely monitored and controlled system of multidisciplinary care. You'll be responsibile for outcomes, length of stay, and use of resources throughout the patient's illness — not just during your shift. And you'll become an expert at scrutinizing and interpreting nursing documentation. These records play a key role in the effect case managers have on a hospital.

Case managers scrutinize the medical record—especially the nursing documenta-

How peer reviewers screen specialized care

When reviewing medical records, peer review organizations (PROs) use special screening criteria to evaluate the intensity of services and the severity of illness. These factors have a direct impact on Medicare and Medicaid reimbursement.

Being familiar with the PRO's criteria can help you document appropriately to demonstrate that patient care complies with Medicare and Medicaid standards. That, in turn, maximizes reimbursement.

Below are the monitoring, medication, and treatment screening criteria that a peer reviewer looks for when verifying that care given in an alcohol or drug detoxification unit meets Medicare and Medicaid standards.

Monitoring criteria
A patient in an alcohol or drug detoxification unit should be monitored every 1 to 2 hours. Monitoring must be appropriate, needed, and ordered.

The caregiver needs to monitor:
• vital signs (pulse and respiratory rates and blood pressure every 1 to 2 hours; temperature at least every 4 hours)
• level of consciousness
• orientation to time and place

• fluid intake and output
• pupillary reaction to light and pupil size
• potential or actual signs and symptoms of withdrawal.

Medication criteria
Reimbursable medications include:
• I.V. medications (excluding vitamins and potassium unless potassium replacement was ordered and administered for documented hypokalemia)
• oral or I.M. medications to control acute withdrawal symptoms (examples include chlordiazepoxide, magnesium sulfate, and thiamine).

Treatment criteria
Besides medication administration, treatment may include:
• I.V. therapy to replace or maintain the patient's fluid volume; the flow rate needs to exceed a keep-vein-open rate and be appropriate for the patient's body mass and condition
• initial need, continuing need, or both, as documented by the doctor, for inpatient detoxification to stabilize the patient's mental and physical condition.

tion—to determine whether a patient's continued hospital and other health care costs and treatment are justified.

Case management is one of the services listed under Comprehensive Omnibus Budget Reconciliation Act (COBRA). This act permits states to apply for waivers and offer community services for patients eligible for nursing home care.

Outside of the health care facility, case managers may be in private practice or employed by home care agencies, family service agencies, hospitals, area agencies on aging, and health maintenance organizations (HMOs).

Quality improvement team efforts

Required for JCAHO accreditation and mandated by the Omnibus Budget Reconciliation Act, quality improvement teams (or committees) are another means by which an organization monitors and evaluates the quality and appropriateness of patient care. Both acute care and long-term care facilities can use the JCAHO 10-step model as a guideline for quality improvement activities.

Quality improvement teams accomplish several tasks, such as:
• generating documentation to confirm that the care provided meets accepted standards
• identifying areas that need improvement
• drawing attention to problems.

Ongoing monitoring and evaluation provides information on the outcome of high-volume and high-risk services, which is required for budget and strategic planning. And examining areas of frequent and infrequent use helps the health care facility to assess various needs. For example, an operating area that handles fewer than five elective neurosurgical cases yearly may use quality improvement data to evaluate the cost-effectiveness of continuing this service.

Other data may provide information that is useful to the community. For example, the health care facility may learn that it's located in a community experiencing a sudden population increase in school-age children. Such demographic data may serve to justify expansion of pediatric health services.

For nurses especially, ongoing quality improvement activities such as monitoring of medication administration serve two purposes: They identify problems and track trends or patterns, and they also evaluate the performance of the individual nurse, who is identified in the data by a numerical code. This enables nurse-managers to assess the performance and competence of the nurses they supervise. (See *Using a quality improvement report.*)

What's more, the documentation gathered by quality improvement teams serves as a self-review for reimbursement eligibility. By applying the screening criteria used by third-party payers, an organization can estimate its projected revenues. Documentation compliance increases the likelihood of reimbursement for services provided.

Quality improvement indicators

When evaluating an organization's performance, quality improvement indicators are key factors.

The JCAHO publishes a series of indicators for use in monitoring patients who receive surgical and obstetrical services. Using these indicators, health care facilities accumulate data to identify areas needing improvement and areas that surpass standards. The data should also show patient outcomes, which the health care facility can use to compare its own results with patient outcomes in other facilities nationwide. (See *Using JCAHO indicators to improve quality of care*, page 54.)

Additional JCAHO indicators are currently in trial use for cardiovascular, oncology, trauma, medication use, infection control, and home-infusion services. A quality improvement indicator is a useful tool for assessing medical records and, consequently, patient care.

Using a quality improvement report

Once you've identified troublesome issues or events, your next step is to complete a report similar to the one below. The quality improvement team may then use it to confirm that patient care meets accepted standards and to identify areas of improvement.

Evaluation period: _11/94_ to _6/95_
Department: _Nursing 3 North_
Report writer: _Sharon Neilson, RN, BSN, Nurse Manager, 3 North_

DATE & ISSUE	January 1995	March 1995
	Patients late for physical therapy appointments. Statistic provided by Rehab Dept.: 252 appointments scheduled for 3 North patients in November, December, and January; 104 (41%) were late for appointments. 59% were on time.	Orders for one-time doses of medication are inconsistently documented on both the physician order sheet and the medication administration record. Rate of compliance for January, February, and March is 62%.
ACTION	Met with department manager of physical therapy and 3 North nurses. Plan: Rehab Dept. will send schedule of appointments to 3 North by 1800 hours the previous day. Physical therapy appointment will be incorporated into the daily nurse assignment.	Reviewed policy with all nurses. Each shift assigned to monitor and submit results to Mary Lake, RN, who is the quality improvement coordinator for 3 North.
FOLLOW-UP	Compliance monitored for February, March, and April. Results: 231 appointments were scheduled. Patients were late for 26 (11%) of the appointments. 89% were on time. Results reflect a 30% improvement.	Compliance monitored for April, May, and June. Results: 81% compliance rate. Results reflect a 19% improvement.
RESOLUTION	Continue to monitor for the next quarter. 90% of patients on time for appointments is an acceptable threshold based on the cooperation level of patients, the transport system, and emergencies on 3 North.	Continue to monitor for next quarter. A compliance rate of 100% is the goal, based on safety and billing issues. Quality improvement coordinator will track by nursing staff.

Using JCAHO indicators to improve quality of care

The Joint Commission on Accreditation of Healthcare Organizations (JCAHO) has published indicators for health care facilities to use when monitoring patients who receive surgical and obstetrical services. Using and documenting these indicators helps a facility accumulate data to measure its performance, compare its performance with similar health care facilities, monitor trends, and enlist feedback from the JCAHO.

The following chart presents four JCAHO indicators and the corresponding patient populations being monitored.

INDICATOR	PATIENT POPULATION
Preoperative patient evaluation, intraoperative and postoperative monitoring, and timely clinical intervention	Patients developing a central nervous system (CNS) complication within 2 days of procedures involving anesthesia administration, subcategorized by the American Society of Anesthesiologists' physical status class, patient age, and CNS- versus non–CNS-related procedures
Preoperative patient evaluation, appropriate surgical preparation, intraoperative and postoperative monitoring, and timely clinical intervention	Patients developing a peripheral neurologic deficit within 2 days of procedures involving anesthesia administration
Prenatal patient evaluation, education, and treatment selection	Patients with vaginal birth after cesarean section
Prenatal patient evaluation, intrapartum monitoring, and clinical intervention	Live-born infants with a birth weight less than 2,500 g

Nursing staff quality

The paper trail accumulated in the medical record and elsewhere in the health care facility describes not only the patient's progress but also the nurse's performance. Data sources, such as indicators that measure clinical outcomes, personnel records, nursing credentials, and other documents, contribute to a full assessment of the quality of the nurse's care and qualifications.

A JCAHO quality standard for nursing care in specialty units states: "The supervision of nursing care in the unit is provided by a designated registered nurse (RN) who has relevant education, training, and experience and who has demonstrated current competence."

Typically, the JCAHO auditors, quality improvement teams, and others judge compliance with this standard by evaluating various kinds of documentation.

Documentation of standards

To confirm the RN requirement, reviewers look for a valid RN license. They also survey staffing schedules and assignment sheets to verify that an RN is designated

CHARTING GUIDELINES

Using documentation to assess specialty nursing competence

The Joint Commission on Accreditation of Healthcare Organizations (JCAHO) publishes standards outlining the documentation needed to verify that a nurse assigned to a special care unit performs competently, thereby ensuring quality care.

According to JCAHO standards, documentation should demonstrate that the supervising nurse can:
• interpret electrocardiograms and recognize significant arrhythmias
• interpret abnormal laboratory test values

• administer routinely used and emergency drugs
• initiate cardiopulmonary resuscitation and other patient safety measures as defined by hospital policy
• perform defibrillation as appropriate
• administer parenteral fluids, blood, and blood components
• provide respiratory and ventilatory care
• coordinate multidisciplinary care
• provide for patient and staff safety
• adhere to infection control policies and procedures.

to supervise nursing care. They validate relevant education, training, and experience by checking references and reviewing the nurse's continuing education units.

The reviewers assess a nurse's current competence by following the intent of JCAHO nursing care standards (NC.2 through NC.2.4.1.1). These standards outline the documentation required to assess the clinical competence of nursing staff members, nursing personnel from outside agencies, and specialty unit nursing staff.

For example, expanded standards for nurses in a special care unit require the nurse to be knowledgeable about the emotional and rehabilitative needs of her patients and able to provide appropriate interventions. Reviewing documentation and patient outcomes enables supervisory personnel to evaluate the competence of nursing staff members. (See *Using docu-*

mentation to assess specialty nursing competence.)

All nurses—not just those in special care units—must competently perform their assigned duties. Again this requirement is defined by the JCAHO. A starting point for defining and documenting the scope of any nurse's responsibilities is a thorough job description.

Specific strategies to achieve quality nursing documentation center on the medical record. Nursing entries verify the quality of patient care, assist caregivers in coordinating treatment, and provide legal protection for the nurse and the employer.

Other resources to consult regarding quality nursing and documentation include the health care facility's risk management office (see Chapter 2, Legal and Ethical Implications of Documentation, for more information), the medical records department, and the utilization management staff.

Documentation and fiscal implications

What the nurse documents in the medical record—and how she documents it—has a direct impact not only on the quality of patient care but also on the health care facility's revenues. The nurse's progress notes, flow sheets, plans of care, and medication administration records are scrutinized by Medicare, Medicaid, and insurance company reviewers in addition to peer reviewers, case managers, and caregiving staff, among others. The quality of care, patient outcomes, and the need for continued treatment are judged according to the documentation.

For example, vital signs, level of consciousness, infusion rates, and administration of injectable medications are all parameters used to determine whether the patient should continue his stay in a health care facility. Failure to provide sufficient documentation may result in denial of reimbursement or transfer of the patient to an alternative health care setting. Unsatisfactory but avoidable outcomes may result in denial of payment.

Obviously, documentation takes on important dimensions. Your records must be clear and concise. They must validate not only care and treatment but also the items that are billed. For example, a bill for 20 suction catheters used in a 24-hour period is unlikely to be paid when nursing documentation indicates that the patient was suctioned as needed during that time. Specific and complete nursing records are the key to ensuring financial reimbursement.

Reimbursement and related structures

Today's health care system includes multiple, complex structures with multiple and complex requirements for receiving reimbursement. Caregivers and health care facilities must deal not only with internal quality improvement teams, case managers, and required reimbursement structures (such as DRGs and COBRA requirements), but also with federal and state agencies, HMOs, preferred provider organizations (PPOs), and independent practice associations (IPAs), among others.

Reviewers from these groups examine the medical record for discrepancies. They look for differences in the treatment ordered and the treatment provided. If a discrepancy can't be explained satisfactorily or reconciled reasonably, payment may be denied.

DRGs

The basis for federal health care reimbursements, the DRG system groups diseases and disorders into specific categories. A DRG includes information about the principal and secondary diagnoses, surgical procedures, and the patient's age, sex, and discharge status. (See *Common DRGs*.)

When Medicare adopted a prospective payment system (PPS), reimbursement regulations changed. Before PPS, Medicare reimbursed a health care provider according to a cost-per-case formula. After PPS, Medicare computed reimbursements prospectively using a formula adjusted for diagnostic groups, symptoms, hospital, re-

Common DRGs

A total of 23 major categories and 470 diagnostic categories constitute the diagnosis-related group (DRG) classification system. A DRG designation may be surgical or medical; either can form the basis for Medicare, Part A, hospital service reimbursement.

Common surgical and medical DRGs appear in the table. Typically, the DRG number and description appear on the patient's bill.

MAJOR DIAGNOSTIC CATEGORY	DRG NUMBER	DESCRIPTION
Diseases and disorders of the nervous system	6	Carpal tunnel release
	14	Specific cerebrovascular disorders, except for transient ischemic attack
Diseases and disorders of the circulatory system	106	Coronary artery bypass with cardiac catheterization
	127	Heart failure and shock
Diseases and disorders of the respiratory system	78	Major chest procedures
	88	Chronic obstructive pulmonary disease

gion, wage levels, and other relevant factors—the DRG system.

Today, health care facilities must ensure meticulous compliance with DRG preadmission and continued-stay criteria to ensure reimbursement. Likewise, they must adhere to the details of the DRG coding process.

The medical record must contain documentation verifying the DRG and supporting the appropriateness of care in the health care facility. What's more, nursing documentation needs to support the diagnoses and indicate that appropriate patient and family teaching and discharge planning were provided.

COBRA

One feature of a federal law known as COBRA allows employees to temporarily carry their employer-provided health insurance benefits when they would otherwise lose them because of terminated employment or another qualifying event, such as reduction in work hours or retirement.

Providing care for patients insured under COBRA makes precise documentation essential. COBRA requires health care facilities receiving federal funds to evaluate any patients admitted to the emergency department. Specifically, the law states that a patient's condition must be stable before he's transferred to another health care facility. If the patient is in labor, her labor must be controlled before she is transferred to another health care facility.

To make sure that health care facilities comply with the law, COBRA and the JCAHO both require that all facilities thoroughly document their actions concerning patient transfers. This documentation must include the chronology of the event, measures taken or treatment implemented, the patient's response to treatment, and the results of the measures taken to prevent the patient's condition from worsening.

HMOs

An HMO is an organized system that provides an agreed-upon set of comprehensive inpatient and outpatient health services to a voluntarily enrolled population in exchange for a predetermined, fixed, and periodic payment.

An HMO may contract for beds and services and may build or buy hospitals. Many HMOs feature doctors who work for a salary or in a partnership arrangement. Or, the HMO may contract for medical services from individual doctors and may function as either a profit-making or non-profit organization.

IPAs

Consisting of an independent group of doctors, an IPA offers services to a specified group of patients. Many HMOs contract with IPAs for medical services.

PPOs

A PPO contracts with health care providers, including hospitals, doctors, therapists, pharmacies, and other professional services. The contracted fees are typically lower than customary, with the under-

standing that PPOs will channel patients into empty hospital beds and underutilized services.

Medicare and Medicaid payments

Payments by Medicare and Medicaid represent sources of operating revenue for hospitals. Both have specific requirements for participation and reimbursement.

Initially, a state agency determines whether a health care facility is eligible to participate in the Medicare program. In doing so, the state agency certifies that the hospital:
• holds JCAHO or American Osteopathic Association accreditation
• uses an adequate utilization review plan that is, or will be, in effect on the first day of the hospital's participation
• meets statutory requirements or, if not, proposes reasonable plans to correct deficiencies and demonstrates evidence of adequate patient care despite any shortcomings.

Medicare certifies hospitals for a 2-year period. Certification guidelines can be used to evaluate the function of all hospital services. Medicare also examines compliance with state and local laws and JCAHO standards. Health care facilities can use the steps for Medicare certification as preparation for JCAHO accreditation.

How documentation affects costs

Nursing documentation provides the data that examiners need to justify reimbursement for health care expenses. Besides studying the records to estimate revenues, examiners use the records to calculate nursing care costs.

Calculating nursing care costs

Traditionally, the cost of nursing care was included in the patient's daily room rate. Now, however, health care facilities are applying standard cost accounting techniques to nursing care.

First, nurses estimate the number of nursing hours required to provide a quality patient outcome. Then, financial management personnel estimate the cost of that nursing time. A major component in providing patient care, the cost of nursing care is directly related to the type and level of care provided. Health care facilities typically factor nursing care costs into the financial and strategic planning process.

Some facilities bill patients separately for nursing care, using pricing systems that charge only for care the patient actually receives. Determining the cost of nursing time requires detailed documentation so appropriate charges can be billed and validated. Nursing documentation then becomes a detailed financial record.

Calculating skilled care costs

Provided by RNs or by licensed practical nurses under an RN's supervision, skilled nursing care involves continuous use of the nursing process, technologically complex monitoring, and patient teaching. It also includes planning, organizing, and managing the plan of care with the doctor and other health care professionals.

What's more, skilled nursing care requires specialized education and the ability to document competently. It differs from custodial care (which may be provided by nonskilled personnel) and fo-cuses on assistance with the activities of daily living, such as eating, dressing, bathing, and ambulation.

Examples of skilled nursing care activities include the following:
• managing central venous lines
• administering I.M., S.C., or I.V. fluids or medications
• treating infected or extensive pressure ulcers
• administering oxygen
• providing nasopharyngeal suctioning
• managing enteral feedings
• changing sterile dressings.

How documentation affects revenues

Medicare Part A provides coverage for skilled nursing care; Part B, for durable medical equipment and supplies. Payment for services to patients insured by Medicare is based on their documented need for skilled nursing care and covers supplies and equipment used during that care.

Continued payment depends on *daily* documentation demonstrating the patient's ongoing need for skilled care. Obviously, the quality of documentation in this area directly affects the amount of Medicare payments and other insurance reimbursements as well.

In fact, revenue disbursements depend on documentation confirming that the nursing staff meets various care standards, such as:
• adhering to the nursing process
• recording changes in the patient's condition and care needs in a timely way
• using medical equipment (such as bedpans, nebulizers, indwelling catheters, and

Avoiding inconsistent documentation

Inconsistencies in documentation leave both you and your health care facility open to accusations of incompetence and fiscal irresponsibility. What's more, a medical record containing inconsistencies can be difficult or impossible to defend in court. To avoid inconsistencies, follow these guidelines.

Be precise
For example, exactly describing the size and location of a pressure ulcer (such as "2.5 cm × 2 cm × 3 cm deep, right elbow") minimizes guesswork when reviewing the patient's progress, whereas an approximation (such as "small, deep pressure ulcer on the patient's arm") may be judged inconsistent if previous or later descriptions differ.

Be specific
For example, describing an object or process in quantifiable terms, such as "500 ml of tea-colored urine" clearly specifies characteristics, whereas "about 400 or 500 ml of discolored urine" leaves room for later misinterpretation and inconsistencies.

Be thorough—and avoid summarizing
For example, a reviewer who encounters a complete outcome evaluation of teaching effectiveness, such as "Patient can correctly remove colostomy bag, clean the ostomy site, and apply new bag without assistance," is less likely to question your patient-teaching performance than the reviewer who encounters an evaluation stating "Patient handles own colostomy care."

walkers) judiciously and appropriately to meet the patient's needs
• adequately teaching the patient about his condition and treatment plan.

Finally, examiners search the documentation carefully for any inconsistencies that may hinder reimbursement (see *Avoiding inconsistent documentation*).

Importance of the nursing process
The nursing process involves the problem solving and decision making that nurses do to provide patient care. It's a simple, systematic process made up of five steps: assessment, problem identification (or nursing diagnosis), planning, implementation, and evaluation. The steps are always sequential and the process is cyclical. The

completion of the fifth step returns you to the first step for reassessment. The nursing process stops when the patient is discharged.

The nursing process serves as a valuable planning tool that can be used by the entire health care team. The standard bearer of nursing care, the nursing process is evident throughout JCAHO requirements and regulations.

Correctly used, the nursing process occurs daily and permeates every aspect of nursing documentation. Every patient event and assessment is recorded. The five-step process ensures compliance with plan of care requirements. The plan of care is mandated by both acute care and long-term care standards and regulations.

The hospital's accreditation status and insurance reimbursement again depend on nursing documentation.

Changes in condition and care

When a patient's condition changes, documentation becomes a quality, reimbursement, and legal issue. An improvement in the patient's condition may signal a successful outcome and the need for discharge. A deterioration demands concise, factual recording of events.

A baseline assessment is recorded when each patient is admitted to the facility. Later changes are evaluated against the presenting symptoms, health history, physical examination, and ancillary test results. Subsequent care is based on the initial data.

Admission, transfer, and discharge notes must accurately reflect changes in the patient's condition. Condition changes justify changes in care and subsequent reimbursement. The appropriateness of admission, transfer, and discharge is also evaluated based on the patient's condition. JCAHO standards provide guidelines for recording changes in the patient's condition and care.

Use of equipment

Nursing documentation can provide evidence that certain equipment is essential to patient care. It verifies that the equipment has been used appropriately and justifies reimbursement.

For example, documentation of a patient's ordered bed rest supports his need for a bedpan. Similarly, documentation of insulin-dependent diabetes supports a patient's need to use a blood glucose monitor. Likewise, documentation of a respiratory impairment qualifies the patient to use a nebulizer. Examiners require this documentation before approving reimbursement.

Patient education

JCAHO standards require comprehensive patient education. Patient teaching can verify whether a patient is ready for discharge. Documented teaching outcomes can also protect a health care facility and its nurses from legal problems.

According to the JCAHO guidelines, patient teaching is required for many topics, including:
• medication use
• medical equipment use
• potential food and drug interactions
• rehabilitation techniques
• community resources
• further treatment.

Patient teaching must be interdisciplinary and related to the plan of care. And arrangements must be made to communicate all discharge instructions to the person or organization responsible for continuing the patient's care.

Inconsistencies

Nursing documentation must be consistent to maximize reimbursement. Charting based on a central problem list or interdisciplinary plan of care produces uniform data. Inconsistencies occur when nurses use different baseline criteria or record imprecise information.

Keep in mind that Medicare and other insurance examiners will always request an explanation for conflicting medical record data. And retrospectively, it may be difficult to obtain the details requested. Denial of payment could result.

Selected references

Berman, H.J., et al. *The Financial Management of Hospitals,* 8th ed. Ann Arbor, Mich.: Health Administrators Press, 1993.

Joint Commission on Accreditation of Healthcare Organizations. *1994 Accreditation Manual for Hospitals.* Oakbrook Terrace, Ill.: Joint Commission on Accreditation of Healthcare Organizations, 1993.

St. Anthony's DRG Working Guidebook. Alexandria, Va.: St. Anthony's Publishing, 1994.

Yura, H., and Walsh, M. *The Nursing Process: Assessing, Planning, Implementing, Evaluating,* 5th ed. New York: Appleton & Lange, 1989.

Quality Improvement
& Reimbursement

Documentation Systems

Although each health care facility determines its own requirements for documentation and evaluation, its requirements must comply with legal, accreditation, and professional standards.

Similarly, a nursing department can select the documentation system it wants to use as long as the system demonstrates adherence to standards and care requirements. For example, the system known as charting by exception (CBE) requires you to document only significant or abnormal findings. If the standard requires all patients' vital signs to be taken every 4 hours, you don't need to document that you performed this activity but you do need to document any abnormal vital signs.

Regardless of the type of documentation system used, specific policies and procedures describing a facility's documentation requirements must be in place and known. Understanding these requirements will help you document care accurately. It will also serve you well when evaluating or modifying your documentation system or when selecting a new one.

System selection

As health care facilities strive for greater efficiency and quality of care, you may need to participate in the decision about whether your current documentation system needs a simple revision, a total overhaul, or no change at all. Your aim: a system that reflects not only the patient's response to care but also the quality of care (which must meet the profession's recognized minimum

acceptable level of care). See *Evaluating your documentation system.*

Measuring up to standard

The committees that set up continuous quality improvement programs (mandated by the state and Joint Commission on Accreditation of Healthcare Organizations [JCAHO] regulations) choose well-defined, objective, and readily measurable indicators that help them assess the structure, process, and outcome of patient care. They use these indicators to monitor and evaluate the contents of a patient's medical record. Both shorter hospital stays and the need to verify the use of supplies and equipment in patient care have placed greater emphasis on nursing documentation as a yardstick for measuring not only the provision of patient care but also its quality.

To verify that treatment was required and provided or that medical tests and supplies were used, third-party payers (the insurers) review nursing documentation carefully. As a result, nurses now document more than ever before, including such data as every I.V. needle used to start an infusion, each use of an I.V. pump to deliver a specific volume of medication, and every test that the patient undergoes. (See Chapter 1, Nursing Documentation and the Medical Record, and Chapter 3, Quality Improvement and Reimbursement, for more information about standards and regulations concerning nursing documentation.)

Evaluating your documentation system

When reviewing the usefulness of your current documentation system, consider the following questions. If you answer no to any of them, you might recommend a closer evaluation of your system. After all, an incomplete, disorganized, or confusing record will not stand up to later scrutiny in case of a lawsuit or formal review.

Documenting interventions and patient progress
• Does your current system reflect the patient's progress and the interventions based on recorded evaluations? Look for records that describe the patient's progress, actual interventions, and evaluations of provided care.
• Does the record include evidence of the patient's response to nursing care? For example, does it report the effectiveness of analgesics or the patient's response to I.V. medications? Does it show that care was modified according to the patient's response to treatment? For example, does it show what action was taken if the patient tolerated only half of a prescribed tube feeding?
• Does the record note continuity of care or do unexplained gaps appear? If gaps appear, are notes entered later that document previous happenings? If late entries appear in the nursing notes on subsequent days, do you have to check the entire record to validate care?
• Are daily activities documented? For example, do the notes include evidence that the patient bathed himself or indicate that the patient could independently transfer himself to a wheelchair?

Documenting the health care team's actions
• Does the record portray the nursing process clearly? Look for actual nursing diagnoses, written assessments, interventions, and evaluation of the patient's responses to them.
• Does the current documentation system facilitate and show communication among health care team members? Check for evidence that telephone calls were made, that doctors were paged and notified of changes in a patient's condition, and that actions reflected these communications.
• Is discharge planning clearly documented? Do the records show evidence of interdisciplinary coordination, team conferences, completed patient teaching, and discharge instructions.
• Does the record reflect current standards of care? Does it indicate that caregivers and administrators follow hospital policies and procedures? If not, does the system provide for explanations of why a policy wasn't implemented or was implemented in an alternative manner?

Checking for clarity and comprehensiveness
• Are all portions of the record complete? Are all flow sheets, checklists, and other forms completed according to hospital policy? Are all necessary entries apparent on the medication forms? If not, does the record describe why a medication wasn't given as ordered and who was informed of the omission if necessary?
• Does the documentation make sense? Can you track the patient's care and hospital course on this record alone?

Evaluating your current system

Whether you're selecting a new documentation system or modifying an existing one, ask the following questions:
• What are the specific positive features of our current documentation system?
• What are the specific problems or limitations of our current documentation system? How can they be solved?
• How much time will we need to develop a new system, educate the staff, and implement the changes?
• How much will changing our current system cost? (Consider the costs of time, staff education, and new equipment.) Will the result eventually save money?
• How will changing the documentation system affect other members of the health care team, including the business office personnel and medical staff? How will we handle resistance to the proposed changes?

Selecting a new system

If assessing your current system leads you to conclude that you need a new system, begin by organizing a committee (or task force) composed of members from all departments that the change will affect. This committee should research all available systems; consult other health care facilities about systems that work or don't work for them; assess the costs, time commitment, and effects of the change on staff members; and evaluate each possible system in light of how well it satisfies professional standards and regulation requirements.

Once the committee selects a system, the next step is to initiate training sessions to familiarize staff members with the new system. Consider implementing change in one unit or area at a time. Then select or design the appropriate forms, and allow enough time for the transition to take place.

Revising an existing system

Altering a documentation system usually involves changing the way you collect, enter, and retrieve information, but it rarely affects the content of the information. If the content of your existing system is lacking in some way, changing formats probably won't solve the problem. Content problems usually stem from sources outside of the system—for example, inadequate objectives or guidelines or insufficient time to document properly.

Following the system format

Depending on the policies of your health care facility, you'll use one or more documentation systems to record your nursing interventions and evaluations and the patient's response.

Some health care facilities elect to use traditional narrative charting systems. Others choose alternative systems—among them, problem-oriented medical record (POMR), problem-intervention-evaluation (PIE), focus, charting by exception (CBE), FACT, core (with DAE), and outcome documentation systems. (See *Comparing charting systems.*) And increasingly, others are using computerized charting systems.

Of the many systems in current use, each has special features and distinct advantages and disadvantages.

Comparing charting systems

SYSTEM	USEFUL SETTINGS	PARTS OF RECORD	ASSESSMENT	PLAN OF CARE	OUTCOMES AND EVALUATION	PROGRESS NOTES FORMAT
Narrative	• Acute care • Long-term care • Home care • Ambulatory care	• Progress notes • Flow sheets to supplement plan of care	• Initial: history and admission form • Ongoing: progress notes	• Plan of care	• Progress notes • Discharge summaries	• Narration at time of entry
POMR	• Acute care • Long-term care • Home care	• Data base • Plan of care • Problem list • Progress notes • Discharge summary	• Initial: data base and plan of care • Ongoing: progress notes	• Data base • Nursing plan of care based on problem list	• Progress notes (section E of SOAPIE and SOAPIER)	SOAP, SOAPIE, SOAPIER
PIE	• Acute care	• Assessment flow sheet • Progress notes • Problem list	• Initial: assessment form • Ongoing: assessment form every shift	• None; included in progress notes (section P)	• Progress notes (section E)	• Problem • Intervention • Evaluation
Focus	• Acute care • Long-term care	• Progress notes • Flow sheets • Checklists	• Initial: patient history and admission assessment • Ongoing: assessment form	• Nursing plan of care based on problems or nursing diagnoses	• Progress notes (section R)	• Data • Action • Response
CBE	• Acute care • Long-term care	• Plan of care • Flow sheets, including patient-teaching records and patient discharge notes • Graphic record	• Initial: data base assessment sheet • Ongoing: nursing-medical order flow sheet	• Nursing plan of care based on nursing diagnoses	• Progress notes (section E)	• SOAPIE or SOAPIER
FACT	• Acute care • Long-term care	• Assessment sheet • Flow sheets • Progress notes	• Initial: baseline assessment • Ongoing: flow sheet and progress notes	• Nursing plan of care based on nursing diagnoses	• Flow sheet (section R)	• Data • Action • Response

Documentation Systems

Comparing charting systems *(continued)*

SYSTEM	USEFUL SETTINGS	PARTS OF RECORD	ASSESSMENT	PLAN OF CARE	OUTCOMES AND EVALUATION	PROGRESS NOTES FORMAT
Core (with DAE)	• Acute care • Long-term care	• Kardex • Flow sheets • Progress notes	• Initial: baseline assessment • Ongoing: progress notes	• Plan of care	• Progress notes (section E)	• Data • Action • Evaluation
Outcome	• Acute care • Long-term care • Home care • Ambulatory care	• Progress notes • Flow sheets • Nursing plan of care • Data base • Teaching plan	• Initial: baseline assessment • Ongoing: progress notes	• Data base • Plan of care	• Outcome-based plan of care	• Evaluative statements • Expected outcomes • Learning outcomes

Traditional narrative

In this approach to charting, you'll document ongoing assessment data, nursing interventions, and patient responses in chronological order. Today, few facilities rely only on the narrative system. Rather they combine it with other systems, primarily the source-oriented record.

Narrative format and components

Narrative charting consists of a straightforward chronologic account of the patient's status, the nursing interventions performed, and the patient's response to those interventions. The nurse usually records the data on the progress notes, with flow sheets commonly supplementing the narrative notes. (See *Charting with the narrative format.*)

Knowing when to document, what to document, and how to organize the data are the key elements of effective narrative notes.

When and what to document

Current JCAHO standards direct all health care facilities to establish policies about the frequency of patient reassessment. So you must assess your patient as often as required by your facility's policy, if not more, and then document your findings.

However, if you find yourself writing repetitious, meaningless notes, you may be documenting too often. In such a case, double-check your facility's written policy. You may find that you're following a time-consuming, unwritten standard initiated by staff members, not by your health care

Charting with the narrative format

This progress note provides an example of the narrative documentation format.

Date	Time	Notes
1/12/95	1100	Removed three 4" x 4" gauze pads saturated with blood-tinged, nonodorous drainage from Ⓛ lower leg wound. Wound measures 6 cm x 6 cm wide x 1 cm deep. Surrounding skin reddened and tender. Redressed wound with four 4" x 4"s and one 4" x 8" dressing and hypoallergenic tape. Will check wound q 1 hr to assess for continued drainage. Will monitor pt.'s T q 4 hr. T-98.8R; BP-122/84; P-86; R-22. Pt. reports pain in Ⓛ lower leg at 8 on a scale of 1 to 10, with 10 being the worst he can imagine. Administered two Percocet tablets and repositioned pt. from back to Ⓛ. side. Will give Percocet ½ hr before subsequent dressing changes. Instructed pt. in dressing change procedure. Pt. stated, "I know that it's important to wash my hands before I do anything so I don't get germs in my wound." Pt. demonstrated sufficient manual dexterity to put on gloves and handle all dressing supplies. Instructed pt. in proper hand-washing technique, dressing removal and disposal, opening and positioning dressing supplies, and signs and symptoms of wound infection and the importance of reporting them. Pt. demonstrated acceptable hand-washing technique and ability to remove dressings but needed instruction on positioning the leg so he could reach the wound. ———————————————— Carol Witt, R.N.
1/12/95	1200	Ⓛ lower left wound dressing dry and intact. Pt. reports pain in leg at 2 on scale of 1 to 10. ———————————————— Carol Witt, R.N.

Documentation Systems

Using military time

To promote accurate charting, many institutions use military time equivalents. Such use avoids confusion over a.m. and p.m. entries.

0100 =	1 a.m.	1300 =	1 p.m.
0200 =	2 a.m.	1400 =	2 p.m.
0300 =	3 a.m.	1500 =	3 p.m.
0400 =	4 a.m.	1600 =	4 p.m.
0500 =	5 a.m.	1700 =	5 p.m.
0600 =	6 a.m.	1800 =	6 p.m.
0700 =	7 a.m.	1900 =	7 p.m.
0800 =	8 a.m.	2000 =	8 p.m.
0900 =	9 a.m.	2100 =	9 p.m.
1000 =	10 a.m.	2200 =	10 p.m.
1100 =	11 a.m.	2300 =	11 p.m.
1200 =	12 p.m.	2400 =	12 a.m.

facility. To guard against this, review the policy at least every 6 months.

Besides documenting simply by policy, be sure to record specific and descriptive narrative notes whenever you observe any of the following:
• a change in the patient's condition (progression, regression, or new problems). For example, write, "The patient can walk 300 feet assisted by one person."
• a patient's response to a treatment or medication. For example, write, "The patient states that right leg pain is unrelieved 1 hour after receiving medication. He's still grimacing and rubbing the site."
• a lack of improvement in the patient's condition. For example, write, "No change in size or condition of leg wound after 5 days of treatment. Dimensions and condition remain as stated in 4/20/94 note."
• a patient or family member's response to teaching. For example, write, "The patient performed a return demonstration of wound care and correctly stated that he should do it three times a day."

Document exactly what you hear, observe, inspect, do, or teach. Include as much specific, descriptive information as possible. For example, if your patient has lower leg edema, include ankle and mid-calf measurements and skin characteristics as well. Always document how the patient responds to your care and the extent of his progression toward a desired outcome.

How to write meaningful notes
• Read the narrative notes written by other health care professionals before you write your own.
• Read the notes recorded by nurses on other shifts and make additional comments on their findings. This demonstrates continuity of care.
• If policy permits, use flow sheets to document repetitious procedures or measurements and summarize the information in the narrative notes.
• Include specific information when you observe a change in your patient's condition, a lack of progress in his condition, or a response to treatment, medication, or patient teaching. Also record the exact time these events occurred. (See *Using military time.*)
• When possible, document an event immediately after it occurs. If you wait until the end of your shift, you may forget some important information. If you can't document at the time of an event, make notes on a piece of paper to help you remember details.

How to organize your notes

Before you write anything, organize your thoughts so your paragraphs will be coherent. If you have difficulty deciding what to write, refer to the patient's plan of care to review unresolved problems, prescribed interventions, and expected outcomes. Then comment on the patient's progress in relation to these items.

If you still have trouble organizing your thoughts, use this sequence of questions to order your entry:
• How did I first become aware of the problem?
• What has the patient said about the problem that's significant?
• What have I observed that's related to the problem?
• What's my plan for dealing with the problem?
• What steps have I taken to intervene?
• How has the patient responded to my interventions?

To make your notes as coherent as possible, discuss each of the patient's problems in a separate paragraph; don't lump them together.

Or use a head-to-toe approach to organize your information. Be sure to notify the doctor of significant changes that you observe. Then document this communication, the doctor's responses, and any new orders to be implemented.

Advantages

The most flexible of all the documentation systems, narrative charting suits any clinical setting and strongly conveys your nursing interventions and your patients' responses.

Because narration is the most common form of writing, the training time needed for new staff members is usually brief. And because narrative notes are in chronological order, other team members can review the patient's progress on a day-to-day basis.

What's more, the narrative format easily lends itself to presenting information collected over an extended period.

Another timesaver is the ease with which narrative notes combine with other documentation devices, such as flow sheets—again helping to decrease charting time.

Disadvantages

Narrative charting can be weak when it comes to recording patient outcomes because you must read the entire record to arrive at the outcome. Even then, you may have trouble determining the outcome of a particular problem because the same information may not be consistently documented.

Tracking problems and identifying trends in the patient's progress can be difficult also—and for the same reason: You have to read the entire record to arrive at an overall impression of the patient's condition and a complete account of his treatment course.

Because the narrative format offers no inherent guide to what's important to document, the tendency is to document "everything." The result: a long, rambling, repetitive, subjective, and time-consuming record.

The narrative format also lends itself to vague or inaccurate language—for example, many records contain phrases such as "appears to be bleeding" or "small amount." Some problems may be documented briefly and others may be docu-

AIR: A new narrative format

A charting format called AIR may help you organize and simplify your charting. The AIR format synthesizes major nursing events while avoiding repetition of information found elsewhere in the medical record. Combined with nursing flow sheets and the nursing plan of care, the AIR format can clearly and concisely document your care.
   Here's how it works:

Assessment
Summarize your physical assessment findings. Rather than simply describing the patient's current condition, you'll document trends and record your impression of the problem. Begin by titling each specific issue that you address, such as nursing diagnosis, admission note, and discharge planning.

Intervention
Summarize your actions and those of other caregivers in response to the assessment data. The summary may include a condensed nursing plan of care or plans for additional patient monitoring.

Response
Summarize the outcome or the patient's response to the nursing interventions. Because a response may not be evident for hours or even days, this documentation may not immediately follow the entries. In fact, it may be recorded by another nurse, which is why titling each of your assessments and interventions is so important.

mented at length for no clear reason. (See *AIR: A new narrative format*.)

Problem-oriented medical record

Alternatively called the problem-oriented record (POR), the problem-oriented medical record (POMR) system focuses on specific patient problems. It was originally developed by doctors and later adapted by nurses. In following the format of this documentation system, you'll describe each problem on multidisciplinary patient progress notes, not on progress notes containing only nursing information. (See *Writing a problem-oriented progress note.*)

POMR format and components
The POMR has five components: data base, problem list, initial plan, progress notes, and discharge summary. You'll record your interventions and evaluations in the progress notes and the discharge summary only. But to gain a full understanding of the POMR, briefly review all five components.

Data base
Most commonly completed by a nurse, the data base (or initial assessment) forms the foundation for the patient's plan of care. A collection of subjective and objective information about the patient, this initial assessment includes the reason for hospitalization, medical history, allergies, medication regimen, physical and psychosocial findings, self-care ability, educational needs, and other discharge

Writing a problem-oriented progress note

Here's the nursing portion of a problem-oriented progress note. The nurse used the SOAP framework in the sample below.

Date	Time	Notes
11/8/94	1000	#1 Altered cerebral tissue perfusion R/T transient decrease in blood flow.
		S: Pt.: I can't remember from one minute to the next.
		O: Pt. states she has no idea what day or time it is. ® pupil 3 mm and sluggish to react. Ⓛ pupil 3 mm and reacts briskly to light. Unsteady gait noted. Otherwise neurologic assessment normal.
		A: Pt. disoriented to time and has abnormal pupillary reaction in response to light.
		P: Notify the Dr. Orient pt. to time, place, and person q 1 hr. Assess the pt.'s ability to retain bilaterally equal motor function q 1 hr. Assess the patient for sensory deficits q 1 hr. Assess pupillary reaction to light q 1 hr. Assess the pt.'s BP q 1 hr. Assess pt's speech and memory for deficits q 1 hr. ——— Marianne Evans, RN
	1000	#2 High risk for injury R/T sensory and motor deficits.
		S: Pt.: I feel dizzy and off balance.
		O: Pt.'s eyes fluttering; pt. holding onto bedside table.
		A: Pt. experiencing dizziness and loss of balance similar to previous episode of TIA.
		P: Assist pt. back to bed and place side rails up. Modify environment to prevent injury. ——— Marianne Evans, RN
	1000	#3 Anxiety R/T possible CVA.
		S: Pt. reports being scared of what will happen to her if she has a stroke—who will take care of her?
		O: Pt. clutching onto side rails and hyperventilating.
		A: Pt. becoming increasingly anxious.
		P: Discuss pt.'s anxiety and feelings about her illness. Help pt. identify the source of her anxiety. Identify and use effective coping mechanisms with the pt. Assure pt. that she will be monitored closely. Marianne Evans, RN

planning concerns. This information becomes the foundation for a problem list.

Problem list

After analyzing the data base, you, the doctor, and other relevant health care team members will identify and list the patient's current problems in chronological order according to the date each was identified—not in order of acuteness or priority. Originally, this system called for one interdisciplinary problem list. You may still see this format used, but usually nurses and doctors keep separate problem lists with problems stated as either nursing or medical diagnoses. This problem list provides an overview of the patient's health status.

Try to number each problem so you can use the numbers to refer to the problems in the rest of the POMR. Make every entry on the patient's initial plan, progress notes, and discharge summary correspond to a number, and file the numbered problem list at the front of the patient's chart. Keep the problem list current by adding new numbers as new problems arise.

Once a problem has been resolved, draw a line through it. Or show that it's inactive by retiring the problem number and highlighting the problem with a colored felt-tip pen. Don't use the problem number again for the same patient.

Initial plan

After constructing the problem list, write an initial plan for each problem. This plan should include the expected outcomes, plans for further data collection (if needed), and patient care and teaching plans. Mutual goal setting is essential to patient compliance and the effectiveness of your interventions.

Progress notes

One of the most prominent features of the POMR system is the structured way in which narrative progress notes are written by all team members, using the SOAP, SOAPIE, or SOAPIER format.

SOAP format

If you use the SOAP format, you'll document the following information for each problem:
• Subjective data: Information the patient or family members tell you, such as the chief complaint and other impressions.
• Objective data: Factual, measurable data you gather during assessment, such as observed signs and symptoms, vital signs, and laboratory test values.
• Assessment data: Conclusions based on the collected subjective and objective data and formulated as patient problems or nursing diagnoses. This dynamic and ongoing process changes as more or different subjective and objective information becomes known.
• Plan: Your strategy for relieving the patient's problem. This plan should include both immediate or short-term actions and long-term measures.

SOAPIE format

Some facilities use the SOAPIE format, adding:
• Intervention: Measures you've taken to achieve an expected outcome. As the patient's health status changes, you may need to modify these interventions. Be sure to document the patient's understanding and acceptance of the initial plan in this section of your notes.
• Evaluation: An analysis of the effectiveness of your interventions. If expected outcomes fall short, use the evaluation

process as a basis for developing alternative interventions.

SOAPIER format

The SOAPIER format includes revision to allow for the documentation of alternative interventions.

• Revision: Document any changes from the original plan of care in this section. Interventions, outcomes, or target dates may need to be adjusted to reach a previous goal.

Typically, you must write a complete SOAP, SOAPIE, or SOAPIER note every 24 hours on any unresolved problem or whenever the patient's condition changes. When doing so, be sure to specify the appropriate number of the problem you're discussing. Keep in mind that you don't need to write an entry for each SOAP or SOAPIE component every time you document. If you have nothing to record for a component, either omit the letter from the note or leave a blank space after it, depending on your facility's policy.

If your facility uses the SOAP format, record your nursing interventions and evaluations on flow sheets. If you use the SOAPIE format, provide explanations as needed in your progress notes under I and E.

Discharge summary

Completing the POMR format, the discharge summary covers each problem on the list and notes whether it was resolved. Discuss any unresolved problems in your SOAP or SOAPIE note, and specify your plan for dealing with the problem after discharge. Note any communications with other facilities, home health care agencies, and the patient.

Advantages

POMR documentation organizes information about each problem into specific categories understandable to all health care teammates, thereby promoting interdisciplinary communication and data retrieval. The problems serve as an index to the medical record.

POMR documentation also illustrates the continuity of care, unifying the plan of care and progress notes into a full record of the care actually planned and delivered. This information is easily incorporated into care planning because the caregiver addresses each problem or nursing diagnosis in the nursing notes. What's more, the POMR format promotes documentation of the nursing process, facilitates more consistent documentation, and eliminates documentation of nonessential data. This format is most effective in acute care or long-term care settings.

Disadvantages

A drawback of POMR documentation is its emphasis on the chronology of problems as opposed to their priority, and teammates may disagree about which problems should be listed. Analyzing trends with this format can be difficult because information may be buried in the daily narrative.

The POMR format commonly produces repetitive charting of assessment findings and interventions, especially with the SOAPIE format. That's because both your assessments and interventions commonly apply to more than one problem. The resulting overlap makes the POMR system time-consuming to perform and to read. And because the format emphasizes problems, routine care may remain undocumented unless flow sheets are used.

The POMR format isn't well suited for settings with rapid patient turnover (for example, the postanesthesia care unit, short procedure unit, or emergency department).

Furthermore, difficulties may arise if teammates fail to keep the problem list current or if they're confused about which problems should be listed. The considerable time and cost of training new personnel to use the SOAP, SOAPIE, or SOAPIER method may also be a disadvantage.

PIE

The problem-intervention-evaluation (PIE) documentation system was developed to simplify the documentation process. PIE charting organizes information according to patients' problems as defined by a group of nurses at Craven Hospital in New Bern, N.C., in 1985. As its name indicates, this problem-oriented documentation approach considers three categories: problem (P), intervention (I), and evaluation (E). To follow this format, you'll need to keep a daily patient assessment flow sheet and progress notes.

By integrating the plan of care into the nurses' progress notes, the PIE format eliminates the need for a separate plan of care. The intention is to provide a concise, efficient record of patient care that has a nursing—not a medical—focus. (See *Using the PIE format.*)

PIE format and components

To implement the PIE documentation system, first assess the patient and document your findings on a daily patient assessment flow sheet. This flow sheet lists defined assessment terms under major categories (such as respiration), along with routine care and monitoring (such as providing hygiene and monitoring breath sounds). The flow sheet typically includes space to record pertinent treatments.

Initial only the assessment terms on the flow sheet that apply to your patient and mark abnormal findings with an asterisk. Record detailed information in your progress notes.

Problem

After performing and documenting an initial assessment, use the collected data to identify pertinent nursing diagnoses. You can use the list of nursing diagnoses accepted by your facility, which usually corresponds to the diagnoses approved by the North American Nursing Diagnosis Association (NANDA).

If you can't find a nursing diagnosis on an approved list, write the problem statement yourself using accepted criteria. Document all nursing diagnoses or problems in the progress notes, labeling each as "P" with an identifying number (for example, P #1).

This labeling system allows you to refer later to a specific problem by label only, eliminating the need to redocument the problem statement. Some facilities also use a separate problem-list form to keep a convenient running account of the nursing diagnoses for a particular patient.

Using the PIE format

This sample shows how to write progress notes using the problem-intervention-evaluation (PIE) format.

Date	Time	Notes
11/22/94	1600	P#1: High risk for ineffective breathing pattern related to possible smoke inhalation.
		IP#1: Assessed respiratory rate and breath sounds q 1 hr to R/O pulmonary edema and bronchospasm. Taught pt. how to perform deep-breathing and coughing exercises and taught use of incentive spirometer. O_2 applied @ 2 L/min via nasal cannula.
		EP#1: Pt. maintains patent airway and normal RR and depth. Pt. understands the importance of performing deep-breathing and coughing exercises q 1 hr. Pt. has normal ABG levels. ————— Deborah Ryan, RN
11/22/94	1600	P#2: High risk for decreased CO R/T reduced stroke volume as a result of fluid loss through burns.
		IP#2: Teach pt. to report any restlessness, diaphoresis, or light-headedness, which may indicate shock. Evaluate VS and hemodynamic readings at least q 2 hr. Monitor urine output q 1 hr. Monitor ABG levels. Provide and monitor I.V. therapy.
		EP#2: Pt. maintains normal VS and stable hemodynamic status. ABGs WNL. Pt. has adequate urine output. Pt. verbalizes signs and symptoms of shock. Pt. receiving adequate replacement through I.V. therapy. ———— Deborah Ryan, RN
11/22/94	1630	P#3: Pain related to second-degree burns over 20% of body.
		I.P#3: Assess pain q 2 hr and medicate q 3 to 4 hr with morphine, as ordered.
		EP#3: Pt. reports a decrease in pain rating from 8 to 2 on a scale of 1 to 10, with 10 being the worst pain imaginable. ———— Deborah Ryan, RN

Documentation Systems

Intervention

In this step, document the nursing actions taken for each nursing diagnosis. Document each intervention on the progress sheet, labeling each as "I" followed by the assigned problem number. (To refer to an intervention for the first nursing diagnosis, for instance, you'd use IP #1.)

Evaluation

After charting your interventions, document the related effects in your progress notes. Use the label "E" followed by the assigned problem number (for example, EP #1).

Make sure that you or another nurse evaluates each problem at least every 8 hours. After every three shifts, review the notes from the previous 24 hours to identify the patient's current problems and responses to interventions.

Document continuing problems daily, along with relevant interventions and evaluations. Cross out any resolved problems from the daily documentation.

Advantages

Using the PIE format ensures that your documentation includes nursing diagnoses, related interventions, and evaluations. This format also encourages you to meet JCAHO requirements, provides an organizing framework for your thoughts and writing, and simplifies documentation by incorporating your plan of care in your progress notes.

What's more, this method improves the progress notes' quality by highlighting care interventions and requiring a written evaluation of the patient's response to those interventions.

Disadvantages

The PIE format may require in-depth training for staff members. The requirement that you reevaluate each problem each shift is time-consuming and leads to repetitive entries (some problems simply don't need such frequent evaluation).

The PIE format omits documentation of the planning step in the nursing process. And this step, which addresses expected outcomes, is essential to evaluating the patient's responses.

Finally, PIE charting doesn't incorporate multidisciplinary charting.

Focus

Developed by nurses at Eitel Hospital in Minneapolis, Minn., who found the SOAP format awkward, focus charting encourages you to organize your thoughts into patient-centered topics, or foci of concern, and then to document precisely and concisely. The format encourages you to use assessment data to evaluate these patient care concerns. It also helps you identify necessary revisions to the plan of care as you document each entry. It works well in acute care settings and in areas where the same care and procedures are repeated frequently.

Focus format and components

To implement focus documentation, you'll use a progress sheet with categories for date, time, focus, and progress notes. (See *Charting with focus.*) Then identify the foci by reviewing your assessment data.

BETTER CHARTING

Charting with focus

This sample shows how to write progress notes using the focus charting format.

Date	Time	Focus	Progress notes
12/18/94	0900	Ineffective breathing pattern R/T decreased energy.	D: Pt. dyspneic and faint after bathing at bedside. Skin reddened. T-99.0, R; P-94; R-30; BP-142/86. Pt. reports that the dyspnea disrupts her sleep and she's lost 20 lb in 3 months. Pt. states she feels hot and is having difficulty catching her breath.——— A: Auscultation reveals decreased vesicular breath sounds, prolonged expiration, and scattered expiratory wheezes in both lung bases. O₂ applied at 2 L/min via nasal cannula. Dr. Miller notified and will examine pt. within 10 min. Explained the purpose of patterned breathing to pt.; demonstrated correct breathing techniques and had the pt. demonstrate them. ——— EU Thimes, RN
12/18/94	0900	Anxiety R/T difficulty in breathing.	D: Pt. shaking and grabbing my hand and stating she is scared.——— A: Spent time with pt. providing support. Discussed importance of and demonstrated diaphragmatic pursed-lip breathing techniques. Allowed pt. to verbalize feelings once dyspnea improved.——— R: Pt. states she feels less anxious and she appears calmer. ——— EU Thimes, RN
12/18/94	0900	Knowledge deficit R/T disease process and its treatment.	D: Pt. reports smoking history of 40 pack years (2 packs x 20 years). Currently smokes one pack per day. Denies exposure to respiratory irritants. A: Reviewed the most common signs and symptoms associated with the disease: dyspnea, especially with exertion; fatigue; cough; occasional mucus production; weight loss; rapid heart rate; irregular P and use of accessory muscles to help with breathing from limited diaphragm function. Provided information about smoking cessation groups. Urged pt. to avoid fumes, temperature extremes, and people with infections. ——— EU Thimes, RN

Documentation Systems

Nursing diagnosis

Typically, you'll write each focus as a nursing diagnosis (such as decreased cardiac output or fluid volume deficit). However, the focus may also refer to a sign or symptom (such as hypotension or chest pain), a patient behavior (such as inability to ambulate) or special need (such as a discharge need), an acute change in the patient's condition (such as loss of consciousness or increase in blood pressure), or a significant event (such as surgery).

Progress notes content

In the progress notes column, you'll organize information using three categories: data (D), action (A), and response (R). In the data category, include subjective and objective information that describes the focus.

In the action category, include immediate and future nursing actions based on your assessment of the patient's condition. This category also may encompass any changes to the plan of care you deem necessary based on your evaluation.

In the response category, describe the patient's response to any aspect of nursing or medical care.

Using all three categories ensures complete documentation based on the nursing process. Be sure to record routine nursing tasks and assessment data on your flow sheets and checklists.

Advantages

Focus charting is flexible and can be adapted to fit any clinical setting. It centers on the nursing process, and the data-action-response format provides cues that direct the recording in a process-oriented way.

By separating the focus statement from the narrative of the progress note, this format makes it easy to find information on a particular problem, thereby promoting communication among health care team members.

The format also highlights the nursing process in the documentation of daily patient care, encourages regular documentation of patient responses to nursing and medical therapy, and ensures adherence to JCAHO requirements for documenting patient responses and outcomes.

You can use this format to document many topics without being confined to those on the problem list or plan of care. What's more, the focus format helps you organize your thoughts and document succinctly and precisely.

Disadvantages

Learning the focus documentation system may require in-depth training—especially for staff members used to other systems. Additionally, the system requires you to use many flow sheets and checklists, which can lead to inconsistent documentation and cause difficulty in tracking a patient's problems. Then, too, the focus format can become a narrative note if you neglect to include the patient's response to interventions.

CBE

The charting by exception (CBE) documentation system was designed by nurses at St. Luke's Hospital in Milwaukee, Wis., to overcome long-standing charting problems, such as lengthy and repetitive notes, poorly organized information, difficult-to-retrieve data, and a high risk of errors of omission. To avoid these pitfalls, the CBE format radically departs from traditional systems by requiring documentation of only significant or abnormal findings. It also uses military time to help prevent misinterpretations.

CBE format and components

To use CBE documentation effectively, you must know and adhere to established guidelines for nursing assessments and interventions. The CBE nursing assessment format has printed guidelines for each body system, and the format relies on written standards of practice that identify the nurse's basic responsibilities to patients. For example, care standards for patient hygiene might include your responsibility to ensure that a patient has a complete linen change every 3 days, or sooner if necessary.

Because the standards are clear and concise, all charting related to routine nursing care—or any other care outlined in the standards—is eliminated. You document only deviations from the standards, thereby omitting repetitive charting of routine procedures.

Interventional guidelines for the CBE system stem from these sources:
• nursing diagnosis–based standardized plans of care. These plans identify patient problems, desired outcomes, and interventions.
• patient care guidelines. These guidelines consist of standardized interventions established for specific patient populations—patients with a nursing diagnosis of pain, for example. They outline the nursing in-terventions, treatments, and time frame for repeated assessments.
• doctor's orders. These are prescribed medical interventions.
• incidental orders. These are usually one-time, miscellaneous nursing or medical orders or interdependent interventions related to a protocol or a piece of equipment.
• standards of nursing practice. These standards define the acceptable level of routine nursing care for all patients. They may describe the essential aspects of nursing practice for a specific unit or for all clinical areas.

The CBE format includes a nursing diagnosis-based standardized plan of care and several types of flow sheets, including the nursing-medical order flow sheet, graphic record, patient-teaching record, and patient discharge note. In certain cases, you may need to supplement your CBE documentation by using nurses' progress notes.

Nursing diagnosis-based standardized plans of care
Use these preprinted plans of care whenever you identify a nursing diagnosis. Use a separate form for each pertinent diagnosis. Keep in mind that the forms have spaces that allow you to individualize them as needed. You can, for example, include expected outcomes and major plan of care revisions. Place the completed forms in the nurses' progress notes section of the clinical record.

Nursing–medical order flow sheet
Use this form to document your assessments and interventions. Each flow sheet is designed for a 24-hour period of care

Using a nursing–medical order flow sheet

Here are the typical features of a nursing–medical order flow sheet.

NURSING-MEDICAL ORDER FLOW SHEET

Date *1/22/95*

ND #/DO	Assessments and interventions	0800*	0830*		
ND 1	*ICP Assessment*	*0800**	*0830**		
ND 1	*Physical Assessment for elevated ICP*	*0800**	*0830**		
ND 2	*Injury Assessment R/T seizures*	*1000*			
DO	*Discontinue peripheral I.V.*	*1230* ✓			
Initials		*MED*	*MED*		

KEY
DO = doctor's orders   → = no change in condition
ND = nursing diagnosis   * = abnormal or significant finding
✓ = normal findings   (See Comments section.)

ND #/DO	Time	Comments	Initials
ND 1	*0800*	*ICP 18 mm Hg. Dr. Morris notified. HOB elevated to 30°. Will*	
		reassess at 0830. ————————————	*MED*
ND 1	*0800*	*LOC WNL. Pt. c/o slight headache. acetaminophen gr X p.o.*	*MED*
ND 1	*0830*	*ICP 16 mm Hg.* ————————————	*MED*
ND 1	*0830*	*No c/o headache.* ————————————	*MED*

Initials	Signature
MED	*Mary Ellen Davis, RN*

for one patient. (See *Using a nursing–medical order flow sheet.*)

The flow sheet uses a specific set of key abbreviations to record care:
• ND indicates nursing diagnosis
• DO indicates a doctor's orders
• a check mark (√) indicates a completed medical order or nursing assessment with no abnormal findings
• an asterisk (*) indicates an abnormal finding on an assessment or an abnormal response to an intervention

• an arrow (→) indicates that the patient's status remains unchanged since the previous entry.

The top part of the flow sheet contains the orders for assessments and interventions. Each nursing order includes a corresponding nursing diagnosis, labeled ND 1, ND 2, and so on; medical orders are labeled DO.

After completing an assessment, compare your findings with the normal parameters defined in the printed guidelines on the back of the form. If the findings are within normal parameters, place a check mark in the appropriate category box. If the findings are not within the normal range, put an asterisk in the category box. Then explain your findings in the comments section on the form.

Remember, a finding that's not defined in the guidelines may be normal for a particular patient. For example, unclear speech may be a normal finding in a patient with a long-standing tracheostomy. Reference this note by nursing diagnosis number or doctor's order and time. If the patient's condition hasn't changed from the last assessment, draw a horizontal arrow from the previous category box to the current one.

Document interventions similarly. Use a check mark to indicate a completed intervention and an expected patient response. Indicate significant findings or abnormal patient responses with an asterisk, and write an explanation in the comments section. When the patient's response is unchanged, use an arrow.

After you document an entire column in the assessments and interventions section, initial it at the bottom. Also initial all your entries in the comments section, and sign the form at the bottom of the page.

Some facilities use a nursing care flow sheet that combines all the necessary sections, such as the graphic sheet, a daily activities checklist, and a patient care assessment section. (See *Using a combined nursing care flow sheet,* pages 84 to 86.)

Graphic record

Use this flow sheet or section of a flow sheet to document trends in the patient's vital signs; weight; intake and output; and stool, urination, appetite, and activity levels. As with the nursing–medical order flow sheet, use check marks and asterisks to indicate expected and abnormal findings, respectively. Record information about abnormalities in the nurses' progress notes or on the nursing–medical order flow sheet.

In the box labeled routine standards, check off the established nursing care interventions you performed—providing hygiene, for example. Don't rewrite these standards as orders on the nursing–medical order flow sheet. Refer to the guidelines on the back of the graphic record for complete instructions.

Patient-teaching record

Use this form or section on the form to identify the knowledge, psychomotor skills, and social or behavioral measures that your patient or his caregiver must learn by a predetermined date. The patient-teaching record includes teaching resources, dates of patient achievements, and other pertinent observations. You may use more than one form for a patient with multiple learning needs.

(Text continues on page 87.)

Using a combined nursing care flow sheet

This sample shows a portion of a nursing care flow sheet that combines a graphic record, a daily nursing care activities checklist, and a patient care assessment form.

Name *Harold Kravitz*

Date		11/29/94											
Hour		0700	0800	0900	1000	1100	1200	1300	1400	1500	1600	1700	1800
Temperature													
°C	°F												
40.4	105												
40.0	104												
39.4	103												
38.9	102												
37.8	100												
37.2	99												
36.7	98												
36.1	99												
35.6	96												
Pulse		84	80	82	78	76	78	78	82	84	82	80	78
Respiration		16	20	20	22	24	24	18	20	22	20	18	24
BP	Lying												
	Sitting	136/82	130/80	126/74	132/82	132/80	140/82	136/74	130/70	138/78	140/80	132/78	136/76
	Standing												
Intake	Oral	400					300						100
	Tube												
	I.V.												
	Blood												
8-Hour total		700											
Output	Urine	300					200						
Other													
Other													
8-Hour total		500											
Teaching		Skin care. s/s of UTI. Safety.											
Signature		*Carol With, RN.* 0700 – 1500								*Donald Baron, RN* 1500 – 2300			

Using a combined nursing care flow sheet *(continued)*

Hour		0700	0800	0900	1000	1100	1200	1300	1400	1500	1600	1700
ACTIVITY	Bed rest	CW							→	DB		→
	OOB											
	Ambulate (assist)											
	Ambulatory											
	Sleeping											
	BRP											
	HOB elevated	CW							→	DB		→
	Cough, deep-breathe, turn		CW								DB	
	ROM: Active / Passive		CW								DB	
HYGIENE	Bath		CW									
	Shave		CW									
	Oral		CW									
	Skin care											
	Perianal care											
NUTRITION	Diet	soft — no added salt										
	% Eating			90%				60%				90%
	Feeding											
	Supplemental											
	S-Self, A-Assist, F-Feed			S				S				S
BLADDER	Catheter	indwelling urinary #18 Fr.										
	Incontinent											
	Voiding	QS–clear, yellow urine										
	Intermittent catheter											
BOWEL	Stools (OB⁺, OB⁻)											
	Incontinent											
	Normal	Small, soft, formed brown stool										
	Enema											
SPECIAL TREATMENTS	Special mattress	Low–pressure airflow mattress applied 0900										
	Special bed											
	Heel and elbow pads											
	Antiembolism stockings											
	Traction: + = on, − = off											
	Isolation type											

(continued)

Documentation Systems

Using a combined nursing care flow sheet *(continued)*

ASSESSMENT FINDINGS

KEY: ✓ = normal findings
✱ = significant findings

	Day	Evening	Night	
Neurologic	✱ CW	✱ DB		Limited ROM ⓛ shoulder. Pt. states, "I have arthritis and my shoulder is always stiff."
Cardiovascular (CV)	✓ CW	✓ DB		
Respiratory	✱ CW	✓ DB		Decreased breath sounds at ⓡ base posteriorly at 0800 + 1400. Lungs clear at 1600 + 2000.
GI	✓ CW	✓ DB		
Genitourinary (GU)	✓ CW	✓ DB		
Surgical dressing and incision	N/A	N/A		
Skin integrity	✱ CW	✱ DB		Poor skin turgor; dry, flaky skin. 4cm X 4cm area of redness at sacral area.
Psychosocial	✓ CW	✓ DB		
Educational	✱ CW	✱ DB		Taught pt. safety, skin care, and signs and symptoms of UTI.
Peripheral vascular	✓ CW	✓ DB		

NORMAL ASSESSMENT FINDINGS

Neurologic
- Alert and oriented to time, place, and person
- Speech clear and understandable
- Memory intact
- Behavior appropriate to situation and accommodation
- Active range-of-motion (ROM) of all extremities; symmetrically equal strength
- No paresthesia

CV
- Regular apical pulse
- Palpable bilateral peripheral pulses
- No peripheral edema
- No calf tenderness

Respiratory
- Resting respirations 10 to 20 per minute, quiet and regular
- Clear sputum
- Pink nail beds and mucous membranes

GI
- Abdomen soft and nondistended
- Tolerates prescribed diet without nausea or vomiting
- Bowel movements within own normal pattern and consistency

GU
- No indwelling catheter in use
- Urinates without pain
- Undistended bladder after urination
- Urine clear, yellow to amber color

Surgical dressing and incision
- Dressing dry and intact
- No evidence of redness, increased temperature, or tenderness in surrounding tissue
- Sutures, staples, Steri-Strips intact
- Sound edges well approximated
- No drainage present

Skin integrity
- Skin color normal
- Skin warm, dry, and intact
- Moist mucous membranes

Psychosocial
- Interacts and communicates in an appropriate manner with others

Educational
- Patient or significant others communicate understanding of the patient's health status, plan of care, and expected response
- Patient or significant others demonstrate ability to perform health-related procedures and behaviors as taught

Peripheral vascular
- Affected extremity pink, warm, and movable within average ROM
- Capillary refill time < 3 seconds
- Peripheral pulses palpable
- No edema; sensation intact without numbness or paresthesia
- No pain on passive stretch

Patient discharge note

Similar to other discharge forms, the patient discharge note is a flow sheet for documenting ongoing discharge planning. Follow the instructions printed on the back of the form.

Progress notes

Another component of the CBE format, the progress notes are used to document plan of care revisions and interventions that don't lend themselves to the nursing–medical order flow sheet. Because the CBE format permits you to document most assessments and interventions on the nursing–medical order flow sheet, your progress notes typically contain little assessment and intervention data.

Advantages

The CBE format has several important advantages. By including only information that deviates from the expected, it decreases the amount of documentation needed, eliminates redundancies, and clearly identifies abnormal data. The use of well-defined guidelines and standards of care promotes uniform nursing practice. What's more, the flow sheets let you easily track trends.

Guidelines, including normal findings, are printed on the forms for ready reference. Abnormal findings are highlighted to help you quickly pinpoint significant changes and trends in a patient's condition. Documentation of routine care is eliminated through the use of nursing care standards.

Patient data are immediately written on the permanent record so you don't have to keep temporary notes and then later transcribe them to the patient's chart. Other

caregivers always have access to the most current data. Assessments are standardized so all caregivers evaluate and document findings consistently. Information that's already been recorded isn't repeated. For instance, you don't have to write a long entry in a patient's chart each time you assess him if his condition remains the same.

One more point: All flow sheets are kept at the patient's bedside, where they serve as a ready reference. This location tends to encourage immediate documentation.

Disadvantages

The chief drawback of the CBE format is the major time commitment needed to develop clear guidelines and standards of care. To ensure a legally sound patient record, these guidelines and standards must be in place and understood by all nursing staff members before the format can be implemented. This radical departure from traditional documentation systems takes time for people to learn, accept, and use correctly. Consistent use of the appropriate documenting procedures is vital.

If your health care facility uses multiple forms rather than one form that combines all the CBE components, the documenting process can be confusing and the records incomplete. Narrative notes may be too brief and an evaluation of a patient's response may not be fully described.

This CBE system was developed for registered nurses. If licensed practical nurses will be using the system, it must be evaluated and modified to meet their scope of practice. CBE complies with legal principles but it may be questioned in court until the system becomes more widely known.

FACT

Named for its comprising elements, the FACT documentation system incorporates many CBE principles. It was designed to avoid the documentation of irrelevant data, redundant and repetitive notes, and inconsistencies among departments and to reduce the amount of time spent charting.

FACT format and components

This system has four key elements:
• Flow sheets individualized to specific services
• Assessment features standardized with baseline parameters
• Concise, integrated progress notes and flow sheets documenting the patient's condition and responses
• Timely entries recorded when care is given.

To implement FACT documentation, begin with a complete initial baseline assessment on each patient using standardized parameters. The system requires that you document only exceptions to the norm or significant information about the patient. It eliminates detailed charting of normal findings and incorporates each step of the nursing process. (See *Documenting with FACT*.)

You'll complete a baseline assessment for each patient. The FACT format uses an assessment-action flow sheet, a frequent assessment flow sheet, and progress notes. The content of the flow sheets and notes may be individualized to some extent.

The flow sheets cover a 24- to 72-hour time span, and you'll need to date, time, and sign all entries.

Assessment-action flow sheet

Use this form to document ongoing assessments and interventions. Normal assessment parameters for each body system are printed on the form, along with the planned interventions. The flow sheet may be individualized according to the patient's needs.

Frequent assessment flow sheet

Use this form to chart vital signs and frequent assessments. On a surgical unit, for example, this form would include a postoperative assessment section.

Progress notes

This form includes an integrated progress record where you'll use narrative notes to document the patient's progress and any significant incidents. As in focus charting, write narrative notes using the data-action-response method. Update progress notes related to patient outcomes every 48 hours.

Advantages

The computer-ready FACT charting system has several advantages. It eliminates repetition and encourages consistent language and structure. The system is outcome oriented and communicates patient progress to all health care team members. It permits immediate recording of current data and is readily accessible at the patient's bedside. The system also eliminates the need for many different forms and reduces the time spent writing narrative notes.

Documenting with FACT

Developed in 1987 at Abbott Northwestern Hospital in Minneapolis, Minn., FACT records nursing assessment findings and interventions that are exceptions to the norm. This sample shows portions of an assessment flow sheet and a postoperative flow sheet using the FACT format.

ASSESSMENT AND ACTION RECORD

	Date Time	12/18/94 1300	12/18/94 1800	12/18/94 2400
Neurologic Alert and oriented to time, place, and person. PEARL. Symmetry of strength in extremities. No difficulty with coordination. Behavior appropriate to situation. Sensation intact without numbness or paresthesia.		✓	✓	✓
Orient patient.				
Refer to neurologic flow sheet.				
Pain No report of pain. If present, include patient's statements about intensity (1 to 10 scale), location, description, duration, radiation, and precipitating and alleviating factors.		Abdominal incision pain 8 – "severe pain"	✓	2 – Incisional pain – "It hurts."
Location		RLQ		RLQ
Relief measures		Percocet ĩ p.o.		Percocet ĩ p.o.
Pain relief: Yes/ No		Y		Y
Cardiovascular Apical pulse 60 to 100. S_1 and S_2 present. Regular rhythm. Peripheral (radial, pedal) pulses present. No edema or calf tenderness. Extremities pink, warm, movable within patient's ROM.		✓	✓	✓
I.V. solution and rate		D5½ NSS @ 125 ml/hr.	D5½ NSS @ 125 ml/hr.	D5½ NSS @ 125 ml/hr
Respiratory Respiratory rate 12 to 20 at rest, quiet, regular and non-labored. Lungs clear and aerated equally in all lobes. No abnormal breath sounds. Mucous membranes pink.		✓	↓BS RUL	✓
O₂ therapy				
TCDB/Incentive spirometer		✓	✓	✓
Musculoskeletal Extremities pink, warm, and without edema; sensation and motion present. Normal joint ROM, no swelling or tenderness. Steady gait without aids. Pedal, radial pulses present. Rapid capillary refill.		✓	✓	✓
Activity (describe)		bed rest	OOB in chair	bed rest
Nurse's signature and title		Cindy Wier RN	Dave Shaw RN	Lynn Fata, RN

KEY   ✓ = Meets assessment criteria

(continued)

Documenting with FACT (continued)

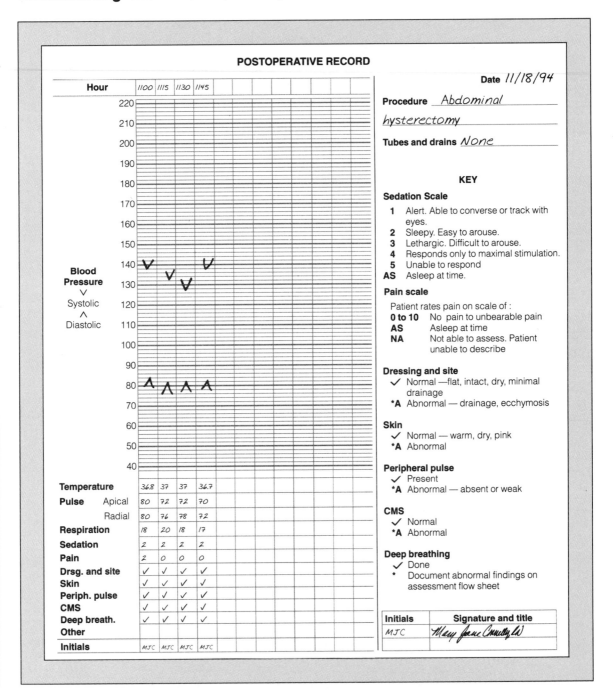

POSTOPERATIVE RECORD

Date 11/18/94

Procedure _Abdominal hysterectomy_

Tubes and drains _None_

KEY

Sedation Scale

1 Alert. Able to converse or track with eyes.
2 Sleepy. Easy to arouse.
3 Lethargic. Difficult to arouse.
4 Responds only to maximal stimulation.
5 Unable to respond
AS Asleep at time.

Pain scale

Patient rates pain on scale of :
0 to 10 No pain to unbearable pain
AS Asleep at time
NA Not able to assess. Patient unable to describe

Dressing and site

✓ Normal —flat, intact, dry, minimal drainage
*A Abnormal — drainage, ecchymosis

Skin

✓ Normal — warm, dry, pink
*A Abnormal

Peripheral pulse

✓ Present
*A Abnormal — absent or weak

CMS

✓ Normal
*A Abnormal

Deep breathing

✓ Done
* Document abnormal findings on assessment flow sheet

Hour	1100	1115	1130	1145							
Temperature	36.8	37	37	36.7							
Pulse Apical	80	72	72	70							
Radial	80	76	78	72							
Respiration	18	20	18	17							
Sedation	2	2	2	2							
Pain	2	0	0	0							
Drsg. and site	✓	✓	✓	✓							
Skin	✓	✓	✓	✓							
Periph. pulse	✓	✓	✓	✓							
CMS	✓	✓	✓	✓							
Deep breath.	✓	✓	✓	✓							
Other											
Initials	MJC	MJC	MJC	MJC							

Blood Pressure ∨ Systolic ∧ Diastolic

Initials	Signature and title
MJC	Mary Jane Connelly, RN

Disadvantages

FACT charting requires a major time commitment to develop standards and implement the system across all hospital or health care facility services. Narrative notes may be too brief, and the nurse's perspective on the patient may be overlooked. The nursing process framework may be difficult to identify in this system as well.

Core (with DAE)

The core documentation system focuses on the nursing process—the *core,* or most important part, of documentation.

Core format and components

Consisting of a data base, plans of care, flow sheets, progress notes, and discharge summary, core charting requires you to assess and record a patient's functional and cognitive status within 8 hours of admission to the hospital. (See *Using core charting,* pages 92 to 95.)

Data base and plans of care

This initial assessment focuses on the patient's body systems and activities of daily living and includes a summary of the patient's problems and appropriate nursing diagnoses. The completed data base and the plan of care are then entered on the patient's medical record card (Kardex).

Flow sheets

Use flow sheets to document the patient's activities and response to nursing interventions, diagnostic procedures, and patient teaching.

Progress notes

On the progress sheet, record the following information (DAE) for each problem:
• Data
• Action
• Evaluation or response.

Discharge summary

This component of core documentation incorporates information related to nursing diagnoses and patient teaching. The discharge summary also includes recommended follow-up care.

Advantages

This system is useful in acute care and long-term care facilities. Core documentation incorporates the entire nursing process in one system. Complemented by the DAE component, the core documentation system groups nursing diagnoses and functional status assessments together, allowing various solutions to be considered. Even more, the system promotes concise documenting with minimal repetition. Furthermore, it promotes the daily recording of psychosocial information.

Disadvantages

Core documenting may require in-depth training for staff members who are used to other documenting systems. Developing forms may be costly and time-consuming, and the DAE format doesn't always present information chronologically, making it difficult to perceive the patient's progress quickly. What's more, the progress notes may not always relate to the plan of care so you'll need to monitor carefully to ensure a record of quality care.

(Text continues on page 96.)

Using core charting

Developed in 1986 by the nurses at St. Joseph's Hospital in Hamilton, Ontario, core charting focuses on the key elements of the nursing process. This sample shows the features of an initial assessment and plan of care.

INITIAL ASSESSMENT

General	Physical	*immobile and severe headache*
Appearance	Skin	☐ Clear ☐ Dry ☑ Intact
	Hygiene	*good*
Cardiopulmonary		*tachycardia and tachypnea*
Mobility	*unable to stand or walk*	Aided by *wheelchair*
Vision	*good*	Aided by
Hearing	*good*	Aided by
Speech	Language	*English*
	Impediment	*none* Aided by
Appetite, diet	*fair, regular*	
	Dentures	☐ Upper ☐ Lower ☐ Partial ☑ None
Urination	*good – voids freely*	Aided by *urinal*
Bowel routine	*daily*	Aided by *laxatives*
Sleep and rest	*poor, secondary to pain*	Aided by *analgesics*
Pain and discomfort	*severe pain Ⓡ temporal area*	Aided by *Percocet*
Reproduction and sexuality	*normal*	
Mental status (orientation, memory)	*oriented X3*	
Emotional status (mood, attitude)	*agitated*	
Religion	*Catholic*	
Nationality	*Irish*	
Lifestyle habits		
	☑ alcohol *occasional beer*	☐ drugs *none*
	☐ tobacco *none*	☐ other
Occupation	*construction worker*	**Hobbies** *sports*

Patient's concerns for discharge   *Pt. states that he's concerned about when will he be able to return to work. States that if he requires surgery no one will be home to help him because his wife works.*

Signature   *Pam Watts, RN*

Date and time   *1/8/95   0200*

Using core charting (continued)

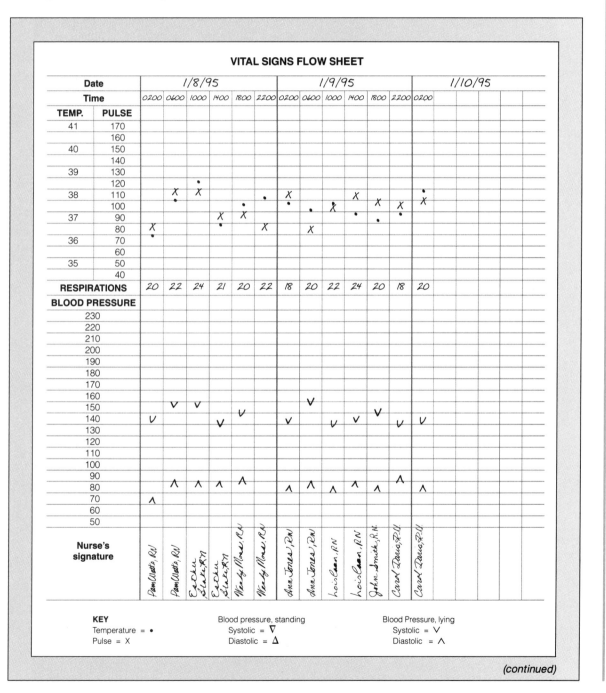

(continued)

Using core charting *(continued)*

24-HOUR FLUID BALANCE FLOW SHEET

Date 1/8/95 Time	INTAKE							OUTPUT						
	Oral or tube feeding	Intravenous D5½ NSS		TPN Travasol	Lipid	Blood & blood products	Total	Urine	NG tube	Emesis	Stool	Drainage	Total
0800	250							500					
0900	100												
1000	250												
1100								500					
1200	400												
1300													
1400	250							1000					
1500													
Sub-total	1250	800					2050	2000					2000
1600								400					
1700	300												
1800													
1900	100							500					
2000													
2100													
2200								400					
2300													
Sub-total	400	800					1200	1300					1300
2400													
0100								200					
0200	100												
0300													
0400								400					
0500													
0600								400					
0700	100												
Sub-total	200	800					1000	1000					1000
Total	1850	2400					4250	4300					4300

Nurse's signature	Day 0800–1500	Pam Watts, RN	24-Hour intake 0800–0700	4250	ml
	Evening 1600–2300	Esther Blake, RN	24-Hour output 0800–0700	4300	ml
	Night 2400–0700	Wendy Moss, RN	Balance ±	−50	ml

Using core charting (continued)

PATIENT CARE PLAN

Date	Nurse's initials	NURSING DIAGNOSES	EXPECTED OUTCOMES	Dead-line	Chart	NURSING INTERVENTIONS	Date Resolved	Nurse's Initials
						Monitor VS &	1/8/95	PW
						neuro. VS q1 hr		
						Monitor CSF out-		
						put q1 hr		
						Observe for signs		
						of rebleeding.		
		Safety needs						
1/8/95	PW	High risk for injury	Pt. will remain			Raise the bed side		
		related to altered	free of injury			rails. Avoid using		
		LOC				restraints, which		
						may raise ICP.		
		Psychosocial needs						
		Fear related to un-				Provide emotional	1/8/95	PW
		known prognosis				support to pt. and		
						family. Minimize		
						stress by encour-		
						aging pt. to verbal-		
						ize feelings.		
		Spiritual, cultural needs						

PATIENT-TEACHING PLANS	DISCHARGE PLANNING
−Teach pt. and family about condition	Expected discharge date 11/12
−Explain all tests, neurologic exams, treatments, and	Home situation
procedures to pt.	Discharge resources involved
−Explain cerebral aneurysm precautions and their purpose.	Publlic health
−Explain physical rehab. plan to pt. and family.	Home care
−Provide nutrition guidelines to pt.	Social work
	Placement Cedar Crest Rehab.
	Other

Nurse's signature	Initials	Nurse's signature	Initials	Nurse's signature	Initials
Pam Watts, RN	PW				

Outcome

Focused on the patient's behaviors and his responses to nursing care, the outcome documentation system is process-oriented. It presents the patient's condition in relation to predetermined outcomes on the plan of care, focusing on desired outcomes rather than problems.

Outcome format and components

This documentation system makes use of progress notes, flow sheets, and plans of care for documentation. Typically combined with another documentation system, it features three components: a data base, a plan of care, and expected outcome statements.

Data base

Obtain an initial information base that includes subjective and objective data identifying the patient's problems. This collected information serves as a foundation for ongoing evaluations of the patient's status.

Plan of care

Using the information in the initial data base, develop a patient plan of care that establishes priorities, identifies expected outcomes and nursing interventions, and documents the plan. This plan gives the health care team a central source of information about the patient's needs and goals.

These four types of plans of care include expected outcomes:

• traditional handwritten plans of care for an individual patient

• standardized plans of care with pre-printed categories, such as nursing diagnoses, outcome statements, and recommended interventions, as well as blank spaces for individualization of the plan

• patient care guidelines that include specific sequential instructions for treating patients with a specific problem

• critical paths or health care maps that outline expected outcomes on a timeline and provide key interventions for a patient with a specific diagnosis.

Expected outcome statements

Also known as goals or objectives, expected outcome statements are drawn from the patient's nursing diagnoses. Expected outcomes describe the desired results of nursing care and serve as the basis for identifying nursing actions to help the patient achieve goals. They also provide a means to evaluate the effectiveness of nursing care and patient teaching.

Because a single nursing diagnosis may have many expected outcomes, you'll need to be specific when stating an expected outcome. Then you'll need to establish specific criteria to determine whether the outcome has been achieved. (See *Writing expected outcomes and outcome criteria.*)

Outcome criteria

The standards by which you objectively evaluate outcomes include these four components:

• specific behaviors that show the patient has progressed toward or reached his goal

• a standard for measuring the patient's behaviors—how much he does and for how long, for example

• the conditions under which the behavior should occur

Writing expected outcomes and outcome criteria

Here are two examples of how to develop patient-focused outcomes and outcome criteria based on selected nursing diagnoses.

Nursing diagnosis	Expected outcomes	Outcome criteria
Ineffective breathing pattern related to incisional pain	Patient will demonstrate an effective breathing pattern by the end of the shift.	• Patient's respiratory rate is 16 to 20 breaths/minute and regular. • Patient uses no accessory muscles. • Patient demonstrates the ability to breathe easily.
Pain related to effects of surgery	Pain will be reduced by time of discharge.	• Patient rates less pain using a numerical scale (for example, if patient had rated pain as 8 on scale of 1 to 10, any reduction in pain would be a rating of less than 8). • Patient expresses pain relief. • Patient can perform self-care activities without assistance. • Patient shows no facial mask of pain. • Patient doesn't guard incision site.

• a target date or time by which the behaviors should occur (short-term goals and long-term goals are identified by their target dates).

When writing outcome criteria, consider the following:
• Make the statement specific. For example, don't write "within a short time" to target an outcome; rather, write "within 3 days."
• Focus on the patient's behavior, not on a nursing action.
• Encourage the patient to participate in developing the outcomes.
• Adapt the outcome to the patient. For example, consider his age, developmental stage, and coping ability. (See Chapter 6,

Documentation of the Nursing Process, for more information on writing outcomes.)

Learning outcomes

The patient-teaching plan identifies what a patient needs to learn, how you will teach him, and ways to evaluate what he has learned. Some teaching plans are part of the patient's plan of care, but many health care facilities require a separate teaching plan. This is because of the emphasis the JCAHO and other regulatory bodies place on documenting a patient's response to teaching.

Learning outcomes should describe measurable and observable behavior and must focus on the patient. A patient's learning behaviors fall into three categories: cognitive (related to knowledge), affective (related to attitudes), and psychomotor (related to movement and coordination). (See *How to write a concise learning outcome.*)

Evaluation

Evaluating expected outcomes includes gathering assessment data, comparing the finding with the outcome criteria, determining the extent of the goals achieved (goals met, partially met, or not met), writing evaluation statements, and revising the plan of care. If the patient meets his goals and the problem is resolved, then you can discontinue the plan of care or teaching plan. If not, continue the plan but set new target dates.

Factors that may work against successful goal completion include unrealistic outcome statements, unrealistic target dates, outcomes that are unacceptable to the patient, and ineffective strategies.

Advantages

With outcome documentation, you use and record all phases of the nursing process, making this system ideal for determining continuous quality improvement. Additionally, the system fosters mutual goal setting and clear documentation of the patient teaching performed and learning achieved.

Disadvantages

If you fail to use the nursing process consistently, carrying out outcome documentation adequately will be difficult.

Computerized charting

Computerization can significantly reduce the time you spend on documentation. Besides facilitating accurate and speedy documentation, computers can also help you complete nurse management reports, provide patient classification data, and make staffing projections. They can identify patient education needs and supply data for nursing research and education. And some bedside terminals can measure vital signs electronically.

In addition to the mainframe computer, most health care facilities locate personal computers or terminals at workstations throughout the facility, allowing departmental staff quick access to vital information. Some hospitals place terminals at patients' bedsides, making data even more accessible.

To enter a patient's computerized clinical record, a health care team member first must enter a special code or codes. Depending on the system, the code may even specify the type of information that a particular team member may have. For example, a dietitian may be assigned a code that allows her to see dietary orders and the patient's nutrition history but not the patient's physical therapy information. Although these codes can help maintain a patient's privacy, if they're misused, his rights can still be violated.

To use a computerized system for documentation, you simply enter a special code, the patient's name, or his account number to bring the patient's electronic chart to the screen. Then you choose the function you want to perform.

For example, you can enter new data on the nursing plan of care or progress notes.

Or you may want to scan the record—for example, for vital signs data or intake and output records for comparison. With a computerized system you can usually obtain information more quickly than you can from traditional documentation.

Systems and functions

Depending on which type of computer and software your health care facility has, you may access information by using a keyboard, a light pen, a touch-sensitive screen, a mouse, or even your voice.

Most computerized documentation or plans of care systems provide a menu of words or phrases you can choose from to individualize documentation on standardized formats. Some systems permit you to use a series of phrases to quickly create a complete narrative note. You can then elaborate on a problem or clarify flow sheet documentation in the comment section of a computerized form by entering standardized phrases or typing in comments. Specialized nursing information systems can increase your efficiency in all phases of documentation. (See *Using computers in the nursing process,* page 100.)

Among current computerized systems are the Nursing Information System (NIS), the Nursing Minimum Data Set (NMDS), and voice-activated systems.

NIS

Currently available NIS software programs allow you to record nursing actions in the electronic record, making nursing documentation easier. These systems reflect most or all of the components of the nursing process so they can meet the standards of the American Nurses' Association (ANA) and the JCAHO. What's more, each

How to write a concise learning outcome

When writing a learning outcome statement for your patient-teaching plan, save time by being concise and clear. Use the representative action verbs below to describe three kinds of learning behaviors and the desired outcomes.

DESCRIPTIVE VERBS	LEARNING OUTCOMES
Cognitive	
Recognize Describe State Discuss Identify List Explain	• The patient will identify three signs of wound infection. • The patient will describe the relationship between a high-fat diet and coronary artery disease.
Affective	
Express Exhibit Relate Communicate Report Verbalize	• The patient will verbalize his feelings regarding loss of independence. • The patient will exhibit positive interaction with family members.
Psychomotor	
Demonstrate Perform Practice Administer Measure Inject	• The patient will correctly measure and record his apical-radial pulse rate before taking digoxin. • The patient will demonstrate the proper technique for dressing his wound.

NIS provides different features and can be customized to conform to a facility's documentation forms and formats.

Currently, most NISs manage information passively. They collect, transmit, organize, format, print, and display informa-

Documentation Systems

Using computers in the nursing process

A computer information system can be either a stand-alone system or a subsystem of a larger hospital system. Nursing information systems (NISs) can increase efficiency and accuracy in all phases of the nursing process— assessment, nursing diagnosis, planning, implementation, and evaluation—and can help nurses meet the standards established by the American Nurses' Association and the Joint Commission on Accreditation of Healthcare Organizations. In addition, an NIS can help you spend more time meeting the patient's needs. Consider the following uses of computers in the nursing process.

Assessment

Use the computer terminal to record admission information. As data are collected, enter further information as prompted by the computer's software program. Enter data about the patient's health status, history, chief complaint, and other assessment factors. Some software programs prompt you to ask specific questions and then offer pathways to gather further information. In some systems, if you enter an assessment value that's outside the usual acceptable range, the computer will flag the entry to call your attention to it.

Nursing diagnosis

Most current programs list standard diagnoses with associated signs and symptoms as references; you must still use clinical judgment to determine a nursing diagnosis for each patient. With this information, you can rapidly obtain diagnostic information. For example, the computer can generate a list of possible diagnoses for a patient with selected signs and symptoms, or it may enable you to retrieve and review the patient's records according to the nursing diagnosis.

Planning

To help nurses begin writing a plan of care, newer computer programs display recommended expected outcomes and interventions for the selected diagnoses. Computers can also track outcomes for large patient populations and general information to help you select patient outcomes. You can use computers to compare large amounts of patient data, help identify outcomes the patient is likely to achieve based on individual problems and needs, and estimate the time frame for reaching outcome goals.

Implementation

Use the computer to record actual interventions and patient-processing information, such as transfer and discharge instructions, and to communicate this information to other departments. Computer-generated progress notes automatically sort and print out patient data (such as medication administration, treatments, and vital signs), making documentation more efficient and accurate.

Evaluation

During evaluation, use the computer to record and store observations, patient responses to nursing interventions, and your own evaluation statements. You may also use information from other members of the health care team to determine future actions and discharge planning. If a desired patient outcome has not been achieved, record interventions taken to ensure such desired outcomes. Then reevaluate the second set of interventions.

tion that you can use to make a decision. But most NISs don't suggest decisions for you.

Some of the newer systems, however, can suggest nursing diagnoses based on predefined assessment data that you enter. The more sophisticated systems provide you with standardized patient status and nursing intervention phrases that you can use to construct your progress notes. These systems let you change the standardized phrases, if necessary, and allow room for you to add your own notes.

New developments

The most recent NISs interact with you, prompting you with questions and suggestions about the information you enter. Ultimately, this computerized sequential decision-making format should lead to more effective nursing care and documentation. Such a system requires you to enter only a brief narrative. The questioning and diagnostic suggestions the system provides make your documentation thorough — and quick. Yet the program allows you to add or change information so that your documentation fits your patient.

NMDS

The NMDS program attempts to standardize nursing information. It contains three categories of data: nursing care (nursing diagnoses and interventions, for example), patient demographics (the patient's name, birthdate, gender, race and ethnicity, and residence), and service elements (length of hospitalization, for example).

Nursing benefits

The NMDS allows you to collect nursing diagnosis and intervention data and identify the nursing needs of various patient populations. It also lets you track patient outcomes and describe nursing care in various settings, including the patient's home. The system helps establish accurate estimates for nursing service costs and provides data about nursing care that may influence health care policy and decision making.

With the NMDS, you can compare nursing trends locally, regionally, and nationally, allowing you to compare nursing data from various clinical settings, patient populations, and geographic areas.

But the NMDS does more than provide valuable information for research and policy making. It also helps you provide better patient care. For instance, examining the outcomes of patient populations will help you set realistic outcomes for an individual patient. Plus, the NMDS can help you formulate accurate nursing diagnoses and plan interventions.

The standardized format of the NMDS also encourages more consistent nursing documentation. All data are coded, making documentation and information retrieval faster and easier. Currently, NANDA assigns numerical codes to all nursing diagnoses so they can be used with the NMDS.

Voice-activated systems

Some hospitals have instituted voice-activated nursing documentation systems — most useful in hospital departments that have a high volume of structured reports, such as the operating room.

The software system uses a specialized knowledge base — nursing words, phrases, and report forms, combined with automated speech recognition (ASR) technology. This system allows the user to record prompt and complete nursing notes by voice. The ASR system requires little or no keyboard use; you simply speak into a telephone handset and the text appears on the computer screen.

The software program includes information on the nursing process, nursing theory, nursing standards of practice, report forms, and a logical format. The system uses trigger phrases, which cue the system to display passages of report text. For example, you can use the text displayed to design an individualized plan of care or fill in standard hospital forms.

Although voice-activated systems are designed to work most efficiently with these trigger phrases, word-for-word dictation and editing are possible. The system increases the speed of reporting and frees the nurse from paperwork so that more time can be spent at the bedside.

Advantages

Computerized documenting procedures make storing and retrieving information fast and easy. The systems themselves store valuable data on patient populations that can help improve the quality of nursing care. They allow for efficient and constant updating of information and help link diverse sources of patient information. Because the computer system uses standard terminology, computerized documentation promotes better communication among health care disciplines and promotes more accurate comparisons. It also makes information legible.

Finally, computerized documentation allows you to send request slips and patient information from one terminal to another quickly and efficiently and can help provide confidentiality.

Disadvantages

Used improperly, a computer may scramble patient information and may threaten a patient's right to privacy if appropriate security measures are neglected. Also, a computer can restrict the accuracy or completeness of information if it uses standardized, limited vocabulary or phrases.

Besides, the computer system may break down, making information temporarily unavailable. Using the computer can take extra time if too many nurses are trying to chart on too few terminals. Finally, the cost of implementing a computerized documentation system may be prohibitive.

Selected References

Gryfinski, J.J., and Lampe, S.S. "Implementing Focus Charting: Process and Critique," *Clinical Nurse Specialist* 4(4):201-205, Winter 1990.

Holmes, S.B., et al. "Development of a Nursing Automated Documentation System," *Orthopedic Nursing* 11(1):55-70, January-February 1992.

Iyer, P.W., and Camp, N.H., *Nursing Documentation: A Nursing Process Approach*, 2nd ed. St. Louis: Mosby–Year Book, Inc., 1995.

Lower, M.S., and Nauert, L.B. "Charting: The Impact of Bedside Computers," *Nursing Management* 23(7):40-42, 44, July 1992.

Mosher, C., et al. "Upgrading Practice with Critical Pathways," *AJN* 92(1):41-44, January 1992.

Documentation Methods

If you're like most nurses, you probably feel discouraged—even overwhelmed—by the number of forms you have to complete each day. Undeniably, paperwork takes time away from your chief priority—patient care. But being familiar with all the forms your health care facility requires and knowing how to use them efficiently have major benefits.

A medical record with well-organized, completed forms will help you communicate patient information to the health care team, garner accreditation and reimbursements, and protect yourself and your employer legally. In the long run, taking the time initially to commit patient information to a standard, easy-to-use format will free you to spend more time providing direct patient care.

On the following pages, you'll find the charting forms and methods commonly used in hospital, home health care, and long-term care settings.

Documentation in hospital settings

Among the forms and notations commonly found in the medical record of a hospitalized patient are the nursing admission assessment, progress notes, Kardexes, graphic forms, flow sheets, critical pathways, patient-teaching documents, discharge summary–patient instruction forms, and others. Dictated documentation, patient self-documentation, and adapted or newly developed forms may also be included.

Nursing admission assessment form

Also known as a nursing data base, the nursing admission assessment form documents your initial patient assessment data. You'll take this step in the nursing process when you first meet the patient. Completing the form itself involves collecting relevant information from various sources and analyzing it to portray a complete picture of the patient. (For more information on documenting nursing assessments, see Chapter 6, Documentation of the Nursing Process.)

The nursing admission assessment form may be constructed in various ways. Some facilities use a form organized by patient responses, such as relating, choosing, exchanging, communicating, and so on. Others use a form organized by body systems (see *Completing the nursing admission assessment*) or other design.

The nursing admission assessment form records your nursing observations, the patient's health history, and your physical examination findings. It includes data on the patient's medications; known food, drug, and other allergies; nursing findings related to activities of daily living (ADLs); impressions of the patient's support systems; and documentation of the patient's advance directives, if any.

How you complete this form depends on your health care facility. You may need to fill in blanks, check off boxes, or write narrative notes.

Advantages
Carefully completed, the form provides pertinent physiologic, psychosocial, and cultural information. It contains both subjective and objective data about the pa-

(Text continues on page 109.)

Completing the nursing admission assessment

Most health care facilities use a combined checklist and narrative admission form like the one below.

NURSING ADMISSION ASSESSMENT

Name *Mary Adams*
Address *101 Shea Lane, Milltown, CO*
Soc sec # *022-22-2222*   D.O.B. *11-9-21*
Religion *Roman Catholic*

Date Admitted *12/15/94*
Time Admitted *1300*

VITAL SIGNS

Temperature	Pulse	Resp.	BP	Height	Weight	Pre-admission testing done ☐
98.6°F	*88*	*14*	*132/86*	*5'5"*	*175 lb.*	

Mode of access

☑ SDA   ☐ DR   ☐ ED
☐ CRISIS   ☐ DIRECT
☐ Unaccompanied
Accompanied by: *daughter—Mary*

Informant
☐ Patient
☑ Other

Admitted via:
☑ Wheelchair
☐ Stretcher
☐ Ambulatory

Reason for admission, according to patient or family *Patient states she is here for a Ⓛ knee replacement*
Special needs (cultural or spiritual) *Requesting Sacrament of the Sick*
Religious preference *Roman Catholic*

ADVANCE DIRECTIVE

Does patient have advance directive?   ☑ Yes   ☐ No   ☑ Written   ☐ Verbal
Is copy of advance directive on file?   ☑ Yes   ☐ No   Date of written directive   *12/93*

ALLERGIES

☐ Food   ☑ Medications   ☐ Other   Uncertain   ☐ None   (specify) *PCN—rash*

MEDICATIONS

List patient's medications (name, dose, route, frequency).
Atenolol 25 mg ↑P.O. qd, ibuprofen 200 mg
ⅱ P.O. t.i.d. prn pain Ⓛ knee, ferrous sulfate
325 mg P.O. t.i.d.
Indicate medications taken today and time administered.
Atenolol 0900 hours, ibuprofen 0900 hours,
ferrous sulfate 0900 hrs.

Did patient bring medications to hospital?   ☐ Yes   ☑ No
If yes, disposition: ☐ Sent home   ☐ Sent to pharmacy
                    ☐ Placed in safety deposit box

Describe personal health, family, medical, surgical, and psychiatric history pertinent to this hospitalization.
Rheumatoid arthritis x 10 years   ☐ Check if none
Anemia x 5 years

BLOOD HISTORY

Previous transfusion   ☐ Yes   ☑ No   ☑ Autologous blood donation
Previous reaction   ☐ Yes   ☑ No   No. of units *2*

(continued)

Completing the nursing admission assessment *(continued)*

INFECTION CONTROL

Precautions initiated other than universal *None*
☐ Type (specify) _____
Other pertinent infection control info. _____

Patient and/or family received explanation?
    ☐ Yes   ☐ No
If no, explain. _____

SAFETY

Patient safety parameters ☑ ID band   ☑ Oriented to unit

Falls risk?   ☑ Yes   ☐ No

Are there specific patient safety or observation needs?
Specify: *Unsteady gait. Pt. needs assistance of cane to ambulate.*

Location of valuables			
	Home	Patient	Safe Dep. Box
Money	✓		
Ring	✓		
Watch	✓		
Other			

FUNCTIONAL STATUS

Daily living habits

Smoking (type/pattern) _____ ☑ None
Informed of smoking policy ☑ Yes
Alcohol (type/pattern) _____ ☑ None
Last drink (time/amount) _____

Regular diet _____
Special diet (specify) *Low salt, low fat*
Sleep pattern *Gets up 3x during night to void*
Substance use (type/pattern) _____ ☑ None

General appearance

Note any unusual skin color, abrasions, pressure ulcers, and so on. Also note the patient's body type and manner of dress.
73 y.o. white female, pale, overweight, not looking as old as her stated years. Favors Ⓛ leg and ambulatory with assistance of cane. Appears to rely on daughter to help with answering questions during assessment. Daughter is a nurse.

General behavior and mental status

☐ Calm   ☑ Anxious   ☐ Agitated   ☐ Comatose   ☐ Lethargic   Oriented?   ☐ Yes   ☐ No (describe below)

Impairments or disabilities

☐ Denies concerns

	Yes
Impaired hearing	☐
Impaired vision	☑

	Yes	With Patient
Hearing aid	☐	☐
Glasses or contact lenses	☑	☑
Lower dentures	☑	☑
Upper dentures	☑	☑

Independent for:
ADLs	☑
Walking	☐
Transfers	☑
Prosthesis	_____
Assistive devices	*cane*

Completing the nursing admission assessment *(continued)*

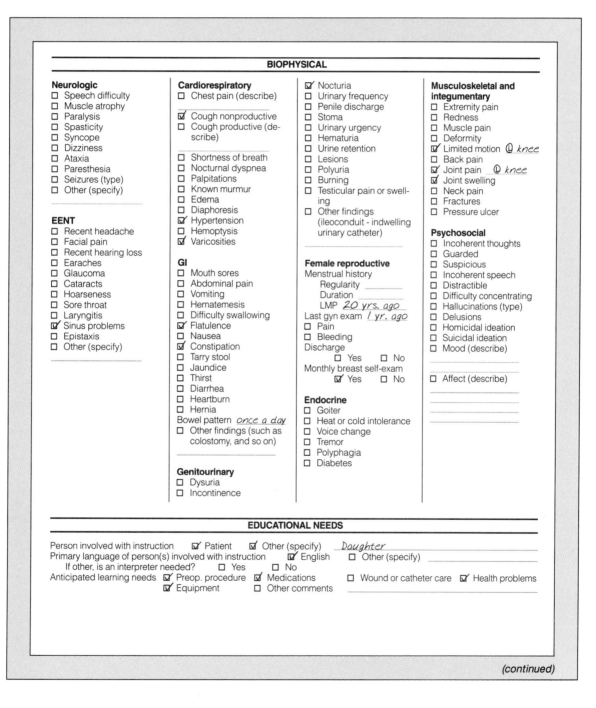

BIOPHYSICAL

Neurologic
- ☐ Speech difficulty
- ☐ Muscle atrophy
- ☐ Paralysis
- ☐ Spasticity
- ☐ Syncope
- ☐ Dizziness
- ☐ Ataxia
- ☐ Paresthesia
- ☐ Seizures (type)
- ☐ Other (specify)

EENT
- ☐ Recent headache
- ☐ Facial pain
- ☐ Recent hearing loss
- ☐ Earaches
- ☐ Glaucoma
- ☐ Cataracts
- ☐ Hoarseness
- ☐ Sore throat
- ☐ Laryngitis
- ☑ Sinus problems
- ☐ Epistaxis
- ☐ Other (specify)

Cardiorespiratory
- ☐ Chest pain (describe)
- ☑ Cough nonproductive
- ☐ Cough productive (describe)
- ☐ Shortness of breath
- ☐ Nocturnal dyspnea
- ☐ Palpitations
- ☐ Known murmur
- ☐ Edema
- ☐ Diaphoresis
- ☑ Hypertension
- ☐ Hemoptysis
- ☑ Varicosities

GI
- ☐ Mouth sores
- ☐ Abdominal pain
- ☐ Vomiting
- ☐ Hematemesis
- ☐ Difficulty swallowing
- ☑ Flatulence
- ☐ Nausea
- ☑ Constipation
- ☐ Tarry stool
- ☐ Jaundice
- ☐ Thirst
- ☐ Diarrhea
- ☐ Heartburn
- ☐ Hernia
- Bowel pattern *once a day*
- ☐ Other findings (such as colostomy, and so on)

Genitourinary
- ☐ Dysuria
- ☐ Incontinence

- ☑ Nocturia
- ☐ Urinary frequency
- ☐ Penile discharge
- ☐ Stoma
- ☐ Urinary urgency
- ☐ Hematuria
- ☐ Urine retention
- ☐ Lesions
- ☐ Polyuria
- ☐ Burning
- ☐ Testicular pain or swelling
- ☐ Other findings (ileoconduit - indwelling urinary catheter)

Female reproductive
Menstrual history
- Regularity _____
- Duration _____
- LMP *20 yrs. ago*
- Last gyn exam *1 yr. ago*
- ☐ Pain
- ☐ Bleeding
- Discharge
  - ☐ Yes　　☐ No
- Monthly breast self-exam
  - ☑ Yes　　☐ No

Endocrine
- ☐ Goiter
- ☐ Heat or cold intolerance
- ☐ Voice change
- ☐ Tremor
- ☐ Polyphagia
- ☐ Diabetes

Musculoskeletal and integumentary
- ☐ Extremity pain
- ☐ Redness
- ☐ Muscle pain
- ☐ Deformity
- ☑ Limited motion *Ⓛ knee*
- ☐ Back pain
- ☑ Joint pain *Ⓛ knee*
- ☑ Joint swelling
- ☐ Neck pain
- ☐ Fractures
- ☐ Pressure ulcer

Psychosocial
- ☐ Incoherent thoughts
- ☐ Guarded
- ☐ Suspicious
- ☐ Incoherent speech
- ☐ Distractible
- ☐ Difficulty concentrating
- ☐ Hallucinations (type)
- ☐ Delusions
- ☐ Homicidal ideation
- ☐ Suicidal ideation
- ☐ Mood (describe)

- ☐ Affect (describe)

EDUCATIONAL NEEDS

Person involved with instruction　☑ Patient　☑ Other (specify) *Daughter*
Primary language of person(s) involved with instruction　☑ English　☐ Other (specify) _____
　If other, is an interpreter needed?　☐ Yes　☐ No
Anticipated learning needs　☑ Preop. procedure　☑ Medications　　☐ Wound or catheter care　☑ Health problems
　　　　　　　　　　　☑ Equipment　☐ Other comments _____

(continued)

Completing the nursing admission assessment *(continued)*

DISCHARGE PLANNING

Support systems and continuing care

Was patient independent for self-care before hospitalization?　☑ Yes　　☐ No (explain) _____

Does patient have family or friend available to assist with and/or manage postdischarge care if needed?
　　☑ Yes　☐ No　Who? *Daughter* _____

Signature/time/date *Elaine Marister, RN*　　*1430 hours*　*12/15/94*　　Unit　*4 North* _____

PLAN OF CARE

Knowledge deficit related to preop and postop routines　　EB

Pain related to arthritis　　EB

Signature *Elaine Marister, RN* _____

tient's current health status and clues about actual or potential health problems. It reveals the patient's ability to comply with treatments, his expectations for treatment, and details about lifestyle, family relationships, and cultural influences.

Using this information can guide you through the nursing process by helping you readily formulate nursing diagnoses, create patient problem lists, and construct plans of care.

As you complete the form, keep in mind that the Joint Commission on Accreditation of Healthcare Organizations (JCAHO), quality improvement groups, and other parties use admission assessment information to continue accreditation, justify requests for reimbursement, and maintain or improve the standards of quality patient care. The recorded data also serve as a baseline for later comparison with the patient's progress.

Another advantage of this form is its usefulness in describing the patient's living arrangement, caregivers, resources, support groups, and other relevant information needed for discharge planning.

Disadvantages
Sometimes, through no fault of your own, you'll be unable to complete the nursing admission assessment form. Or the information you record may be inaccurate, especially if the patient is too sick to answer questions or a family member can't answer for him.

Documentation style
Until recently, admission assessment forms always followed a medical format, emphasizing the patient's initial symptoms and a comprehensive review of body systems. Although many facilities still follow this for-

mat, others have opted for formats that reflect the nursing process. (See Chapter 6, Documentation of the Nursing Process.) Regardless of which format you now use, admission assessments are documented in one or a combination of three styles: narrative, open-ended, and closed-ended.

Narrative notes
Handwritten or computer generated, narrative notes summarize information obtained by general observation, the health history interview, and a physical examination. They allow you to list your findings in order of importance. They can be quite time-consuming, both to write and to read, because they require you to remember and record all significant information in a detailed, logical sequence. (See *Writing a narrative admission assessment*, pages 110 to 112.)

Standard open-ended style
In this style, the assessment form has standard fill-in-the-blank pages with preprinted headings and questions. Information is organized into specific categories so you can easily record and retrieve it. Use phrases and approved abbreviations to complete this form.

Standard closed-ended style
Arranged categorically with preprinted headings, checklists, and questions, a closed-ended admission assessment form requires you simply to check off the appropriate responses. This eliminates the problem of illegible handwriting and makes reviewing documented information easy. The form also clearly establishes the type and amount of information required by the health care facility.

(Text continues on page 112.)

Writing a narrative admission assessment

Here's an example of a nursing admission assessment form documented in narrative style. The data begin with the patient's health history.

Patient's name: James McGee

Address: 20 Tomlinson Road, Elgin, IL 60120

Home phone: (555) 203-0704

Work phone: (555) 203-0177

Sex: Male   **Age:** 44

Birth date: 5/11/50

Social security no.: 001-00-0001

Place of birth: Waterbury, CT

Race: Caucasian

Nationality: American

Culture: Irish-American

Marital status: Married, Susan, age 42

Dependents: James, age 14; Gretchen, age 12

Contact person: Wife (same address as patient) or Clare Hennigan, sister, 1214 Ridge Road, DeKalb, IL 60115; phone (555) 203-1212

Religion: Roman Catholic

Education: M.S.

Occupation: Chemistry teacher, Park Ridge High School

CHIEF HEALTH COMPLAINT

Pt. states, "I've had several episodes of gnawing pain in my stomach, and I feel very tired. My doctor examined me and told me I should have some tests to find out what's wrong."

HEALTH HISTORY

Pt. has been feeling unusually tired for about a month. States he lost 12 lb last month and about 5 lb before that without trying. States that he's busier at work than usual. He thinks his fatigue may be caused more by his schedule than by physical problems.

Past health: Had measles, mumps, chicken pox as child. Hospitalized at age 6 for tonsillectomy and adenoidectomy. Had a concussion and a fractured left leg at age 17 from a football accident. Has had no complications from that. Immunizations are up-to-date. Last tetanus shot 5 years ago; received hepatitis B vaccine 1 year ago.

Functional health: Describes himself as having a good sense of humor. Feels good about himself; gets along well with people.

Cultural and religious influences: Pt. says he has strong religious background, goes to church regularly—important part of his life.

Family relationships: Because he's enrolled in a doctorate program at night, pt. regrets he doesn't get to spend much time with wife and children. Jimmy and Gretchen get along well together, but sometimes compete for time with him. Pt. says he is usually easygoing but lately blows up at the kids when stress and deadlines from school have him tied in knots.

Describes relationship with wife, father, and sister as good (mother deceased).

Sexuality: Says he and wife had a decent (adequate) sex life before he started work toward PhD. Now he is too tired.

Social support: Has many close friends who live in his neighborhood. Would like to socialize more but schoolwork claims most of his time.

Other:

Writing a narrative admission assessment (continued)

Personal health perception and behaviors: _Smokes cigarettes—between 1 and 2 packs/d. Never used recreational drugs. Takes vitamin and mineral supplements and occasional nonprescription cold medicines. Diet is eat and run—usually goes to fast-food place for dinner before night class. Drinks 1 or 2 glasses of beer a week when he has time for dinner at home. Drinks 6 to 8 cups black coffee daily._

Rest and sleep: _Describes himself as a morning person. Gets up at 0630, goes to bed between 2330 and 2400. Likes to get about 8 hours of sleep, but rarely does. Needs to study at night after kids are asleep._

Exercise and activity: _Says he'd like to be more active but can't find the time. Occasionally takes a walk in the evening but has no regular exercise regimen._

Nutrition: _24-hour recall indicates deficiency in iron, protein, and calcium. Takes vitamin and mineral supplements. Skips lunch often. States he's been losing weight without trying._

Recreation: _Likes swimming, hiking, and camping. Tries to take family camping at least once each summer. Wishes he had more time for recreation._

Coping: _Describes his way of coping as avoiding problems until they get too big. Feels he copes with day-to-day stresses O.K. Says job is busy and stressful most days. Says he's feeling a lot of pressure trying to juggle family, career, and educational responsibilities._

Socioeconomic: _Earns around $57,000 a year. Has health insurance and retirement benefits through job. Wife Susan is a chemical engineer earning $60,000._

Environmental: _No known environmental hazards. Lives in 4-bedroom house in town._

Occupational: _Works 10–12 hr./d. Gets along well with coworkers. Feels pressure to attain doctorate to advance his career into educational administration. Has had present position for 12 years._

FAMILY HEALTH HISTORY

Maternal and paternal grandfathers are deceased. Both grandmothers are alive and well at ages 87 and 91. Father is alive and well at age 68; mother is deceased (at age 59, of breast cancer). Younger sister is alive and well.

PHYSICAL STATUS

General health: _Complains of recent stomach pain and fatigue. Had two head colds last winter. No other illnesses or complaints._

Skin, hair, and nails: _Pallor, no skin lesions. Hair receding, pale nails._

Head and neck: _Headaches occasionally, relieved by acetaminophen. No history of seizures. Reports no pain or limited movement._

Nose and sinuses: _No rhinorrhea. Has occasional sinus infections; no history of nosebleeds._

Mouth and throat: _Last dental exam and cleaning 6 months ago._ (continued)

(continued)

Writing a narrative admission assessment (continued)

<hr>

PHYSICAL STATUS (continued)

Eyes: Last eye exam 3 years ago. Reports 20/20 vision.

Ears: Reports no hearing problems. No history of ear infections. Last hearing evaluation 2 years ago.

Respiratory system: No history of pneumonia, bronchitis, asthma, or dyspnea.

Cardiovascular system: No history of murmurs or palpitations. No history of heart disease or hypertension.

Breasts: Flat

GI system: Frequent episodes of indigestion, sometimes relieved by several doses of an antacid (usually Mylanta). Currently complains of gnawing stomach pain. Regular bowel movements but recently noticed dark, tarry stools.

Urinary system: No history of kidney stones or urinary tract infections. Voids clear, yellow urine several times a day without difficulty.

Reproductive system: No history of sexually transmitted disease. Is currently sexually active, though tired. States that sexual relationship with marriage partner is fine.

Nervous system: Denies numbness, tingling, or burning in extremities.

Musculoskeletal system: Reports no muscle or joint pains or stiffness.

Immune and hematologic systems: Pt. says doctor told him his hemoglobin was low. Reports no lymph gland swelling.

Endocrine system: No history of thyroid disease.

Documentation guidelines

Acute illness, short hospital stays, and staff shortages sometimes make conducting a thorough and accurate initial interview difficult. In certain circumstances, you can ask the patient to complete a questionnaire about his past and present health status and use this to document his health history. If he's too ill to be interviewed and family members aren't available, base your initial assessment on your observations and physical examination. Just be sure to document on the admission form why you couldn't obtain complete data.

Conduct an interview and record the complete information on the admission form or progress notes as soon as possible, noting the date and time of the entry. Remember that new information may require you to revise the plan of care accordingly.

Before completing the admission assessment form, consider the patient's ability and readiness to participate. For example, if he's sedated, confused, hostile, angry, or having pain or breathing problems, ask only the most essential questions. You can perform an in-depth interview later when his condition improves. In the meantime, try to find secondary sources (relatives, for example) to provide needed information. Be sure to document your source.

During your interview, try to alleviate as much of the patient's discomfort and

Keeping standard progress notes

Use the following example as a guide for completing your progress notes.

PROGRESS NOTES

Date	Time	Comments
12/20/94	0900	Notified Dr. Watts re Ⓛ lower lobe crackles and ineffective cough. R 40 and shallow. Skin pale. Nebulizer treatment ordered.————————— Ruth Bullock, R.N.
12/20/94	1030	Skin slightly pink after nebulizer treatment. Lungs clear. R 24. Showed pt. how to do pursed-lip and abdominal breathing.——————— Ruth Bullock, R.N.
12/20/94	1400	Ⓛ leg dressing and irrigation done using 1:1 hydrogen peroxide solution and sterile 0.9% sodium chloride solution followed by sterile 0.9% sodium chloride solution flush. Ⓛ leg wound 3 cm x 1 cm wide x 1 cm deep. Small amount of pink-yellow, nonodorous drainage noted on dressing. Surrounding skin reddened and tender. 2 sterile 4" x 4" gauze pads placed over wound and taped in place with hypoallergenic tape.————Ruth Bullock, R.N.
12/20/94	1930	Pt. instructed about upper GI test. Pt. related correct understanding of test purpose and procedure. ——————————————— Doris Kohnsler, R.N.

anxiety as possible. Also try to create a quiet, private environment for your talk.

Progress notes

After you've completed your nursing assessment and devised an initial plan of care, use progress notes to record the patient's status and track changes in his condition. Progress notes describe, in chronological order, patient problems and needs, pertinent nursing observations,

nursing reassessments and interventions, patient responses to interventions, and progress toward meeting expected outcomes.

They promote effective communication among all members of the health care team and continuity of care. Standard progress notes have a column for the date and time and a column for detailed comments. (See *Keeping standard progress notes.*)

Advantages

Because progress notes are written chronologically and usually reflect the patient's problems (the nursing diagnoses), retrieving information can be easy. Also, progress notes contain information that doesn't fit into the space or format of other forms.

Disadvantages

If the notes aren't well organized, you may have to read through the entire form to find what you're looking for. Nurses also may waste time recording information on progress notes that they've already recorded on other forms. In addition, the notes may contain insignificant information because the documenter feels compelled to fill in space.

Documentation guidelines

When writing a progress note, include the date and time of the care given or your observations, what prompts the entry, changes in the patient's condition, and other pertinent data.

Some progress notes are designed to focus on the nursing diagnoses. If your facility uses this type of progress note, be sure to record each nursing diagnosis, problem, goal, or expected outcome that relates to your entry. For example, the nursing diagnosis *Pain* and related problems, such as pain relief and the effectiveness of analgesics, may be the focus of a nursing progress note (see *Using nursing diagnoses to write progress notes*).

Chart times

Be sure that every progress note has the specific time of the care given or the observation noted. Don't record entries in blocks of time ("1500 to 2330 hours," for example). Years ago, when nurses were

required to write progress notes every 2 hours, charting blocks of time was common. Today, however, most nurses use a flow sheet to chart how often they check on a patient. Together, flow sheets and progress notes usually provide adequate evidence of nursing care.

Chart changes in condition

Be sure to document new patient problems ("onset of seizures," for example); resolution of old problems (such as "no complaint of pain in 24 hours"); or deteriorations in the patient's condition (for example, "Pt. has increasing dyspnea, causing him to remain on bed rest. ABG values show PO_2 of 52. O_2 provided by rebreather mask as ordered.").

Record observations

Document your observations of the patient's response to the plan of care. If the patient's behaviors are similar to agreed-upon objectives, document that the goals are being met. If the reverse is true, document that the goals aren't being met. For example, you might record:

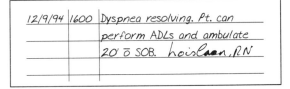

| 12/9/94 | 1600 | Dyspnea resolving. Pt. can perform ADLs and ambulate 20' c̄ SOB. *Lois Caan, RN* |

or you might write:

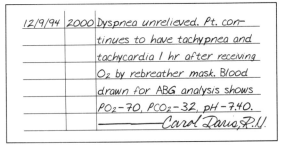

| 12/9/94 | 2000 | Dyspnea unrelieved. Pt. continues to have tachypnea and tachycardia 1 hr after receiving O_2 by rebreather mask. Blood drawn for ABG analysis shows $PO_2 - 70$, $PCO_2 - 32$, $pH - 7.40$. *Carol Davis, R.N.* |

Using nursing diagnoses to write progress notes

Progress notes can be written using a nursing diagnosis, as the example below shows.

Patient Identification Information John Adams 111 Oak St. Centerville, CA (202) 123-4560	Centerville Hospital, Centerville, CA

PROGRESS NOTES

Date and time	Nursing diagnosis and related problems	Notes
1/9/95 – 2300	Pain related to pressure sore on Ⓛ elbow	Pt. rates pain an 8 on a scale of 1 to 10, with 1 being no pain and 10 being the worst pain ever experienced. Pt. frowning when pointing to wound. BP 130/84; P 96. Pain aggravated by dressing change @ 2200. Percocet ↑ P.O. given and pt. repositioned on Ⓡ side. ——— Anne Curry, R.N.
1/9/95 – 2330	Pain related to pressure sore on Ⓛ elbow	Pt. states that pain is relieved. Will give Percocet 1/2 hr. before next dressing change and before future dressing changes.——— Anne Curry, R.N.

Don't repeat yourself

Generally, avoid including information that's already on the flow sheet. The exception: a sudden change in the patient's condition, such as a decreased level of consciousness, a change in skin condition, or swelling at an I.V. site.

Be specific

When you write a progress note, remember to avoid vague wording. For example, if you use a phrase such as "appears to be," you are indicating that you're not sure about what you're charting. Phrases such as "no problems" and "had a good day" are also ambiguous and subject to interpretation. Instead, chart specifics, such as the details found in the following example:

1/06/95	1000	Pt. ate 80% of breakfast and 75% of lunch; OOB to bathroom and walked in hall-way 3 times for a distance of 10' . ———— John Smith, R.N.

Respond to needs or complaints

Sometimes, nurses document a problem but fail to describe what they did about it. Outline your interventions clearly—how and when you notified the doctor, what his orders were, when you followed through, and how and when you followed through on a request for nursing orders, information, or services. Here's an example:

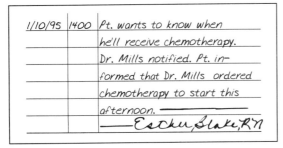

1/10/95	1400	Pt. wants to know when he'll receive chemotherapy. Dr. Mills notified. Pt. informed that Dr. Mills ordered chemotherapy to start this afternoon. ———— Esther Blake, RN

Kardexes

In use for decades, the patient care Kardex (sometimes called the nursing record or nursing Kardex) gives a quick overview of basic patient care information. A Kardex typically contains boxes for you to check off what applies to each patient as well as current orders for medications, patient care activities, treatments, and tests (see *Components of a patient care Kardex*). You'll refer to the Kardex during change-of-shift reports and throughout the day. Kardexes come in various shapes, sizes, and types. They may also be computer generated.

Kardexes include the following information:
• the patient's name, age, marital status, and religion (usually on the address stamp)
• medical diagnoses, listed by priority
• nursing diagnoses, listed by priority
• current doctors' orders for medication, treatments, diet, I.V. therapy, diagnostic tests, procedures, and other measures
• consultations
• results of diagnostic tests and procedures
• permitted activities, functional limitations, assistance needed, and safety precautions.

A Kardex can be made more effective by tailoring the information to the needs of a particular setting. For instance, a home health care Kardex should have information on family contacts, doctors, other services, and emergency referrals. Some facilities have eliminated the Kardex and incorporated the information into the patient's plan of care.

Some health care facilities use Kardexes specifically to document medication information (or other data, such as test results or nonnursing information, which avoids duplicating what's already written in the nursing plan of care). And some facilities rely on computer-generated Kardexes.

Medication Kardex

If your health care facility uses a separate medication Kardex on acute care units, you'll find this document on the medication cart. The medication Kardex may include the medication administration record (MAR), with medications usually listed at the top of the form. If you don't

BETTER CHARTING

Components of a patient care Kardex

Below you'll find the kind of information that might be included on the cover sheet of a patient care Kardex for a medical-surgical unit. Inside the Kardex, which is folded in half horizontally, you'll find additional patient care information.

Keep in mind that the categories, words, and phrases on a Kardex are brief and intended to quickly trigger images of special circumstances, procedures, activities, or patient conditions.

Care status
- Self-care ☐
- Partial care with assistance ☐
- Complete care ☑
- Shower with assistance ☐
- Tub ☐
- Active exercises ☑
- Passive exercises ☑

Special care
- Back care ☑
- Mouth care ☑
- Foot care ☐
- Perineal care ☑
- Catheter care ☑
- Trach care ☐
- Other (specify) _____

Condition
- Satisfactory ☐
- Fair ☑
- Guarded ☐
- Critical ☐
- No code ☑
- Advanced directive?
  - Yes ☑
  - No ☐
- Date: _12/18/94_

Prosthesis
- Dentures
  - upper ☑
  - lower ☑
- Contact lenses ☐
- Glasses ☑
- Hearing aid ☐
- Other (specify): _____

Isolation
- Strict ☐
- Wound and skin ☐
- Respiratory ☐
- Hepatitis ☐
- Enteric ☐
- Other (specify): _____

Diet
- Type: _2 gm Na_
- Force fluids ☐
- NPO ☐
- Assist with feeding ☑
- Isolation tray ☐
- Calorie count ☑
- Supplements: _____

Tube feedings ☐
- Type: _____
- Rate: _____
- Route: _____
  - NG ☐
  - G tube ☐
  - J tube ☐

Admission
- Height: _6'1"_
- Weight: _161 lb. (73 kg)_
- BP: _118/84_
- TPR: _99.6 P.O. – 101 – 21_

Frequency
- BP: _q 4hr._
- TPR: _q shift_
- Apical pulses:
- Peripheral pulses: _q shift_
- Weight: _daily_
- Neuro check:
- Monitor:
- Strips:
- Turn: _q 2 hr._
- Cough: _q shift_
- Deep breathe: _q shift_
- Central venous
  pressure:
- Other (specify): _____

GI tubes
- Salem sump ☐
- Levin tube ☐
- Feeding tube ☐
- Type (specify): _____
- Other (specify): _____

Activity
- Bed rest ☐
- Chair _t.i.d._ ☑
- Dangle ☐
- Commode ☐
- Commode with assist ☑
- Ambulate ☐
- BRP ☐
- Fall-risk category (specify): _#1_ ☑
- Other (specify): _____

Mode of transport
- Wheelchair ☑
- Stretcher ☐
- With oxygen ☐

I.V. devices
- Heparin lock ☐
- Peripheral I.V. ☑
- Central line ☐
- Triple-lumen CVP ☐
- Hickman ☐
- Jugular ☐
- Peripherally inserted ☐
- Parenteral nutrition ☐
- Irrigations: _____

Dressings
- Type:
- Change:

(continued)

Components of a patient care Kardex   *(continued)*

Respiratory therapy
Pulse oximetry
   SpO$_2$ level (%):
Oxygen   ☑
Liters/minute: *2 L/min*
Method
   Nasal cannula   ☑
   Face mask   ☐
   Venturi (Venti) mask   ☐
   Partial rebreather mask   ☐
   Nonrebreather mask   ☐
   Trach collar   ☐
Nebulizer   ☐
Chest PT   ☑
Incentive spirometry   ☑
T-piece   ☐
Ventilator   ☐
   Type:
   Settings:
Other (specify): _____

Drains
Type: _____
Number: _____
Location: _____

Urine output
I & O   ☑
Strain urine   ☐
Indwelling catheter   ☐
Date inserted: _____
Size: _____
Intermittent catheter   ☐
   Frequency: _____

Side rails
Constant   ☐
PRN   ☐
Nights   ☐

Restraints
Date: _____
Type: _____

Specimens and tests
ACCU check q 6 h

24-hour collection
Other (specify): _____

Stools

Special notes
Evaluate pain level q/hr

Social services
Started 12/18/94

The format and specific information on a Kardex will vary with the needs of the patient population. For instance, the cover sheet of a patient care Kardex on a critical care unit would include the same basic information already shown plus information specific to the unit, including the following:

Monitoring
Hardwire   ☐
Telemetry   ☐

Pulmonary artery catheter   ☐
   Pulmonary artery
   pressure: _____
   Pulmonary artery
   wedge pressure: _____
Arterial line   ☐
Other (specify): _____

Mechanical ventilation
Type: _____
Tidal volume: _____
FIO$_2$: _____
Mode: _____
Rate: _____

On an obstetrics unit, you might find the following additional information on the Kardex cover sheet:

Delivery
Date: _____
Time: _____
Type of delivery: _____

Special procedures
Perianal rinse   ☐
Sitz bath   ☐
Witch hazel compress   ☐
Breast binders   ☐
Ice   ☐
Abdominal binders   ☐
Other (specify)

Mother
Due date: _____
Gravida: _____
Para: _____
Rh: _____
Blood type: _____
Membranes ruptured: _____
Episiotomy   ☐
Lacerations   ☐
RhoGAM studies?
   Yes   ☐
   No   ☐
Rubella titer?
   Yes   ☐
   No   ☐

Infant
Male   ☐
Female   ☐
Full term   ☐
Premature   ☐
   Weeks
Apgar Score   ☐
Nursing   ☐
Formula   ☐
Condition (specify): _____
Other (specify): _____

use a medication cart, the medication sheet needn't be kept separate from the Kardex. (For a sample of a completed medication Kardex, see Chapter 7, Documentation of Everyday Events.)

Computer-generated Kardex
Typically used to record laboratory or diagnostic test results and X-ray findings, a computerized Kardex usually includes information regarding medical orders, referrals, consultations, specimens (for example, for culture and sensitivity tests or for blood glucose analysis), vital signs, diet, activity restrictions, and so forth (see *Characteristics of a computer-generated patient care Kardex,* pages 120 and 121).

Advantages
A patient care Kardex provides quick access to data about task-oriented interventions, such as medication administration and I.V. therapy. Although it duplicates information, the plan of care may be added to the Kardex to provide all the necessary data for patient care.

Disadvantages
Kardexes are only as useful as nurses make them. A Kardex won't be effective if it doesn't have enough space for appropriate data, if it's not updated frequently, if it's not completed, or if the nurse doesn't read it before giving patient care.

Documentation guidelines
The most effective Kardexes are designed for specific units and reflect the needs of the patients on those units. Keep in mind that you should record information that helps nurses plan daily interventions (for example, the time a particular patient prefers to bathe, his food preferences before

and during chemotherapy, and which analgesics or positions are usually required to ease pain).

If you're documenting on a medication Kardex, here are some tips:
• Be sure to include the date, the administration time, the medication dose, route, and frequency, and your initials.
• Indicate whenever you administer a stat dose and, if appropriate, the specific number of doses, as ordered, or the stop date.
• Write legibly, using only standard abbreviations. When in doubt about how to abbreviate a term, spell it out.
• After giving the first dose of a medication, sign your full name, your licensure status, and your initials in the appropriate space.
• After withholding a medication dose, document which dose wasn't given (usually by circling the time it was scheduled or by drawing an asterisk) and the reason it was omitted (for example, withholding oral medications from a patient the morning of scheduled surgery).

If you administer all medications according to the plan of care, you don't need further documentation. However, if your MAR doesn't have space for information, such as the parenteral administration site, the patient's response to medications given as needed, or deviations from the medication order, you'll need to record this information in the progress notes. Here's an example:

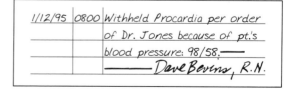

(Text continues on page 122.)

Characteristics of a computer-generated patient care Kardex

In the computer-generated Kardex shown below, you'll find a detailed list of medical orders and other patient care data.

```
11/10/94   1539                                    PAGE 001
= = = = = = = = = = = = = = = = = = = = = = = = = = = = = = = =
Stevens, James                                        M 65
MR#: 000310593                            ACCT#: 9400037290
DR: J. Carrio                                    2/W 204-01
DX: Unstable angina                          DATE:11/10/94
= = = = = = = = = = = = = = = = = = = = = = = = = = = = = = = =
SUMMARY: 11/10   0701 to 1501

PATIENT INFORMATION
     11/10          ADVANCED DIRECTIVE: No.
                    Advance directive does not exist
     11/10          ORGAN DONOR: Unknown
     11/10          ADMIT DX: Unstable angina
     11/10          MED ALLERGY: None known
     11/10          ISOLATION:

MISC. PATIENT DATA

NURSING PLAN OF CARE PROBLEMS
     11/10          Alteration in comfort R/T: Anginal pain

ALL CURRENT MEDICAL ORDERS

  NURSING ORDERS:
     11/10          Activity, OOB, Up as tol.
     11/10          Routine V/S Q8H
     11/10          Telemetry
     11/10          IF 1800 PTT <50, increase heparin drip to 1200
                    units/hr, IF 50 - 100, maintain 1000 units/hr,
                    IF > 100, reduce to 900 units/hr
     11/10          Please contact M. Sweeney to see pt.
                    regarding-diabetic management and insulin
                    treatment

  DIET:
     11/10          Diet: Diabetic: 1600 cal., start with lunch
                    today

  IVS:
     11/10          Peripheral line #1....Start D5/W, 250ml,
                    heparin 25,000 units: rate, 1000 units/hr
```

Characteristics of a computer-generated patient care Kardex *(continued)*

```
11/10/94  1539                                    PAGE 002

= = = = = = = = = = = = = = = = = = = = = = = = = = = = = =
Stevens, James                              M 65
MR#: 000310593                    ACCT#: 9400037290
DR: J. Carrio                          2/W 204-01
DX: Unstable angina                   DATE:11/10/94
= = = = = = = = = = = = = = = = = = = = = = = = = = = = = =
SUMMARY:           0701 to 1501

  SCHEDULED MEDICATIONS:
     11/10          Nitroglycerin oint 2%, 1.5 inches, apply to
                    chest wall, Q8H, starting on 11/10, 1800 hrs.
     11/10          Diltiazem tab 90 mg, #1, P.O., Q6H 0800, 1400,
                    2000, 0200
     11/10          Furosemide tab 40mg, #1, P.O., daily 0900
     11/10          Potassium chloride tab 10meq #1, P.O. daily
                    0900
     11/10          Labetalol tab 100mg, #1/2, P.O. bid 0900, 1800

  STAT/NOW MEDICATIONS:
     11/10          Furosemide tab 40mg, #1, P.O., today
     11/10          Potassium chloride tab 10 meq, #1, P.O., today

  PRN MEDICATIONS:
     11/10          Procardia nifedipine cap 10mg, #1, subling.
                    Q6H, prn SBP > 170 or DSBP > 105
     11/10          Acetaminophen tab 325mg, #2, P.O., Q4H, prn
                    pain
     11/10          Tamazepam cap 15mg, #1, P.O., QHS, prn
     11/10          Alprazolam tab 0.25mg, #1/2, P.O., Q8H, prn

  LABORATORY:
     11/10          CK & MB 1800 today
     11/10          CK & MB 0200 tomorrow
     11/10          Urinalysis floor to collect
     11/10          PTT 1800 today

  ANCILLARY:
     11/10          Stress test persantine, prep H1, Patient
                    handling: wheelchair, Schedule: tomorrow

                          Last page
```

Graphic forms

Used for 24-hour assessments, graphic forms usually have a column of data printed on the left side of the page, times and dates printed across the top, and open blocks within the side and top borders. You'll use graphic forms to plot various changes—in the patient's vital signs, weight, intake and output (stools, urine, and vomitus), appetite, and activity level, for instance.

Advantages

Graphic forms present information at a glance, allowing a more visual comparison of data than the numerical comparisons used in narrative-style forms. For example, blood pressure that rises, falls, or fluctuates over time can be detected much more readily on a graph than in a narrative accounting of raw numbers. Besides, health care personnel such as licensed practical nurses are permitted to document measurements on a graphic form, thereby saving registered nurses valuable time.

Disadvantages

Data placed on the graph must be accurate, legible, and complete. Every vital sign you take should be transcribed onto this form. If these guidelines aren't followed, the form loses its value. For accuracy, double-check the graph after transcribing any information onto it.

Avoid using the information on a graph alone; instead, combine it with narrative documentation to present a complete picture of the patient's clinical condition.

Documentation guidelines

For greater accuracy, try to chart on graphic forms at the same time each day. Document the patient's vital signs on both the graphic form and the progress notes when you administer an analgesic, antihypertensive, or antipyretic drug, for example. This provides a record of the patient's response to a drug that may produce a change in a particular vital sign.

Also document vital signs on both forms—when a patient has chest pain, chemotherapy, a seizure, or a diagnostic test—to indicate the patient's condition at that time, for example.

Be sure to chart legibly, to put data in the appropriate time line, and to make the dots on the graph large enough to be seen easily. Connect the dots if your facility requires you to do so. (See *Using a graphic record.*)

Flow sheets

Also called abbreviated progress notes, flow sheets have vertical or horizontal columns for recording dates, times, and interventions. You can insert nursing data quickly and concisely, preferably at the time you give care or observe a change in the patient's condition. Because flow sheets provide an easy-to-read record of changes in the patient's condition over time, they allow all members of the health care team to compare data and assess the patient's progress.

Using flow sheets doesn't exempt you from narrative charting to describe your observations, patient teaching, patient responses, detailed interventions, and unusual circumstances. However, flow sheets are handy for charting data related to a patient's ADLs, fluid balance, nutrition,

BETTER CHARTING

Using a graphic record

This partial form illustrates how to use a typical graphic record.

GRAPHIC RECORD

Date		1/10/95						1/11/95						1/12/95		
Hour		0200	0600	1000	1400	1800	2200	0200	0600	1000	1400	1800	2200	0200	0600	1000

Temperature

°C	°F
40.6	105
40.0	104
39.4	103
38.9	102
37.8	100
37.2	99
36.7	98
36.1	97
35.6	96

Pulse		80	82	78	75	90	82	76	90	88	84	80	80	76	74	72
Respiration		20	18	20	16	24	20	18	18	18	16	20	22	20	18	20
Blood pressure		122/70	114/80	116/76	118/82	120/78	118/68	124/80	120/70	124/74	126/84	110/78	112/82	132/80	124/80	126/80

Activity					
2300 to 0700	Sleeping		Sleeping		Sleeping
0700 to 1500	OOB x 3 without assist		OOB as desired		
1500 to 2300	OOB x 2 with assist		OOB x 2 with assist		

pain, and skin integrity. They're also useful for recording nursing interventions.

In response to a request by the JCAHO, nurses are using these forms to document basic assessment findings and wound care, hygiene, and routine care interventions. In addition, many facilities document I.V. therapy and patient education on flow sheets. The style and format of flow sheets may be varied to fit the needs of patients on particular units. (See *Using a flow sheet to record routine care.*)

Advantages

Because of their concise format, flow sheets let you evaluate patient trends at a glance, especially if you keep the forms conveniently near the patient's bedside. The format of flow sheets also reinforces nursing standards of care and allows precise nursing documentation.

Disadvantages

Because flow sheets have little space, they're not well suited for recording unusual events. And overuse of these forms can lead to incomplete or fragmented documentation that obscures the patient's clinical picture. Also, flow sheets may cause legal problems if they're not consistent with the progress notes, which may happen if the nurse hurriedly checks off whatever the nurse on the previous shift checked off and then charts the actual care in the progress notes.

In some cases, the flow sheet format fails to reflect the needs of the patients and the documentation needs of the nurses on each unit. If the flow sheet doesn't take these needs into account, or isn't revised as needs change, it becomes more of a liability than an asset.

In addition, flow sheets add bulk to the medical record, causing handling and storage problems and duplication of documentation.

Documentation guidelines

Ideally, you'll use flow sheets to document all routine assessment data and nursing interventions, such as repositioning or turning the patient, range-of-motion exercises, patient education, wound care, and medication administration. This allows you then to include only the patient's progress toward achieving desired outcomes and any unplanned assessments in your progress notes.

Be sure data on the flow sheet are consistent with data in your progress notes. Of course, all entries should accurately reflect the care given. Discrepancies can damage your credibility and increase your chance of liability.

Sometimes, recording only the information requested isn't sufficient to give a complete picture of the patient's status. In such cases, record additional information in the space provided on the flow sheet. If additional information isn't necessary, draw a line through this space to indicate that further information isn't required.

If your flow sheet doesn't have additional space and you need to record more information, use the progress notes.

Fill out flow sheets completely, using the key symbols provided, such as a check mark, an X, initials, circles, or the time to indicate that a parameter was observed or an intervention was carried out. When necessary, use the abbreviation "N/A" (not applicable) or another abbreviation recognized by your facility.

Don't leave blank spaces—they imply that an intervention wasn't completed, wasn't attempted, or wasn't recognized. If you have to omit something, document the reason.

Critical pathways

A critical pathway integrates the principles of case management into nursing documentation. It outlines the standard of care for a specific diagnosis-related group

(Text continues on page 129.)

Using a flow sheet to record routine care

As this sample shows, a patient care flow sheet lets you quickly document your routine interventions.

PATIENT CARE FLOW SHEET

Date 1/22/95	2300 – 0700	0700 – 1500	1500 – 2300
RESPIRATORY			
Breath sounds	Clear 2330 PW	Crackles LLL 0800 SR	Clear 1600 MLF
Treatments/results	——	Nebulizer 0830 SR	——
Cough/results	ō PW	Mod. amt. tenacious yellow mucus 0900 SR	ō
O₂ therapy	Nasal cannula @ 2 L/min PW	Nasal cannula @ 2 L/min SR	Nasal cannula @ 2 L/min MLF
CARDIAC			
Chest pain	ō PW	ō SR	ō MLF
Heart sounds	Normal S1 and S2 PW	Normal S1 and S2 SR	Normal S1 and S2 MLF
Telemetry	N/A	N/A	N/A
PAIN			
Type and location	Ⓛ flank 0400 PW	Ⓛ flank 1000 SR	Ⓛ flank 1600 MLF
Intervention	meperidine 0415 PW	Repositioned and meperidine 1010 SR	meperidine 1615 MLF
Pt. response	Improved from #9 to #3 in 1/2 hr PW	Improved from #8 to #2 in 45 min. SR	Complete relief in 1 hr MLF
NUTRITION			
Type	——	Regular SR	Regular MLF
Toleration %	——	90% SR	80% MLF
Supplement	——	1 can Ensure SR	——
ELIMINATION			
Stool appearance	ō PW	ō SR	⊤ soft dark brown MLF
Enema	N/A	N/A	N/A
Results	——	——	——
Bowel sounds	Present all quadrants 2330 PW	Present all quadrants 0800 SR	Hyperactive all quadrants 1600 MLF

(continued)

BETTER CHARTING

Using a flow sheet to record routine care *(continued)*

PATIENT CARE FLOW SHEET			page 2
Date 1/22/95	2300 – 0700	0700 – 1500	1500 – 2300
ELIMINATION *(continued)*			
Urine appearance	Clear, amber 0400 PW	Clear, amber 1000 SR	Dark yellow 1500 MLF
Indwelling urinary catheter	N/A	N/A	N/A
Catheter irrigations	——	——	——
I.V. THERAPY			
Tubing change	——	1100 SR	——
Dressing change	——	1100 SR	——
Site appearance	No edema, no redness 2330 PW	No redness, no edema, no drainage 0800 SR	No redness, no edema 1600 MLF
WOUND			
Type	(L) flank incision 2330 PW	(L) flank incision 1200 SR	(L) flank incision 2000 MLF
Dressing change	Dressing dry and intact 2330 PW	1200* SR	2000* MLF
Appearance	Wound not observed PW	See progress note. SR	See progress note. MLF
TUBES			
Type	N/A	N/A	N/A
Irrigation	——	——	——
Drainage appearance	——	——	——
HYGIENE			
Self / partial / complete	——	Partial 1000 SR	Partial 2100 MLF
Oral care	——	1000 SR	2100 MLF
Back care	0400 PW	1000 SR	2100 MLF
Foot care	——	1000 SR	——
Remove/reapply elastic stockings	0400 PW	1000 SR	2100 MLF

Using a flow sheet to record routine care *(continued)*

PATIENT CARE FLOW SHEET			page 3
Date 1/22/95	2300 – 0700	0700 – 1500	1500 – 2300
ACTIVITY			
Type	Bed rest PW	OOB to chair x 20 min 1000 SR	OOB to chair x 20 min 1800 MLF
Toleration	Turns self PW	Tol. well SR	Tol. well MLF
Repositioned	2330 Supine PW 0400 Ⓛ side PW	Ⓛ side 0800 SR Ⓡ side 1400 SR	Self MLF
ROM	───	1000 (active) SR	1800 (active) MLF
		1400 (active) SR	2200 (active) MLF
SLEEP			
Sleeps well	0400 PW 0600 PW	N/A	N/A
Awake at intervals	2330 PW 0400 PW	───	───
Awake most of the time	───	───	───
	───	───	───
SAFETY			
Side rails up	2330 PW 0200 PW 0400 PW	1500 SR	1800 MLF
Call button in reach	2330 PW 0200 PW 0400 PW	0800 SR	1600 MLF
EQUIPMENT			
Type IVAC pump	Continuous 2300 PW	Continuous 0800 SR	Continuous 1600 MLF
TEACHING			
Wound splinting	0400 PW	1000 SR	───
Deep breathing	0400 PW	1000 SR	1600 MLF
Initials / Signature / Title	PW / Pam Watts, RN	SR / Susan Reynolds, R.N.	MLF / Mary La Faye, RN

(continued)

Using a flow sheet to record routine care   *(continued)*

PATIENT CARE FLOW SHEET   page 4

PROGRESS SHEET

Date	Time	Comments
1/22/95	1200	Ⓛ flank dressing saturated with serosang. drng. Dressing removed. Wound edges well-approximated except for 2 cm. Opening noted at lower edge of incision. Small amount serosang. drng. noted oozing from this area. No redness noted along incision line. Sutures intact. Incision line painted with povidone-iodine. Five 4" x 4" gauze pads applied and taped in place. Dr. Wong notified of increased amt. of drng. ——— Susan Reynolds, R.N.
1/22/95	2000	Dr. Wong to see pt. Ⓛ flank drsg. removed. 2-cm opening noted at lower edge of incision. Otherwise, wound edges well-approximated. Dr. Wong sutured opening with one 3-0 silk suture. No redness or drng. noted along incision line. Painted incision line with povidone-iodine and applied two 4" x 4" gauze pads. Taped drsg. in place. — Mary La Farge, RN

(DRG). It incorporates multidisciplinary diagnoses and interventions, such as nursing-related problems, combined nursing and medical interventions, and key events that must occur for the patient to be discharged by a target date.

These events include consultations, diagnostic tests, treatments, medications, procedures, activities, diet, patient teaching, discharge planning, and anticipated outcomes. Other events or interventions may be added and the pathway's categories may be presented in various formats and combinations.

Within the managed care system, critical pathways set the standard for patient progress and track it as well. They provide the nursing staff with necessary written criteria to guide and monitor patient care. In some health care facilities, the nursing diagnosis forms the critical pathway's basis for patient care, although critics believe that structuring the pathway in this way interferes with communication and coordination of care among nonnursing members of the health care team.

A critical pathway is usually organized by categories according to the patient's diagnosis, which dictates his expected length of stay, daily care guidelines, and expected outcomes. The care guidelines specified for each day may be organized into such categories as activity, diet or nutrition, treatments, medications, patient teaching, discharge planning, and so forth.

The structure and categories may vary from institution to institution and depend on which are appropriate for the specific DRG. For an example of a completed critical pathway for the patient and another for the nurse, see *Following critical pathways,* pages 130 to 133.

Advantages

Using a critical pathway form as a permanent documentation tool can eliminate duplicate charting. Narrative notes need only be written when a standard on the pathway remains unmet or when the patient's condition warrants a deviation in care as planned on the pathway.

As long as standardized orders or standing protocols have been determined and accepted, nurses can advance the patient's activity level, diet, and treatment regimens without waiting for a doctor's order. And doctors receive fewer phone calls because nurses have the freedom to make nursing decisions.

Critical pathways improve communication among all members of the health care team because everyone works from the same plan. Proponents of critical pathways believe that shared accountability for patient outcomes also improves the overall quality of care.

Some health care facilities adapt certain critical pathways for distribution to patients, finding that many patients feel less anxiety and cooperate more with therapy because they know what to expect. What's more, some patients seem to recover more quickly and go home sooner than anticipated. A secondary benefit of critical pathways seems to be improved, patient teaching and discharge planning.

Disadvantages

Critical pathways prove most effective for a patient who has only one diagnosis; they're less effective for a patient with several diagnoses or one who experiences complications (because of the difficulty establishing a time line for such a patient). For example, treatment progress is usually

(Text continues on page 134.)

Following critical pathways

A relatively recent outgrowth of quality-improvement and cost-containment efforts, critical pathways constitute standard clinical courses for a particular diagnosis-related group. At any point in a treatment course, a glance at the standard critical pathway serves as a way to compare the patient's prog-

CRITICAL PATHWAY: TOTAL HIP REPLACEMENT

INTERVENTIONS	PREADMISSION	DAY 1	DAY 2 (postop. day 1)
Consultations	Family doctor	Anesthesiologist	
Tests	Blood tests, urinalysis, X-rays, ECG, autologous blood donation	After surgery, X-rays and blood tests done while recovering in the postanesthesia care unit.	Blood tests
Medications		Antibiotics before, during, and after surgery; warfarin to prevent blood clots; pain medication to relieve discomfort	Antibiotics, warfarin, pain medication, stool softener or laxative
Treatment and related activity	• Meet the preadmission nurse. • Meet the operating room nurse. • Meet the unit nurse (from 3 West). • Meet the physical therapist.	• Before surgery, you'll have your hip washed or shaved, a catheter placed in your bladder, and an I.V. line for fluids and medications during surgery. • After surgery, expect blood pressure and pulse checks, an overhead frame and trapeze to pull yourself up in bed, incision drains, ice packs, abductor pillow, and coughing and deep-breathing exercises.	• Perform activities as recommended by your doctor. You may be able to do exercises at bedside or sit in a special hip chair assisted by a physical therapist and a walker. • You may still need a surgical drain, an abductor pillow, and I.V. fluids.
Nutrition	Have breakfast at the hospital.	Before surgery, no food or liquids. After surgery, liquids allowed.	Increase your diet to 50% and eat more of it.
Education			Physical therapy and instruction
Ancillary services	Meet social worker to make discharge and rehabilitation plans.		Continue discharge plans with social worker.
Expected outcome	Discuss or demonstrate: • coughing and deep-breathing exercises • pain control measures • hospital and walking equipment • follow-up treatment • physical therapy.	• Do coughing and deep-breathing exercises and have good pain control. • Learn hip precautions to promote healing and avoid complications. • You may need a blood transfusion.	• Do coughing and deep-breathing exercises and have good pain control. • Review precautions to promote healing, avoid complications, and advance your walking. • You may need a blood transfusion.

ress and your performance as a caregiver with care standards. The following critical pathways are typical examples. The critical pathway for total hip replacement is printed for patient distribution. The one for acute myocardial infarction is for the nurse.

DAY 3 (postop. day 2)	DAY 4 (postop. day 3)	DAY 5 (postop. day 4)
Blood tests	Blood tests	Blood tests
Warfarin, pain medication, stool softener or laxative	Warfarin, pain medication, stool softener or laxative	Warfarin, pain medication, stool softener or laxative
• Your doctor will change your bandages and, possibly, remove your drains and urinary catheter. • Perform activities recommended by your doctor, such as standing and walking with a walker. • Use a raised toilet seat. • Sit in a special hip chair.	Continuing treatment measures include: • wound care • special hip chair, elevated toilet seat, abductor pillow • activity as recommended by doctor • occupational therapy (optional).	Continuing treatment measures include: • wound care • special hip chair, elevated toilet seat, abductor pillow • activity as recommended by doctor • occupational therapy (optional).
Increase your diet to 75%.	Increase your diet to 100%.	Increase your diet to 100%.
Physical therapy	Physical therapy	Physical therapy
Continue plans for discharge and rehabilitation. Investigate suitable facilities.	Coordinate discharge plans.	
Continue hip precautions, use an abductor pillow, have pain under control, and use the bathroom.	Continue hip precautions and use a walker correctly.	Continue hip precautions, understand how to take your prescribed medications, perform wound care at home, and request antibiotic therapy before dental work or any other surgical procedures.

(continued)

Following critical pathways   (continued)

CRITICAL PATHWAY: ACUTE MYOCARDIAL INFARCTION

PROGRESS MARKERS	DAY 1	DAY 2
Diagnostics	• Complete blood chemistry • CBC with differential • Cardiac isoenzymes q 8 hr until peak • PT, PTT, ACT initially and q 6 hr (if on thrombolytic therapy); PTT q 6 hr (only if on heparin) • Beta hCG (if female of childbearing age) • 12-lead ECG daily and per protocol • Chest X-ray	• Complete blood chemistry • CBC • PTT (if on heparin) • Cardiac isoenzymes if not at baseline • 12-lead ECG daily and per protocol • MUGA scan or echocardiogram, if indicated
Assessment and monitoring	• ECG monitoring • HR, RR, BP q 1 hr • Rhythm strip q shift and p.r.n. • Continuous oximetry • Heart sounds, breath sounds q 1- 2 hr and during chest pain episodes • Assess other body systems as needed.	• ECG monitoring • HR, RR, BP q 2 hr • Rhythm strip q shift and p.r.n. • Continuous oximetry • Heart sounds and breath sounds q 2 hr and during episodes of chest pain
Medications	• Heparin I.V. • NTG continuous I.V. infusion • Thrombolytic therapy (if indicated) • Beta blocker • Calcium channel blocker • ACE inhibitor • ASA • Morphine I.V., analgesics • Stool softener • Sedative • Antiemetic	• Heparin I.V. • Titrate and D/C NTG infusion • NTG SL, transdermal, or spray • Beta blocker • Calcium channel blocker • ACE inhibitor • ASA • Analgesics • Stool softener • Sedative
Diet	• Low-salt, low-fat, low-cholesterol, or ADA diet (possible fluid restriction); NPO if patient has chest pain, nausea, or is vomiting	• Low-salt, low-fat, low-cholesterol, or ADA diet
Activity	• Bed rest (semi-Fowler's) with commode or BRP if permitted; assistance with ADLs	• OOB to chair • Assistance with ADLs
Procedures	• I.V. access • Antiembolism stockings • Intake and output • Oxygen 2 liters/min via nasal cannula	• I.V. access • Antiembolism stockings • Intake and output • Oxygen 2 liters/min
Teaching	• Orientation to CCU and hospital routines • Review of critical pathway • Instruction on chest pain scale • Cardiac teaching begins.	• Instruction on diet • Cardiac teaching
Discharge plan	• Social services consultation • Discharge teaching begins.	• Dietary and cardiac rehabilitation consultation • Plan for family teaching.

DAY 3	DAY 4	DAY 5	DAY 6
• Complete blood chemistry • CBC • PTT (if on heparin) • Cardiac isoenzymes if not at baseline • 12-lead ECG daily and per protocol	• Complete blood chemistry • CBC • PTT (if on heparin) • Cardiac isoenzymes if not at baseline • 12-lead ECG daily and per protocol	• Complete blood chemistry • CBC • 12-lead ECG daily and per protocol	• Complete blood chemistry • CBC • 12-lead ECG
• ECG monitoring • HR, RR, BP q 2 hr • Rhythm strip q shift and p.r.n. • D/C oximetry • Assess other body systems as needed.	• ECG monitoring • HR, RR, BP q 4 hr • Rhythm strip q shift and p.r.n.	• ECG monitoring • HR, RR, BP q 4 hr • Rhythm strip q shift and p.r.n. • Assess other body systems as needed.	• ECG monitoring • HR, RR, BP q 4 hr • Assess other body systems as needed.
• Heparin I.V. • NTG SL, transdermal, or spray • Beta blocker • Calcium channel blocker • ACE inhibitor • ASA • Analgesics • Stool softener • Sedative	• D/C heparin • NTG SL, transdermal, or spray • Beta blocker • Calcium channel blocker • ACE inhibitor • ASA • Analgesics • Stool softener • Sedative	• NTG SL, transdermal, or spray • Beta blocker • Calcium channel blocker • ACE inhibitor • ASA • Analgesics • Stool softener • Sedative	• NTG SL, transdermal, or spray • Beta blocker • Calcium channel blocker • ACE inhibitor • ASA • Analgesics • Stool softener
• Low-salt, low-fat, low-cholesterol, or ADA diet	• Low-salt, low-fat, low-cholesterol, or ADA diet	• Low-salt, -fat, -cholesterol, or ADA diet; NPO after 2400 for stress test	• Low-salt, low-fat, low-cholesterol, or ADA diet
• OOB to chair • Assistance with ADLs	• Ambulation with assistance; assist with ADLs.	• Ambulation with supervision	• Ambulation with supervision
• I.V. access • Antiembolism stockings • Intake and output • Possibly D/C O_2	• I.V. access • Transfer to telemetry unit. • Antiembolism stockings • D/C intake and output	• I.V. access • Antiembolism stockings	• Stress test • D/C I.V. access after stress test.
• Orientation to the difference between CCU and telemetry unit • Cardiac teaching	• Cardiac teaching	• Explanation of stress test • Complete cardiac teaching.	• Written instructions: medications, what to report, activity limits, and next appointment
• Discharge teaching	• Discharge teaching	• Discharge teaching • Plan discharge.	• Discharge to home.

predictable for a patient who undergoes a cholecystectomy and is otherwise healthy. However, if the same patient has diabetes and coronary artery disease, the expected treatment course is fairly unpredictable. What's more, the plan of care is likely to change. The result? Lengthy and fragmented documentation.

Documentation guidelines

When developing a critical pathway to distribute to patients, use simple vocabulary and keep your instructions short. Avoid abbreviations and complex medical terminology. Ideally, this version of the pathway should explain the diagnosis, review any tests and care the patient can expect, and inform him about activity restrictions, diet, medications, and home health care services.

When writing a critical pathway, you'll need to collaborate with the doctor and other members of the health care team. Keep in mind that the standardized orders for the critical pathway require the doctor's signature on admission of the patient.

To ensure consistent documentation from shift to shift, review the critical pathway during the change-of-shift report with the nurse who's taking over. Point out any critical events, note any changes in the patient's expected length of stay, and discuss any variances that may have occurred during your shift.

If an objective for a particular day remains unmet, document this fact on the appropriate form. Variances from the plan may result for several reasons: the plan itself, patient complications, or unforeseeable events.

Document variances as justifiable or unjustifiable. For instance, you may have a patient who doesn't walk in the hall as scheduled. If he has a secondary infection that prevents him from walking, the variance is justifiable. If he prefers to stay in bed to read or watch TV, the variance is unjustifiable. You'll need to take steps to correct the problem and then document your interventions.

Patient-teaching documents

A preprinted patient-teaching form lets you clearly and completely document the dates, times, and results of your patient-teaching sessions. The form provides evidence that you implemented a teaching plan and that you're evaluating its effectiveness. Completed, the form also documents the patient's progress toward an acceptable level of self-care or assisted care.

Of course, you'll need to construct a patient-teaching plan before you can perform patient-teaching services, complete patient-teaching forms, or distribute educational materials.

Patient-teaching plans

Because standard-setting and reimbursing bodies require the health care facility to instruct patients about their condition and treatment regimen, you'll need to draw up teaching plans to meet your patient's particular needs.

Beginning with your assessment findings, compile a list of topics and strategies that the patient needs to know or perform to attain his maximum level of health and self-care. These are called learning outcomes or objectives. Next, devise teaching activities, methods, and tools (such as brochures, one-on-one discussions, and videotapes) to convey and reinforce the information. Then design a way to evaluate your teaching effectiveness, such as a written quiz or an oral question-and-answer session (see *Filing a teaching plan,* pages 136 and 137).

Identifying what needs to be learned and how you will teach it constitutes the patient-teaching plan. Translated into reality, the instructive elements and activities should:

• define the patient's condition. If the patient has hypertension, the plan will likely begin with a working definition of normal blood pressure—both systolic and diastolic—and the roles played by the heart and blood vessels. Then the lesson will continue with an explanation of what happens in abnormal blood pressure.

• identify risk factors associated with the patient's condition. General risk factors usually have something to do with family history, age, race, diet, activity patterns, personal habits (such as smoking cigarettes or drinking alcohol), and so forth.

• explain what causes the patient's condition. For example a patient-teaching plan on hypertension would include a simplified lesson on the dynamics of cardiac output and peripheral vascular resistance. (The teacher might use a model blood vessel for illustration.) If appropriate, the teaching plan should include an explanation of variations of the patient's condition (such as essential hypertension or secondary hypertension).

• point out the importance of therapy, emphasizing, if necessary, the consequences of untreated disease. (In untreated hypertension, for example, consequences include cardiovascular disease, stroke, and kidney damage.)

• explain the goals of treatment and identify the components of the treatment plan. In hypertension, for example, the goal of treatment would be stable, normal blood pressure; the components of the treatment plan might include dietary modifications, weight reduction, medications, exercise, stress management, self-monitoring, and regular health care follow-up.

• define the patient's anticipated learning outcomes and provide a time frame. Again using hypertension as an example, some timed learning outcomes might include:

—By discharge, the patient will be able to plan three well-balanced, low-sodium meals from the food list supplied by the nutritionist.

—Within 48 hours, the patient will be able to name his medications, explain their purposes, state how and when to take them, and list related adverse reactions that he should report to the doctor or nurse.

—By discharge, the patient will develop a doctor-approved exercise program.

Advantages

Though the patient-teaching plan doesn't stand alone as a document in the medical record, it is part of the patient's plan of care, which is part of the medical record. The teaching plan tells health care team members at a glance what the patient learned and what he still needs to learn and do about his health condition. It also shows quality-improvement measures in progress and meets professional and accrediting requirements as well.

Disadvantages

Constructing individual teaching plans requires time and thought. Fortunately, some health care facilities have patient education departments that focus on devel-

(Text continues on page 138.)

Documentation Methods

Filing a teaching plan

Your teaching plan should include your assessment findings; projected learning outcomes, along with the activities, methods, and tools needed to accomplish the outcomes; and the techniques you'll use to evaluate the effectiveness of teaching.

The teaching plan below was structured for Harold Harmon, who has congestive heart failure.

Assessment findings	Learning outcomes	Activities
Mr. Harmon needs to understand the action of his medication.	Mr. Harmon will: –explain the action of digoxin. –state when to take the drug.	–Present written brochures. –Discuss content. –Check Mr. Harmon's knowledge.
Mr. Harmon needs to learn how to take his pulse.	Mr. Harmon will take his pulse and come within two beats of his doctor's or nurse's results.	–Show Mr. Harmon a videotape that includes instruction on how to take a pulse. –Instruct him to study printed materials. –Demonstrate the procedure. –Provide feedback and practice time. –Ask Mr. Harmon to demonstrate the procedure.
Mr. Harmon reports feeling increased anxiety. He needs to learn how to cope with this anxiety and to control stress in his life.	Mr. Harmon will explain two techniques that he'll use to help him relax.	–Invite Mr. Harmon to watch a videotape on how to control stress. –Encourage him to read printed materials (booklets, pamphlets) on techniques to reduce stress. –Demonstrate deep-breathing and progressive muscle relaxation techniques. –Role-play a guided imagery scene. –Present a case study on how other people cope with stress.

Teaching methods	Teaching tools	Evaluation methods
−One-on-one discussion	−Printed materials describing digoxin's action	−Question and answer
	−Patient-teaching aid on digoxin	−Written test
	−Illustration of a medication clock	
−Demonstration	−Videotape	−Question and answer
−Supervised practice sessions	−Printed materials	−Return demonstration
−One-on-one discussion	−Photographs or illustrations of key steps in the procedure	
−One-on-one discussion	−Printed materials	−Question and answer
−Group discussion (with family)	−Videotape	−Interview
−Role-playing		−Observation
−Case study		−Return demonstration of re-
−Self-monitoring		laxation techniques

Documentation
Methods

oping and implementing standard teaching plans for many common disorders.

Documentation guidelines

Check your facility's policies and procedures to learn where you're expected to file the patient-teaching plan—for example, within the plan of care, on charts, in progress notes, in the patient education office, or elsewhere.

When writing the teaching plan, be sure to follow the nursing process. Assess the patient's learning needs first, formulate a list of learning diagnoses (or learning outcomes), plan ways to meet the patient's learning needs, implement the plan, and periodically evaluate the results of your teaching.

Be sure to keep the plan succinct and precise. Most important of all, be sure to talk with the patient about the patient-teaching plan and agree on realistic learning outcomes.

Encourage and expect the patient's participation in the plan. Doing so usually increases his cooperation and your effectiveness.

Patient-teaching forms

Despite their similar content, patient-teaching forms vary according to the health care facility. For the most part, they contain general information about the patient's learning abilities, goals to be met, and skills to be acquired by the time of discharge. They may also focus on teaching aspects as they relate to a patient's particular disease. You can document information by filling in blanks, checking boxes, or writing brief narrative notes. (See *Documenting your patient teaching*.)

Additional documentation materials include patient-teaching aids, such as pre-printed instructional materials, illustrations, models, games, dolls, audiocassettes, and videotapes. (See *Meeting patient-teaching standards,* page 143.)

Advantages

Patient-teaching forms make documenting your patient education quicker and easier by creating a record of a patient's outcomes, responses, and level of learning. Correct use of these forms may be your legal defense for many years against charges of inadequate patient care. These forms also prevent duplication of patient-teaching efforts by other staff members. There are no disadvantages of using patient-teaching forms.

Documentation guidelines

Aim to have your completed patient-teaching forms include the patient's learning ability, his response to teaching, and the outcomes. If your facility doesn't have a preprinted form, talk to your supervisor about developing one. In the meantime, document your patient teaching in accurate, detailed progress notes. (See Chapter 6, Documentation of the Nursing Process, for more information on patient-teaching forms.)

Whether you chart on a preprinted form or on progress notes, remember these tips:
• Check your facility's policies and procedures regarding when, where, and how to document your teaching.
• Each shift, ask yourself these questions: What part of the teaching plan did I complete? What other instruction did I give the patient or his family? Then document your answers.

(Text continues on page 142.)

Documenting your patient teaching

Use the model patient-teaching form below—for a patient with diabetes mellitus—as a guideline for documenting your teaching sessions clearly and completely.

PATIENT TEACHING
Instructions for Diabetic Patients

Centerville Hospital, Centerville, MA

Bernard Miller
7 Main St.
Centerville, MA 04872

Admission date: _1/3/95_ **Anticipated discharge:** _1/8/95_ **Diagnosis:** _T I A NIDDM_

EDUCATIONAL ASSESSMENT

Comprehension level
Ability to grasp concepts
☑ High
☐ Average
☐ Needs improvement
Comments: _____

Motivation level
☑ Asks questions
☐ Eager to learn
☐ Anxious
☐ Uncooperative
☐ Disinterested
☐ Denies need to learn
Comments _____
_____

Knowledge and skill levels
Understanding of health condition and how to manage it
☐ High (>75% working knowledge)
☐ Adequate (50% to 75% working knowledge)
☑ Needs improvement (25% to 50% working knowledge)
☐ Low (< 25% working knowledge)
Comments: _____
_____

Learning barriers
☐ Language (specify: foreign, impairment, laryngectomy, other): _____
☐ Vision (specify: blind, legally blind, other): _____
☐ Hearing (impaired, deaf)
☐ Memory
  ☐ Change in long-term memory (specify): _____
  ☐ Change in short-term memory (specify): _____
☐ Other (specify): _____
Instructor's Initials _CW_

ANTICIPATED OUTCOMES

Patient will be prepared to perform self-care at the following level:
☑ High (total self-care)
☐ Moderate (self-care with minor assistance)
☐ Minimal (self-care with more than 50% assistance)

KEY

P = patient taught
F = caregiver or family taught
R = reinforced
N/A = not applicable

A = asked questions
B = nonattentive, poor concentration
C = expressed denial, resistance
D = verbalized recall
E = demonstrated ability

(continued)

Documentation Methods

Documenting your patient teaching   (continued)

Date	1/4/95	1/5/95	1/5/95	1/5/95	1/6/95	1/7/95	1/7/95	1/8/95		
Time	1900	0800	1330	1830	1000	0800	1830	0800		
ASSESSED EDUCATIONAL NEEDS										
Assessment of patient's (or caregiver's) current knowledge of disease (include medical, family, and social histories)	A/CW									
Assessment of learner's reaction to diagnosis (verbal and nonverbal responses)	A/CW									
GENERAL DIABETIC EDUCATION GOALS The patient (or caregiver) will:										
• define diabetes mellitus.	P/A/CW	R/EG	D/ME					D/EG		
• state hormone produced in the pancreas.	P/A/CW	R/EG	D/ME					D/EG		
• identify three signs and symptoms of diabetes.	P/CW	R/EG	D/ME					D/EG		
• discuss risk factors associated with the disease.	P/CW	R/EG	D/ME					D/EG		
• differentiate between Type I and Type II diabetes.	P/A/CW	R/EG	D/ME					D/EG		
SURVIVAL SKILL GOALS The patient (or caregiver) will:										
• identify the name, purpose, dose, and time of administration of medication ordered.		P/EG	R/ME	D/LT				D/EG		
• properly administer insulin.	N/A									
– draw up insulin properly.	N/A									
– discuss and demonstrate site selection and rotation.	N/A									
– demonstrate proper injection technique with needle angled appropriately.	N/A									
– explain correct way to store insulin.	N/A									
– demonstrate correct disposal of syringes.	N/A									
• distinguish among types of insulin.	N/A									
– species (pork, beef, recombinant DNA)	N/A									
– regular	N/A									
– NPH/ultralente (longer acting)	N/A									
• properly administer mixed insulins.	N/A					.				
– demonstrate injecting air into vials.	N/A									

BETTER CHARTING

Documenting your patient teaching   (continued)

Date	1/4/95	1/5/95	1/5/95	1/5/95	1/6/95	1/7/95	1/7/95	1/8/95		
Time	1900	0800	1330	1830	1000	0800	1830	0800		
– draw up mixed insulin properly (regular before NPH).	N/A									
•demonstrate knowledge of oral antidiabetic agents.										
– identify name of medication, dose, and time of administration.		P/EG	A/ME		D/EG	F/EG	R/LT	D/EG		
– identify purpose of medication.		P/EG	A/ME		D/EG	F/EG	R/LT	D/EG		
– state possible adverse effects.		P/EG	A/ME		D/EG	F/EG	R/LT	D/EG		
•name signs and symptoms, causes, implications, and treatments of hyperglycemia and hypoglycemia.		P/EG	A/ME			F/EG		D/EG		
•monitor blood glucose levels satisfactorily.										
– demonstrate proper use of blood glucose monitoring device.				P/LT	E/EG	E/EG	R/LT	E/EG		
– perform fingerstick.				P/LT	E/EG	E/EG	R/LT	E/EG		
– obtain accurate blood glucose reading.				P/LT	E/EG	E/EG	R/LT	E/EG		
HEALTHFUL LIVING GOALS The patient (or caregiver) will:										
•consult the nutritionist about meal planning.			P/ME	R/LT	A/EG			D/EG		
•follow the diet recommended by the American Diabetes Association.			P/ME	R/LT	A/EG			D/EG		
•state importance of adhering to diet.			P/ME	R/LT	A/EG			D/EG		
•give verbal feedback on 1-day meal plan.			P/ME	D/LT	A/EG			D/EG		
•state the effects of stress, illness, and exercise on blood glucose levels.			P/ME	D/LT	A/EG			D/EG		
•state when to test urine for ketones and how to address results.			P/ME	D/LT	A/EG			D/EG		
•identify self-care measures for periods when illness occurs.			P/ME	D/LT	A/EG			D/EG		
•list precautions to take while exercising.			P/ME	D/LT	A/EG			D/EG		
•explain what steps to take when patient doesn't want to eat or drink on proper schedule.			P/ME	D/LT	A/EG			D/EG		
•agree to wear medical identification (for example, a Medic Alert bracelet).			P/ME	A/LT				D/EG		

(continued)

Documenting your patient teaching (continued)

Date	1/4/95	1/5/95	1/5/95	1/5/95	1/6/95	1/7/95	1/7/95	1/8/95		
Time	1900	0800	1330	1830	1000	0800	1830	0800		
SAFETY GOALS The patient (or caregiver) will:										
• state the possible complications of diabetes.	P/CW	R/EG		D/LT		F/EG		D/EG		
• explain the importance of careful, regular skin care.	P/CW	R/EG		D/LT		F/EG		D/EG		
• demonstrate healthful foot care.	P/CW	R/EG		D/LT		F/EG		D/EG		
• discuss the importance of eye care and regular examinations.	P/CW	R/EG		D/LT						
• state the importance of oral hygiene.	P/CW	R/EG		D/LT						
INDIVIDUAL GOALS										

Initial	Signature
CW	Carol Witt, RN, BSN
EG	Ell Thomas RN MSN
ME	Marianne Evans, RN
LT	Lynn Tata, RN, BSN

• Each shift, ask yourself these questions: What part of the teaching plan did I complete? What other instruction did I give the patient or his family? Then document your answers.

• Be sure to document that the patient's ongoing educational needs are being met.

• Before discharge, document the patient's remaining learning needs and note whether you provided him with printed or other patient-teaching aids (see *Using patient-teaching aids,* page 144).

• Be sure to evaluate your teaching. One way is by using a checklist. (See *Evaluating your teaching: The checklist method,* page 145.)

Discharge summary and patient instruction form

To comply with JCAHO requirements related to discharge planning, you must document your assessment of a patient's continuing care needs as well as any referrals for such care. To assist this kind of documentation, many health care facilities combine discharge summaries and patient instructions in one form. This form contains sections for recording discharge documentation, patient assessment, patient education, and detailed special instructions. On such forms, a narrative style coexists with open- and closed-ended styles.

Meeting patient-teaching standards

One way to make sure that you fulfill patient-teaching requirements set forth by the Joint Commission on Accreditation of Healthcare Organizations, Medicaid, and other standard-setting groups is to prepare, print, and dispense patient-teaching aids such as the sample medication teaching aid below. Also be sure to document this teaching measure in the patient's record.

Dear Patient:

Your doctor has prescribed verapamil (also called Calan or Isoptin) to treat your condition. Verapamil helps relax blood vessels, which increases the flow of blood to your heart. In turn, this helps relieve chest pain, heart irregularities, and high blood pressure.

How to take verapamil
Take verapamil only as your doctor directs. If you're taking an extended-release tablet, swallow it whole without crushing or chewing it.

Take verapamil on an empty stomach. Taking extended-release tablets with food may decrease your body's ability to absorb the drug.

Take your medication even if you feel well. Stopping suddenly could cause your condition to worsen.

What to do if you miss a dose
Take it as soon as possible. However, if it's almost time for your next dose, skip the missed dose and take your next dose as scheduled.

What to do about adverse effects
Call your doctor immediately if you develop any of the adverse effects listed here:
- breathing difficulty, coughing, or wheezing
- irregular or fast, pounding heartbeat
- swelling of ankles, feet, or lower legs.

Also notify your doctor if you become constipated, feel faint or unusually tired, or continue to have chest pain.

What you must know about other drugs
Some medications may affect how verapamil works. At the same time, verapamil may interfere with another drug's actions. Therefore, be sure to tell your doctor about any medications you're taking, particularly lithium carbonate (Lithane) or heart medications, or medications for high blood pressure, seizures, tuberculosis, or glaucoma.

Special directions
Because verapamil may cause certain medical conditions to worsen, tell your doctor if you have a history of kidney or liver disease or some other heart or blood vessel disorder.

Eat foods high in fiber, and be sure to drink plenty of fluids (unless your doctor tells you otherwise) to help prevent constipation.

If fatigue is a problem, remember to allow yourself several rest periods during the day.

Important reminder
If you're pregnant or breast-feeding, check with your doctor before taking verapamil.

Additional instructions
_____
_____
_____
_____
_____
_____
_____

Using patient-teaching aids

One way to save time and ensure consistent, thorough teaching is to provide preprinted patient-teaching aids. These materials may be developed by you, your patient education department, drug companies, or other responsible organizations.

Although patient-teaching aids are no substitute for the caring instruction you provide personally, they are an excellent reference tool for the patient who needs to review and reinforce what you've taught him.

Below is an example of a teaching aid developed for patients using patient-controlled analgesia (also known as PCA).

Dear Patient:

Your doctor has prescribed patient-controlled analgesia (PCA) to help relieve your pain and help you feel more comfortable. He'll order the medication, prescribe the dose, and make it possible for you to receive the medication intravenously (I.V.) or epidurally.

You'll be using a PCA pump. This is a computerized device that delivers a preset dose of medication. It's safe and effective and you control when you receive it.

How does PCA work?
Your nurse will explain how PCA works and what it can and can't do. She'll teach you how to change the medication, attach the tubing to the pump, prime the pump, and attach the tubing to your I.V. device. She'll explain how to secure the pump to an I.V. pole or to your belt.

She'll show you how the alarm system works, how to make sure that the pump and I.V. tubing are working correctly, and how to deal with problems. She'll also answer your questions and monitor your condition to evaluate the safety and effectiveness of your therapy.

Essentially, the PCA system delivers a dose of medication when you push the button that activates the pump. It's programmed with a safe time between doses so that you can't give yourself too much medication.

PCA pointers
Here are some tips to help you operate your system easily and safely:
• To make sure that your PCA unit is programmed correctly, match the dose and delay time (interval between infusions) on the pump's display screen with the doctor's orders. Call your nurse in the hospital or your home health care nurse if you notice a difference.
• Use your pump's instruction manual and check the pump carefully to see that all unit parts (including batteries) are connected, correctly positioned, and in working order.
• Keep a record of your comfort level. Give yourself only enough medication to relieve your pain. Then don't give yourself another dose if you start to feel sleepy. Instead try to balance the pain relief against sleepiness.
• Jot down any adverse effects you notice, such as nausea, vomiting, itching, or rashes. Report them to your doctor. At home report them to your home health care nurse. You may need a dosage adjustment.
• Call your nurse in the hospital or your home health care nurse for instructions if infusion problems, such as a leak or blood in the tubing, develop.

Evaluating your teaching: The checklist method

Using a checklist is a simple, quick way of obtaining information, evaluating your patient teaching, and gauging your patient's progress at various learning stages.

Using checklists will give you and the patient clear evidence of which goals he's achieved and which goals remain. To devise a useful checklist, follow these tips:
• Make the list concise but wide-ranging enough to cover all aspects of the skill or activity being evaluated.
• Limit the items on the checklist to a group of related activities, such as the steps in tracheostomy care or the segments of a cardiac rehabilitation plan.
• Arrange items in a logical order—sequentially, chronologically, or in order of importance.
• Identify the essential steps of the activities or behavior you're evaluating.
• Relate items on the list to the patient's learning goals and to your teaching methods.
• Use only one idea or concept for each item.
• Phrase each item succinctly and accurately.
• Test your checklist on at least two patients before adopting it permanently.
• Use the checklist along with other evaluation tools to promote balance and avoid giving it undue importance.

The sample checklist below might be used for evaluating how well a diabetic patient has learned to draw up insulin.

DRAWING UP INSULIN

Yes	No	
☐	☐	Disinfects top of vial thoroughly
☐	☐	Inserts needle into vial without contamination
☐	☐	Injects air into vial
☐	☐	Withdraws proper amount of insulin
☐	☐	Expels air from syringe
☐	☐	Retains exact dose of insulin in syringe
☐	☐	Replaces cap on needle without contamination

(For more information, see *Using a discharge summary–patient instruction form,* pages 146 to 148.)

Advantages
This combined form provides useful information about additional teaching needs and points out whether the patient has the information he needs to care for himself or to get further help. It establishes compliance with JCAHO requirements and helps to safeguard you from malpractice accusations.

There are no disadvantages of using a discharge summary–patient instruction form.

(Text continues on page 149.)

Documentation Methods

Using a discharge summary–patient instruction form

Combining the patient's discharge summary with instructions for his care after discharge fills two requirements with a single stroke of your pen. When using this documentation method, be sure to give one copy to the patient and keep one for the record.

DISCHARGE SUMMARY AND INSTRUCTIONS

Patient stamp and I.D.

Mary Adams
101 Shea Lane
Milltown, CO
PCN - 0006 - 234 - 56

DIET

☑ No restrictions   ☐ Special diet _____

ACTIVITY

☐ No restrictions
☑ Lifting restricted to __5__ lb for ____ week(s) or ⟨until after next office visit⟩
☑ Stair climbing restricted to _2 to 4_ steps/day for ____ weeks(s) or ⟨until after next office visit.⟩
☑ No driving for ____ week(s) or ⟨until next office visit.⟩
☑ Riding in car restricted: _None for 1 week, then 1 hr at a time_
May take: ☐ shower   ☐ tub bath   ☑ sponge bath

☑ Walking/exercise restricted to:
Per instructions from PT
☑ Other restrictions:
use raised toilet seat
May return to work: _N/A_
      ☐ immediately
      ☐ ____ week(s)
      ☐ undetermined

COMFORT LEVEL

☐ No pain   ☐ Minimal discomfort   ☑ Moderate discomfort   ☐ Maximum discomfort

AIDS USED

☐ None   ☐ Cane   ☑ Walker   ☐ Prosthesis   ☐ Wheelchair   ☐ Crutches

HYGIENE AND ACTIVITIES OF DAILY LIVING

☐ Independent   ☑ Needs some assistance   ☐ Needs total assistance   ☐ Other _____

	No Difficulty	Other (explain)
Respiratory	✓	
CV	✓	
Neurologic	✓	
Skin		*wound care to Ⓛ knee incision*
Musculoskeletal		*Ambulates with use of walker*
GI	✓	
Nutrition	✓	

	No Difficulty	Other (explain)
Vision		*Needs glasses at all times.*
Hearing	✓	
Speech	✓	
Reproductive	✓	
Elimination (bladder)	✓	
Elimination (bowel)	✓	

Using a discharge summary–patient instruction form *(continued)*

MENTAL STATUS

☑ Alert ☑ Oriented ☐ Lethargic ☐ Confused

INCISIONAL CARE

☐ No special care required ☑ Other

Paint incision with betadine swabs twice a day. Use three swabs each time: one straight down on top of the incision line; one down the one side of the incision; then the third stick down the other side of the incision. Do not scrub incision back and forth. Dress with non-adhesive dressing.

SPECIAL INSTRUCTIONS FOR MEDICATIONS

Dose/time/route (Do not take any other medications before checking with your physician.)

	Prescription Given	Has at Home
Percocet – one tablet every 4 hr as needed for severe pain.	☑	☐
Tylenol 325 mg, two tablets every 4 hr as needed for mild pain.	☐	☑
Continue taking other medications as before surgery.	☐	☐
	☐	☐
	☐	☐
	☐	☐

PATIENT EDUCATION

	Patient Yes	Patient No	S/O Yes	S/O No	N/A
Verbalizes symptoms of disease process	✓		✓		
Verbalizes activities or exercises	✓		✓		
Verbalizes special diet, if ordered	✓		✓		
Verbalizes medication's adverse effects, if ordered	✓		✓		
Demonstrates ability to perform specialized care or treatment (wound healing, dressings, and so forth)		✓	✓		
Verbalizes when to contact doctor	✓		✓		
Given patient education information	✓		✓		

COMMENTS:

(continued)

Using a discharge summary–patient instruction form *(continued)*

FORMS GIVEN

Prescriptions
Percocet one tablet every 4 hr as needed for
severe pain.
Diet
2 Gram Sodium

Other (specify)

DISCHARGE DESTINATION

☐ home independently
☐ extended care facility

☑ home with home health care
☐ transfer to another facility

REFERRAL SERVICES

Referred to home health care services for:
☑ home health care needs　　☑ follow-up care　　☑ continued learning

---

MODE OF TRANSPORTATION

☐ ambulatory
☑ wheelchair
☐ stretcher

Accompanied by　*Mary Kane*
Relationship　*Daughter*

FOLLOW-UP

Call Dr. *Susan Brown*　　　　　　　at　*(206) 555-5555*
to schedule an appointment in　*2 weeks*
☑ Other　*Schedule appointment with your personal doctor for follow-up of hypertension.*
☐ Other

Physician's signature　*Susan Brown, MD*
Phone　*(206) 555-5555*

Discharge date　*12/18/94*
Discharge time　*1000 hours*

I have received these instructions.
Signature　*Mary Adams*
Date　*12/18/94*

Caregiver (relationship)　*Mary Kane (daughter)*
RN　*Nora Martin*
MD　*Susan Brown*

Writing a narrative discharge summary

Some health care facilities use a narrative-style discharge summary (much like a progress note), such as the one below.

PROGRESS NOTES

Date	Time	
1/19/95	Discharge: 1305 (summary)	36 y.o. white female admitted 1/18/95 with severe LLQ pain. To surgery 1/18 for exploratory laparoscopy and subsequent (L) oophorectomy for ruptured ovarian cyst. Tolerated procedure well. Postop vital signs stable (see flow sheet). Pt. was slow to ambulate but has been OOB walking in the hallway at least twice per shift for the past 24 hours. Pain was controlled for the first 24 hours with meperidine 75 mg I.M. p.r.n. Pt. is currently taking oxycodone 5 mg P.O. q 4 h p.r.n. for incisional pain (prescription sent home with pt.). Incision clean and dry. Pt. instructed to clean wound once daily with povidone iodine swab. No dressing required. Pt. returned demonstration of wound care. Instructed to avoid lifting more than 10 lb. She will call Dr. Jones to make 2-week postop appointment. Instruction sheet given.————Joan Delaney, RN

Documentation guidelines

Remember to give one copy of the form to the patient and put another copy in the medical record for future reference.

Be sure that your discharge summary outlines the patient's care, provides useful information for further teaching and evaluation, and documents that the patient has the information he needs to care for himself or to get further help.

Not all facilities use combined forms. Your facility may use a narrative discharge summary. (See *Writing a narrative discharge summary.*) If it does, be sure to include the following information on the form:

• the patient's status at admission and discharge
• significant highlights of the patient's stay in the health care facility
• outcomes of your interventions
• resolved and unresolved patient problems, continuing care needs for unresolved problems, and referrals for continuing care

• instructions given to the patient, his family, or other caregivers about medications, treatments, activity, diet, referrals, and follow-up appointments, as well as any other special instructions.

Dictated documentation

In some situations, nurses dictate from a nursing unit or clinical setting, and clerical personnel transcribe the information for the written clinical record. This occurs commonly among visiting nurses who may dictate into a recorder or a car phone between patient visits.

Advantages

Convenient and fast, dictated documentation can be performed without the distractions and interruptions encountered in a clinical setting. Using this documentation technique allows the nurse more time for patient care. Dictation can be done at any time of day or night, and studies show that this kind of documentation is highly accurate. What's more, it complies with JCAHO standards and may actually improve the quality of documentation.

Disadvantages

Delays in transcription time can prevent necessary documentation from being readily available to doctors and other health care team members. And supplies for recorded documentation may be more costly than for handwritten charting. Also, the nurse may need time to adjust to this type of documentation.

Documentation guidelines

Before dictating a report, familiarize yourself with the recording equipment. Then review the existing records and the nota-tions you made during contact with your patient. Here are some tips for more effective dictation:

• Refer to your health care facility's policy and procedures manual for dictation guidelines, and consult the transcriptionist if you have related questions.

• Prepare a brief outline of your report so that it illustrates the nursing process.

• At the beginning of your dictation, name the patient and give his identification number, if necessary.

• Tell the transcriptionist when the report begins and ends. Be sure to provide the date of the report and the date of the visit with the patient. Instruct the transcriptionist to provide the date of transcription. At the end of the report, include a summary, evaluation, and recommendations. Discuss your plans for the next time you'll see the patient.

• Use a checklist as you dictate to be sure that you include all the necessary information. For example, state the purpose of your time with the patient, list assessments performed and findings, discuss any new or changing patient problems, list interventions and patient responses, identify future care needs, explain patient teaching provided, and describe the patient's response.

• Try to dictate the information as near to the time that you provided care as possible so that your activities and observations are fresh in your mind.

• Speak clearly and slowly, avoiding unnecessary medical terminology or uncommon abbreviations.

• If you need to add information or change something you've said, give clear and specific directions to the transcriptionist.

Patient self-documentation

Although self-documentation obviously isn't feasible or desirable for every patient, it can be effective for patients who must perform considerable self-care (diabetic patients, for example) or for patients trying to discover what precipitates a problem (such as those with chronic headaches).

In using self-documentation, a diabetic patient may record information on his diet, insulin dose, self-tested blood glucose levels, and activity level. The accumulated information can help him avoid insulin reactions and delay, prevent, or even reverse complications from hyper- or hypoglycemia.

A patient with chronic headaches may be asked to chart, among other things, when a headache occurred, what warning signs he noticed, and what pain relief measures he tried. Analyzing this information may help ward off future headaches. (See *Teaching self-documentation skills,* pages 152 and 153.)

The patient can document entries on preprinted forms or in journal style. Such records can be used in both inpatient and outpatient care settings. Depending on health care facility policies, they may or may not become a permanent part of the medical record (see *Keeping a record of monitored activity,* page 154).

Advantages

Having the patient document data and events related to his own condition teaches him about his problem and its causes, symptoms, and treatment. It also may provide needed clues to the problem's precipitators and suggest solutions to the problem.

Data recorded by the patient may actually be more accurate than data interpreted by someone else. For example, a nurse or doctor may better understand the character of a patient's problem if he describes it in his own words.

Self-documentation also improves therapeutic compliance by making the patient an active participant in his treatment and providing him with some control.

Disadvantages

Self-documentation isn't difficult, but it takes time, patience, planning, motivation, and perseverance—on the part of both the nurse and the patient. The patient needs to understand how to keep careful records, what's important to document, and when to document. Otherwise, the records won't be useful and may even adversely affect his treatment and recovery.

Documentation guidelines

The patient must fully understand what needs to be documented and why it's important. If he will use preprinted forms, take the time to review each aspect of a form with him. If he will use a chart or a graph, show him how to use the form. If possible, show him examples of self-documentation.

Identify the person that the patient can contact if he has questions.

Emphasize the benefits of self-documentation to the patient (increased knowledge about his condition and increased control of his treatment, for example). By doing so, you may help boost his interest in keeping his records updated.

Finally, show him the results of his self-documentation, pointing out how or what the data contribute to his treatment.

Documentation
Methods

Teaching self-documentation skills

For some patients, self-documentation has wide-ranging benefits. By learning to keep a log or a journal, for example, a patient may find out what triggers certain health problems (such as headaches, asthma attacks, or hypoglycemic episodes). Once the trigger emerges, the patient and caregiver can implement preventive strategies.

To help a patient learn self-documentation skills, some health care facilities use individual self-documentation forms like the sample headache log shown at right.

Reviewing instructions

Give the patient instructions and review them with him. Tell him to complete the headache log daily. Inform him that doing so may help him to identify what triggers his headaches (for example, environmental factors, foods, or stress). Explain that information collected in the log may also help him discover effective ways to relieve a headache once it starts.

Instruct the patient to describe the details of each headache in a diary, log, or small notebook.

Checking the boxes

Review these steps with the patient.
• Using the log page at right as a guide, note the date and time of the headache and any warning signs.
• Put a check mark in the appropriate box to indicate the headache's intensity.
• Next, check the box to mark how long you've had the headache.
• Check the appropriate box for any other signs or symptoms that accompany your headache, such as nausea, vomiting, or sensitivity to light.
• Continue by checking the steps you took to relieve the headache (for example, medication, biofeedback, rest), as well as the effectiveness of these measures.

Completing the log

Urge the patient to think carefully about the events that occurred before the headache. For instance, was his headache attack triggered by emotional stress, by drinking a cup of coffee, or by something else? He should write down the details of such potential triggers in his log.

Adapted or new forms

You may find that one or several documentation forms you've been using no longer suit your needs. This may occur because of changes in therapies, patient population, or reimbursement criteria. Duplicated and fragmented documentation data are among the first signs that the forms in use aren't filling current needs.

HEADACHE LOG

Date and time headache began
12/25/94 – 5:00 p.m.

Warning signs
- ☑ Flashing lights
- ☐ Blind spots
- ☐ Colors
- ☐ Zigzag patterns
- ☐ None
- ☐ Other

Intensity
- ☐ Mild
- ☑ Moderate
- ☐ Severe
- ☐ Disabling

Duration
- ☑ 4 hours or less
- ☐ 4 to 7.5 hours
- ☐ 8 to 11.5 hours
- ☐ 12 to 24 hours
- ☐ More than 1 day
- ☐ More than 2 days

Associated signs and symptoms
- ☐ Upset stomach
- ☑ Nausea or vomiting
- ☐ Dizziness
- ☑ Sensitivity to light
- ☐ Sensory, motor, or speech disturbances
- ☐ Other

Measures for relief
- ☑ Medication
- ☐ Rest
- ☑ Sleep
- ☐ Biofeedback
- ☐ Ice pack
- ☐ Relaxation exercises

Extent of relief
- ☐ None
- ☑ Mild
- ☐ Moderate
- ☐ Marked
- ☐ Complete

Possible triggers

Caffeine and sugar

When developing a new form or adapting an old one, remember to ask yourself these questions:
- What problems exist with the old forms?
- What information is really needed?
- What changes would correct these problems?
- Which parts of the old forms remain valuable and need to be retained?

Even if your health care facility uses a computerized documentation system, ask staff members to help design the new form or reprogram the system. To develop an effective form, follow these guidelines:
- If your facility uses a specific nursing theory or framework for delivering nursing care, make sure that the nursing assessment form reflects it.
- If the old nursing assessment form reflects a medical format, change it to highlight the nursing process. For example, reorganize the form according to human response patterns or functional health care designs.
- Ask staff members who'll be using the form to evaluate possible formats and indicate which they prefer. Ask for their ideas about how best to organize and document their data.
- List all information the form must include. Be sure to document this information to comply with professional practice standards published by such organizations as the American Nurses' Association (ANA) and the JCAHO.
- Consider combining documentation styles in one form. Decide which style is most appropriate for each type of information included in the form. For instance, a narrative note may best suit one part of the form, whereas an open-ended style may best convey information on another part.
- After developing the form, write procedural guidelines for its use. Provide clear explanations and completed examples for each section.

Keeping a record of monitored activity

In many situations, your patient can provide more information more accurately than can a member of the health care team. A case in point: a patient who wears a Holter monitor to evaluate the effect of medication on his heart and his daily activities.

Keeping this in mind, some health care facilities prepare patient instructional materials in conjunction with a diary-like chart (such as the example below), which the patient refers to and completes for the medical record.

DATE	TIME	ACTIVITY	FEELINGS
1/15/95	10:30 a.m.	Rode home from hospital in cab	Legs tired, felt short of breath
	11:30 a.m.	Watched TV in living room	Comfortable
	12:15 p.m.	Ate lunch, took propranolol	Indigestion
	1:30 p.m.	Walked next door to see neighbor	Felt short of breath
	2:45 p.m.	Walked home	Very tired, legs hurt
	3:00 to 4:00	Urinated, took nap	Comfortable
	5:30 p.m.	Ate dinner slowly	Comfortable
	7:20 p.m.	Had bowel movement	Felt short of breath
	9:00 p.m.	Watched TV, drank one beer	Heart beating fast for about 1 minute, no pain
	11:00 p.m.	Took propranolol, urinated, and went to bed	Tired
1/16/95	8:15 a.m.	Woke up, urinated, washed face and arms	Very tired, rapid heart beat for about 30 seconds
	10:30 a.m.	Returned to hospital	Felt better

• Ask staff members not involved in developing the form to analyze both the form and the guidelines. This helps identify potentially confusing sections that require more detailed explanation or revision.
• Before adopting the form, have staff members test it to make sure they can use it easily for entering information and retrieving it as well.
• If you expect the form will become a permanent part of the medical record, check the section devoted to form adoptions in your policy and procedures manual. Some health care facilities require a

form to be approved by the medical records committee or certain departments before official use.

Documentation in home health care settings

Like hospitals, rehabilitation centers, and nursing homes, home health care agencies are regulated by state and federal laws and bodies. These standard bearers require accurate and complete documentation as well as standard and quality care from home health care agencies. Without these features, a home health care agency may fail to earn licensure, accreditation, and reimbursement—or may have current licensure, accreditation, and reimbursement withheld.

Accreditation and quality improvement programs are available through the Foundation for Hospice and Homecare, the JCAHO, and the ANA, which instituted the ANA Standards of Home Care Nursing Practice. The nursing process forms the basis of these standards.

Home health care growth

With the speedy discharge of patients from hospitals, the increasing number of elderly people, and the availability of safe, easily operated health care equipment, home health care has a bright future. Services provided range from caretaking and assistance with ADLs to such highly complex and advanced interventions as I.V. therapy delivered by central and peripheral lines, mechanical ventilation, and chemotherapy.

Providing nursing care to patients in their home requires you to assume many roles, including those of skilled-care provider, educator, and communicator. The skilled home care practitioner must be highly competent and well organized—especially in the area of documentation.

In no other health care setting are you as responsible for ensuring reimbursement payments as you are in the home health care setting. Your success or failure virtually depends on your documentation skills. For this reason, home health care organizations have a tightly structured documentation system.

Standardized and required documents

Home health care nurses are bound by all the controls imposed by the professional standards and nurse practice acts that govern nurses in all other settings.

Medicare and Medicaid

By mandate in 1985, the Health Care Financing Administration (HCFA), the watchdog agency for Medicare and Medicaid disbursements, required home health care agencies to standardize and update their record keeping and documentation methods.

Required data for each qualified recipient include a home health certification and plan of treatment form (see *Certifying home health care needs and treatments*, pages 156 and 157) and a medical update and patient information form (see *Providing updated medical and patient information*, page 158).

These data allow Medicare reviewers to evaluate each claim in accordance with the criteria for coverage. Medicare will provide no payment unless the required

Documentation Methods

Certifying home health care needs and treatments

Charged with completing the Medicare document known as "Certification and Plan of Treatment," you'll need to carefully match the correct patient needs, diagnoses, and treatment measures with the preferred terminology and code numbers to speed the health care approval process. The completed example below is for a patient with heart disease and a colostomy.

CERTIFICATION AND PLAN OF TREATMENT

1. Patient's HI claim no. *III–III*	2. Start of care date *01/08/95*		3. Certification period From:*11/7/94* To: *1/7/95*	4. Medical rec. no. *11–2222*	5. Provider no. *30–7051*

6. Patient name, address
John Klein, Main St., Oakland, CA

7. Provider name, address
Home Health Care Agency,
Second St., Oakland, CA

8. Date of birth *01/18/14*	9. Sex *M*	10. Medications: dose/frequency/route

11. Principal procedure code *42731 Atrial fibrillation*	**Date** *11/08/94*

Digoxin 0.25 mg P.O. QD; Lasix 40 mg P.O. QD;
allopurinol 100 mg P.O. B.I.D.; Capoten 12.5 mg P.O.
B.I.D.; Proventil INH 2 PUFFS Q.I.D./P.R.N.; MVI 1
P.O. QD; FESO₄ 325 MG P.O. QD; acetaminophen 500
mg P.O. Q4HR P.R.N.; Albuterol 0.5 ml with 3 ml NS
via nebulizer B.I.D.; Aspirin 325 mg P.O. QD

12. Principal procedure code *0481 Anesthetic injection of* *peripheral nerve*	**Date** *01/03/95*

13. Other diagnosis code *4280 CHF* *496 COPD*	**Date** *01/04/95* *11/29/94*

14. DME and supplies *Colostomy supplies, Cane*	**15. Safety measures** *Prevent falls*

16. Nutritional requirements *Regular*	**17. Allergies** *NKA*

18A. Functional limitations

1 ☐ Amputation
2 ☐ Bowel/bladder
   (incontinence)
3 ☐ Contracture
4 ☐ Hearing
5 ☐ Paralysis
6 ☑ Endurance

7 ☐ Ambulation
8 ☐ Speech
9 ☐ Legally blind
A ☐ Dyspnea with minimal
   exertion
B ☐ Other (specify)

18B. Activities permitted

1 ☐ Complete bed rest
2 ☐ Bedrest BRP
3 ☑ Up as tolerated
4 ☐ Transfer bed/chair
5 ☐ Exercises prescribed
6 ☐ Partial weight bearing
7 ☐ Independent at home

8 ☐ Crutches
9 ☐ Cane
A ☐ Wheelchair
B ☐ Walker
C ☐ No restrictions
D ☐ Other (specify)

19. Mental status

1 ☑ Oriented
2 ☐ Comatose
3 ☐ Forgetful

4 ☐ Depressed
5 ☐ Disoriented
6 ☐ Lethargic

7 ☐ Agitated
8 ☐ Other

20. Prognosis

1 ☐ Poor
2 ☐ Guarded

3 ☐ Fair
4 ☑ Good

5 ☐ Excellent

Certifying home health care needs and treatments (continued)

---

21. Orders for discipline and treatments (specify amount/frequency/duration)

RN: Assess CHF, effects of digoxin, monitor c/o arthritis, pain control; monitor fistula, lower abdomen, help with temp. colostomy. Draw blood as ordered. AI: 2–3wk; assist with personal care and ADLs.

22. Rehabilitation and discharge plans

Pt. needs reinforcement and emotional support with colostomy. Rehab potential good.

23. Nurse's signature and date of verbal SOC where applicable *Cathy Wren RN 1/08/95*	**25. Date HHA received signed POT**
24. Physician's name and address *James P. Spencer, M.D.* *111 Pine St.* *Oakland, CA*	**26.** I certify/recertify that this patient is confined to his/her home and needs intermittent skilled nursing care, physical therapy and/or speech therapy, or continues to need occupational therapy. The patient is under my care, and I have authorized the services on this plan of care and will periodically review the plan.
27. Attending physician's signature and date signed *James P. Spencer MD 1/8/95*	**28.** Anyone who misrepresents, falsifies, or conceals essential information required for payment of federal funds may be subject to fine, imprisonment, or civil penalty under applicable federal laws.

---

forms are properly completed, signed, and submitted. Forms are usually filled out by the nurse assigned to the patient—although the nursing supervisor can complete them also. The data are usually filed after completing a comprehensive nursing assessment and devising a suitable plan of care. Forms must be signed by the nurse and the attending doctor.

Agency assessment forms
Once a patient is referred to the home health care agency, you must complete a thorough and specific assessment of the patient's:
• physical status

• mental and emotional status
• home environment in relation to safety and supportive services and groups such as family, neighbors, and community
• knowledge of his disease or current condition, prognosis, and treatment plan
• potential for complying with the treatment plan.

Plan of care
As in any health care setting, the nursing process forms the basis for developing the plan of care. However, because the patient's care occurs in the home—usually with family participation—you have less control than you would in an institutional

Providing updated medical and patient information

To continue providing reimbursable skilled nursing care to a patient in her own home, the home health care organization must comply with government documentation regulations. An example of required information, known as "Medical Update and Patient Information," appears below.

MEDICAL UPDATE AND PATIENT INFORMATION

1. Patient's HI claim no. *01–1112*	2. Start of care date *07/08/94*	3. Certification period From: *11/08/94* To: *01/07/95*	4. Medical record no. *12–3467*	5. Provider no. *12–3456*

6. Patient's name *Mary Smith, Third Ave., Dover, DE*	7. Provider's name *Vantage Health Care Agency*

8. Medicare covered ☑ Yes ☐ No ☐ Do not know	9. Date physician last saw patient *07/07/94*	10. Date last contacted physician *10/20/94*

11. Is the patient receiving care in an 1861 (J)(1) skilled nursing facility?
☐ Yes ☑ No ☐ Do not know

12.
☐ Certification ☑ Recertification ☐ Modified

13. Specific services and treatments

Discipline	Visits (this bill) rel. to prior cert.	Frequency and duration	Treatment codes	Total visits projected this cert.
SN	OO	2M0203	AOI A06	O7
AI	OO	3WK09	FO4	27

14. Dates of last inpatient stay: Admission *07/01/94* Discharge *07/07/94*	15. Type of facility: A

16. Updated information: New orders/Treatments/Clinical facts/Summary from each discipline

SN A&O x3. Skin warm, dry, pink. Slight dyspnea noted with activity. No dependent edema noted. Lungs clear. No C/o. Improved & increased feeling of well-being demonstrated. Colostomy functioning well with mod amt. soft brown stool present in bag. Meds reviewed. Foot soaked/nails trimmed.
AI pt. seen 2-3x/wk; assisted with shower, colostomy care, and dressing.
Put hair up in curlers, got her mail, and emptied garbage.

17. Functional limitations (Expand from 485 and level of ADLs) Reason homebound/Prior functional status
Pt. needs emotional support; weepy at times. Does not want to be burden to daughter.

18. Supplementary plan of treatment on file from physician other than referring physician:

19. Unusual home/social environment (describe) *N/A*

20. Indicate any time when the Home Health Care Agency made a visit and patient was not home and reason why if ascertainable:	21. Specify any known medical and/or nonmedical reasons the patient regularly leaves home and frequency of occurrence:

22. Nurse or therapist completing or reviewing form *Deborah Ryan, RN*	Date (Mo., Day, Yr.) *01/07/95*

setting. The patient and his family become the decision makers in many aspects and have greater control of the situation. These factors must be addressed realistically when developing the plan of care, and you may need to adjust your interventions, patient goals, and teaching accordingly.

Many agencies use the certification and plan of treatment form as the patient's official plan of care. Other agencies require a separate plan of care, whereas still others see the two plans as redundant and time-consuming.

Progress notes

Each time you visit a patient, you must write a progress note, which documents:
• any changes in the patient's condition
• skilled nursing interventions performed related to the plan of care
• the patient's responses to services provided
• any event or incident in the home that would affect the treatment plan
• vital signs
• education of the patient and home caregiver. (This includes written instructional materials and brochures.)

Nursing summaries

As a home health care nurse, you must compile a summary of the patient's progress (and discharge from home health care, when appropriate). You must also submit a monthly patient progress report to the attending doctor and to the reimburser to confirm the need for continuing services.

When writing these summaries, include the following information:
• current problems, treatments, interventions, and instructions

• care provided by other home caregivers, such as physical therapists and speech pathologists
• reason for any change in services
• patient outcomes and responses—both physical and emotional—to services provided.

Discharge summaries

You'll prepare a discharge summary for the doctor's approval to discharge, for notifying reimbursers that services have been terminated, and for officially closing the case. When preparing this document, summarize:
• the services provided
• the clinical and psychosocial conditions of the patient at discharge
• recommendations for further care
• the patient's response to and comprehension of patient-teaching efforts
• outcomes attained.

Documentation guidelines

Keep a copy of the plan of care in the patient's home for easy reference by the patient and his family. Update the record with any changes in the patient's condition or plan of care and document that you reported these changes to the doctor. Keep in mind that Medicare and Medicaid will not reimburse for skilled services implemented but not reported to the doctor.

Be certain to state in your documentation that the patient is housebound and provide the reason for this. Again, keep in mind that Medicare requires that a patient receiving skilled care in the home must be housebound, although some commercial insurers do not.

If an emergency arises in the home during your presence, accompany the patient to the hospital or emergency unit and stay with him until another professional caregiver takes over. Document all assessments and interventions performed for the patient until you're relieved. Note the date and time of transfer and the name of the caregiver who assumes responsibility for the patient.

To prevent your patient from feeling neglected, do not spend a lot of time charting in his home. Instead, complete your records while the patient sleeps or is otherwise occupied.

Be sure that documentation reflects consistent adherence to the plan of care by all caregivers involved.

Whenever possible, use flow sheets and checklists to record vital signs, intake and output measurements, and nutritional data. Encourage the patient or home caregiver to fill out these forms when appropriate. Doing so involves the patient and family in the patient's progress and increases their feeling of control.

At least once a week, remove documentation materials completed and left in the patient's home. This keeps volumes of paper from piling up or becoming misplaced. It also makes the records available for review by the agency supervisor.

Documentation in long-term care settings

Documenting the status, care, and events affecting patients in a long-term care facility is every bit as important as it is in hospital and home health care settings. The forms and requirements of documentation in these settings share many similarities.

Whether you're an independent practitioner or on staff in a rehabilitation center or a nursing home, accurate and complete records provide your employer with evidence of standard, quality nursing care. The evidence of quality and compliant care, in turn, provides your employer with the validation needed for certification, licensure, reimbursement, accreditation, and the information needed to defend you and your health care facility in court.

In long-term patient care settings, documentation requirements are based on professional standards, state and federal regulations, and the health care facility's policies as well. Long-term care facilities offer varied care that's typically categorized by level. Consider care level a primary factor when documenting patient information.

Among the levels of care are skilled care and intermediate care. In a skilled care facility, patient care requires greater and more specialized nursing skills (I.V. therapy, parenteral nutrition, respiratory care, and mechanical ventilation, for example).

An intermediate care facility focuses on patients who have chronic illnesses but who need less complex care. For example, these patients may simply need assistance with ADLs, such as bathing and dressing.

Residents from either group may need care on a short- or long-term basis and may move from one level to another according to their progress or decline. Many facilities offer both skilled and intermediate care.

Effect of regulatory bodies

Among the government organizations, titled programs, and laws that influence the kind of documentation required in long-term care facilities are the offices of Medicare and Medicaid, the HCFA, and the Omnibus Budget Reconciliation Act (OBRA) of 1987.

Medicare

The Medicare administration provides little reimbursement for services provided in long-term care facilities except for services requiring skilled care, such as chemotherapy or tube feeding.

For such patients, you'll need to supply a stated minimum of daily documentation to substantiate the need for a covered service. If the patient's status changes, you'll need to supply a revised plan of care within 7 days. Of course, you must document the need for any new or continuing skilled services provided.

Medicaid

Residents who are under age 65, who are in long-term care facilities, and who are receiving skilled care are usually paying for the service themselves or, if they have coverage and qualify, are receiving reimbursement through the Medicaid program. To secure Medicaid reimbursement, you must document patient care daily.

Health care for a patient who qualifies for intermediate care must be documented weekly unless his status changes and necessitates a change in services. In such cases, you'll need to chart the change and document the patient's status more frequently.

Additionally, you'll need to perform a monthly reevaluation. Both Medicare and Medicaid require an evaluation of expected outcomes on the plan of care.

HCFA

This branch of the Department of Health and Human Services was developed to ensure compliance (especially by the states) with federal Medicare and Medicaid standards. Accordingly, to comply with regulations for residential long-term care patients, the facility's staff must complete the MDS within 14 days of a patient's admission, review the patient's status every 3 months, and perform a comprehensive reassessment annually.

OBRA

This law requires that a comprehensive assessment be performed within 4 days of a patient's admission to a long-term care facility. The lengthy required form is known as the "Minimum Data Set [MDS] for Resident Assessment and Care Screening." The assessment and care screening process must be reviewed every 3 months and repeated annually—sooner if the patient's condition changes.

A comprehensive nursing assessment and a formulated plan of care must be completed within 7 days of admission.

Standard and required documents

As you would in any other setting, you'll use the nursing process as the basis for documenting care in a long-term facility. Required documents include the MDS, the "Resident Assessment Protocol" (RAP), the "Preadmission Screening Annual Resident Review" (PASARR), the initial nursing assessment form, and nursing summaries.

Documentation
Methods

MDS

Mandated by OBRA, this federal regulatory form must be filled out for every resident admitted to a long-term care facility (see *Documenting health status for long-term care*).

Used to comply with quality improvement and reimbursement requirements, the MDS standardizes information and facilitates communication among all agencies and among members of the health care team. Different sections of this form must be completed and signed by staff members from various professions, including doctors, nurses, medical records personnel, social workers, and others.

RAP

An outgrowth of the MDS, the RAP is another form mandated by federal regulations. Here's a summary of the requirement. Once a completed MDS is coded, computed, and processed, the patient's primary problems should emerge. These problems then serve as the basis for developing the plan of care. For example, if the patient has a stage 2 pressure ulcer documented in section N of the MDS, the RAP summary will indicate the need for a plan of care for a pressure ulcer (see *Identifying the patient's needs,* page 168).

PASARR

Just as a patient's physical status must be documented to qualify for Medicare or Medicaid reimbursement, so must his mental status. Federal regulations require the long-term care facility to perform and document a complete mental status assessment. Required information appears on a form known as PASARR (see *Documenting mental status for long-term care,* pages 169 to 174).

Initial nursing assessment form

Similar to the initial nursing assessment in an acute care facility, the initial nursing assessment must be performed and documented for a patient in any long-term care facility. In this setting, you'll place special emphasis on the patient's activity, hearing and vision, bowel and bladder control, communication, safety, need for adaptive devices to assist dexterity and mobility, family relationships, and the patient's transition from home or hospital to the long-term care facility.

Nursing summaries

Similar to summary documentation required by acute health care facilities, care and status updates in long-term care facilities must be completed regularly.

The nurse usually completes a nursing care summary at least once a week for patients requiring skilled care and every 2 weeks for patients requiring intermediate care. The summary should address such categories as ADLs; nutrition and hydration; needed safety measures such as bed rails, restraints, or adaptive devices; medications and other treatments; and adjustment problems related to the transition from the hospital to the facility or from home to the facility.

Additionally, to comply with Medicare and Medicaid standards, you'll need to complete a nursing assessment summary at least monthly.

ADL checklists or flow sheets

Commonly filled out by the nurses' assistants on each shift, these forms must be reviewed and signed by the nurse. They include data related to such categories as diet, personal and oral hygiene, bowel and

(Text continues on page 175.)

BETTER CHARTING

Documenting health status for long-term care

Residents in long-term care facilities that receive federal funds must have their health status evaluated and a plan of care devised. To ensure compliance, this form must be completed and on file.

MINIMUM DATA SET FOR NURSING HOME RESIDENT ASSESSMENT AND CARE SCREENING (MDS)
BACKGROUND INFORMATION/INTAKE AT ADMISSION

I. IDENTIFICATION INFORMATION

#			
1.	RESIDENT NAME	*Amy* (First) *J.* (Middle Initial) *Gaston* (Last)	
2.	DATE OF CURRENT ADMISSION	1 2 — 0 7 — 1 9 9 4 (Month) (Day) (Year)	
3.	MEDICARE NO. (SOC. SEC. or Comparable No. if no Medicare No.)	0 4 1 2 4 0 0 0 0	
4.	FACILITY PROVIDER NO.	1 2 3 4 5 6 7 8 9 1 0 Federal No. 1 2 3 4 5 6 7 8 9 1 0	
5.	GENDER	1. Male 2. Female	2
6.	RACE/ETHNICITY	1. American Indian/Alaska Native 4. Hispanic 2. Asian/Pacific Islander 5. White, not of 3. Black, not of Hispanic origin Hispanic origin	3
7.	BIRTHDATE	1 1 — 1 0 — 1 9 2 4 (Month) (Day) (Year)	
8.	LIFETIME OCCUPATION	*English Professor*	
9.	PRIMARY LANGUAGE	Resident's primary language is a language other than English 0. No 1. Yes _____ (Specify)	0
10.	RESIDENTIAL HISTORY PAST 5 YEARS	(Check all settings resident lived in during 5 years prior to admission)	
		Prior stay at this nursing home	a.
		Other nursing home/residential facility	b.
		MH/psychiatric setting	c.
		MR/DD setting	d.
		NONE OF ABOVE	e. X
11.	MENTAL HEALTH HISTORY	Does resident's RECORD indicate any history of mental retardation, mental illness, or any other mental health problem? 0. No 1. Yes	0
12.	CONDITIONS RELATED TO MR/DD STATUS	(Check all conditions that are related to MR/DD status, that were manifested before age 22, and are likely to continue indefinitely)	
		Not applicable—no MR/DD (Skip to Item 13)	a. X
		MR/DD with Organic Condition	
		Cerebral palsy	b.
		Down's syndrome	c.
		Autism	d.
		Epilepsy	e.
		Other organic condition related to MR/DD	f.
		MR/DD with no organic condition	g.
		Unknown	h.
13.	MARITAL STATUS	1. Never Married 3. Widowed 5. Divorced 2. Married 4. Separated	3
14.	ADMITTED FROM	1. Private home or apt. 3. Acute care hospital 2. Nursing home 4. Other	3
15.	LIVED ALONE	0. No 1. Yes 2. In other facility	1
16.	ADMISSION INFORMATION AMENDED	(Check all that apply)	
		Accurate information unavailable earlier	a.
		Observation revealed additional information	b. X
		Resident unstable at admission	c.

II. BACKGROUND INFORMATION AT RETURN/READMISSION

#			
1.	DATE OF CURRENT READMISSION	[ ] [ ] — [ ] [ ] — [ ] [ ] [ ] [ ] Month Day Year	
2.	MARITAL STATUS	1. Never Married 3. Widowed 5. Divorced 2. Married 4. Separated	
3.	ADMITTED FROM	1. Private home or apt. 3. Acute care hospital 2. Nursing home 4. Other	
4.	LIVED ALONE	0. No 1. Yes 2. In other facility	
5.	ADMISSION INFORMATION AMENDED	(Check all that apply)	
		Accurate information unavailable earlier	a.
		Observation revealed additional information	b.
		Resident unstable at admission	c.

III. CUSTOMARY ROUTINE (ONLY AT FIRST ADMISSION)

#			
1.	CUSTOMARY ROUTINE (Year prior to first admission to a nursing home)	(Check all that apply. If all information UNKNOWN, check last box only.) **CYCLE OF DAILY EVENTS**	
		Stays up late at night (e.g., after 9 pm)	a.
		Naps regularly during day (at least 1 hour)	b. X
		Goes out 1+ days a week	c. X
		Stays busy with hobbies, reading, or fixed daily routine	d.
		Spends most time alone or watching TV	e. X
		Moves independently indoors (with appliances, if used)	f.
		NONE OF ABOVE	g.
		EATING PATTERNS	
		Distinct food preferences	h.
		Eats between meals all or most days	i. X
		Use of alcoholic beverage(s) at least weekly	j.
		NONE OF ABOVE	k.
		ADL PATTERNS	
		In bedclothes much of day	l.
		Wakens to toilet all or most nights	m. X
		Has irregular bowel movement pattern	n. X
		Prefers showers for bathing	o. X
		NONE OF ABOVE	p.
		INVOLVEMENT PATTERNS	
		Daily contact with relatives/close friends	q.
		Usually attends church, temple, synagogue (etc.)	r. X
		Finds strength in faith	s. X
		Daily animal companion/presence	t. X
		Involved in group activities	u.
		NONE OF ABOVE	v.
		UNKNOWN—Resident/family unable to provide information	w.

END

(continued)

Documenting health status for long-term care *(continued)*

MINIMUM DATA SET FOR NURSING HOME RESIDENT ASSESSMENT AND CARE SCREENING (MDS)
(Status in last 7 days, unless other time frame indicated)

SECTION A. IDENTIFICATION AND BACKGROUND INFORMATION

1. ASSESSMENT DATE
`1 2` – `0 7` – `1 9 9 4`
Month — Day — Year

2. RESIDENT NAME
Amy (First) — J. (Middle Initial) — Gaston (Last)

3. SOCIAL SECURITY NO.
`0 4 1` – `2 4` – `0 0 0 0`

4. MEDICAID NO. (If applicable)

5. MEDICAL RECORD NO.
`M M 0 0 0 9 9 2 2 6 8`

6. REASON FOR ASSESSMENT
1. Initial admission assess.
2. Hosp/Medicare reassess.
3. Readmission assessment
4. Annual assessment
5. Significant change in status
6. Other (e.g., UR)
→ `2`

7. CURRENT PAYMENT SOURCE(S) FOR N.H. STAY *(Billing Office to indicate; check all that apply)*

Medicaid	a.	VA	d.
Medicare	b. X	Self pay/Private insurance	e. X
CHAMPUS	c.	Other	f.

8. RESPONSIBILITY/ LEGAL GUARDIAN *(Check all that apply)*

Legal guardian	a.	Family member responsible	d. X
Other legal oversight	b.	Resident responsible	e.
Durable power attrny./ health care proxy	c. X	NONE OF ABOVE	f.

9. ADVANCED DIRECTIVES *(For those items with supporting documentation in the medical record, check all that apply)*

Living will	a.	Feeding restrictions	f.
Do not resuscitate	b.	Medication restrictions	g.
Do not hospitalize	c.	Other treatment restrictions	h.
Organ donation	d.	NONE OF ABOVE	i. X
Autopsy request	e.		

10. DISCHARGE PLANNED WITHIN 3 MOS. *(Does not include discharge due to death)*
0. No   1. Yes   2. Unknown/uncertain → `0`

11. PARTICIPATE IN ASSESSMENT
a. Resident   0. No   1. Yes → `1`
b. Family   0. No   1. Yes   2. No family →

12. SIGNATURES
Signature of RN Assessment Coordinator
Christine Saslo RN MSN
Signatures of Others Who Completed Part of the Assessment
James Shaw RN BSN
Susan Rowe MSW

SECTION B. COGNITIVE PATTERNS

1. COMATOSE *(Persistent vegetative state/no discernible consciousness)*
0. No   1. Yes *(Skip to SECTION E)* → `0`

2. MEMORY *(Recall of what was learned or known)*
a. Short-term memory OK—seems/appears to recall after 5 minutes
   0. Memory OK   1. Memory problem → `1`
b. Long-term memory OK—seems/appears to recall long past
   0. Memory OK   1. Memory problem → `1`

3. MEMORY/ RECALL ABILITY *(Check all that resident normally able to recall during last 7 days)*

Current season	a.	That he/she is in a nursing home	d.
Location of own room	b.	NONE OF ABOVE are recalled	e. X
Staff names/faces	c.		

= Code the appropriate response   = Check all the responses that apply

SECTION [C. COGNITIVE, continued]

4. COGNITIVE SKILLS FOR DAILY DECISION-MAKING *(Made decisions regarding tasks of daily life)*
0. Independent—decisions consistent/reasonable
1. Modified Independence—some difficulty in new situations only
2. Moderately Impaired—decisions poor; cues/supervision required
3. Severely Impaired—never/rarely made decisions → `2`

5. INDICATORS OF DELIRIUM —PERIODIC DISORDERED THINKING/ AWARENESS *(Check if condition over last 7 days appears different from usual functioning)*

Less alert, easily distracted	a.
Changing awareness of environment	b.
Episodes of incoherent speech	c.
Periods of motor restlessness or lethargy	d.
Cognitive ability varies over course of day	e.
NONE OF ABOVE	f. X

6. CHANGE IN COGNITIVE STATUS
Change in resident's cognitive status, skills, or abilities in last 90 days
0. No change   1. Improved   2. Deteriorated → `2`

SECTION C. COMMUNICATION/HEARING PATTERNS

1. HEARING *(With hearing appliance, if used)*
0. Hears adequately—normal talk, TV, phone
1. Minimal difficulty when not in quiet setting
2. Hears in special situations only—speaker has to adjust tonal quality and speak distinctly
3. Highly impaired/absence of useful hearing → `1`

2. COMMUNICATION DEVICES/ TECHNIQUES *(Check all that apply during last 7 days)*

Hearing aid, present and used	a.
Hearing aid, present and not used	b.
Other receptive comm. techniques used (e.g., lip read)	c.
NONE OF ABOVE	d. X

3. MODES OF EXPRESSION *(Check all used by resident to make needs known)*

Speech	a. X	Signs/gestures/sounds	c.
Writing messages to express or clarify needs	b.	Communication board	d.
		Other	e.
		NONE OF ABOVE	f.

4. MAKING SELF UNDERSTOOD *(Express information content—however able)*
0. Understood
1. Usually Understood—difficulty finding words or finishing thoughts
2. Sometimes Understood—ability is limited to making concrete requests
3. Rarely/Never Understood → `1`

5. ABILITY TO UNDERSTAND OTHERS *(Understanding verbal information content—however able)*
0. Understands
1. Usually Understands—may miss some part/intent of message
2. Sometimes Understands—responds adequately to simple, direct communication
3. Rarely/Never Understands → `2`

6. CHANGE IN COMMUNICATION/ HEARING
Resident's ability to express, understand or hear information has changed over last 90 days
0. No change   1. Improved   2. Deteroriated → `0`

SECTION D. VISION PATTERNS

1. VISION *(Ability to see in adequate light and with glasses if used)*
0. Adequate—sees fine detail, including regular print in newspapers/books
1. Impaired—sees large print, but not regular print in newspapers/books
2. Highly Impaired—limited vision; not able to see newspaper headlines; appears to follow objects with eyes
3. Severely Impaired—no vision or appears to see only light, colors, or shapes → `0`

2. VISUAL LIMITATIONS/ DIFFICULTIES

Side vision problems—decreased peripheral vision (e.g., leaves food on one side of tray, difficulty traveling, bumps into people and objects, misjudges placement of chair when seating self)	a.
Experiences any of following: sees halos or rings around lights; sees flashes of light; sees "curtains" over eyes	b.
NONE OF ABOVE	c. X

3. VISUAL APPLIANCES
Glasses; contact lenses; lens implant; magnifying glass
0. No   1. Yes → `1`

BETTER CHARTING

Documenting health status for long-term care *(continued)*

SECTION E. PHYSICAL FUNCTIONING AND STRUCTURAL PROBLEMS

1. ADL SELF-PERFORMANCE—*(Code for resident's PERFORMANCE OVER ALL SHIFTS during last 7 days—Not including setup)*

   0. *INDEPENDENT* — No help or oversight — OR — Help/oversight provided only 1 or 2 times during last 7 days
   1. *SUPERVISION* — Oversight, encouragement or cueing provided 3+ times during last 7 days — OR — Supervision plus physical assistance provided only 1 or 2 times during last 7 days
   2. *LIMITED ASSISTANCE* — Resident highly involved in activity; received physical help in guided maneuvering of limbs or other nonweight bearing assistance 3+ times — OR — More help provided only 1 or 2 times during last 7 days
   3. *EXTENSIVE ASSISTANCE* — While resident performed part of activity, over last 7-day period, help of following type(s) provided 3 or more times:
      — Weight-bearing support
      — Full staff performance during part (but not all) of last 7 days
   4. *TOTAL DEPENDENCE* — Full staff performance of activity during entire 7 days

2. ADL SUPPORT PROVIDED — *(Code for MOST SUPPORT PROVIDED OVER ALL SHIFTS during last 7 days; code regardless of resident's self-performance classification)*

   0. No setup or physical help from staff
   1. Setup help only
   2. One-person physical assist
   3. Two+ persons physical assist

			(1) SELF-PERF.	(2) SUPPORT
a.	BED MOBILITY	How resident moves to and from lying position, turns side to side, and positions body while in bed	3	3
b.	TRANSFER	How resident moves between surfaces—to/from: bed, chair, wheelchair, standing position (EXCLUDE to/from bath/toilet)	4	3
c.	LOCO-MOTION	How resident moves between locations in his/her room and adjacent corridor on same floor. If in wheelchair, self-sufficiency once in chair	4	2
d.	DRESSING	How resident puts on, fastens, and takes off all items of street clothing, including donning/removing prosthesis	4	3
e.	EATING	How resident eats and drinks (regardless of skill)	2	2
f.	TOILET USE	How resident uses the toilet room (or commode, bedpan, urinal); transfer on/off toilet, cleanses, changes pad, manages ostomy or catheter, adjusts clothes	4	3
g.	PERSONAL HYGIENE	How resident maintains personal hygiene, including combing hair, brushing teeth, shaving, applying makeup, washing/drying face, hands, and perineum (EXCLUDE baths and showers)	4	2

3. BATHING — How resident takes full-body bath/shower, sponge bath, and transfers in/out of tub/shower (EXCLUDE washing of back and hair. *Code for most dependent in self-performance and support. Bathing Self-Performance codes appear below)*

   0. Independent—No help provided
   1. Supervision—Oversight help only
   2. Physical help limited to transfer only
   3. Physical help in part of bathing activity
   4. Total dependence

   a. 4 b. 3

4. BODY CONTROL PROBLEMS — *(Check all that apply during last 7 days)*

Balance—partial or total loss of ability to balance self while standing	a. X	Hand—lack of dexterity (e.g., problem using toothbrush or adjusting hearing aid) g. X
Bedfast all or most of the time	b.	Leg—partial or total loss of voluntary movement h.
Contracture to arms, legs, shoulders, or hands	c. X	Leg—unsteady gait i. X
Hemiplegia/hemiparesis	d.	Trunk—partial or total loss of ability to position, balance, or turn body j.
Quadriplegia	e.	
Arm—partial or total loss of voluntary movement	f.	Amputation k.
		NONE OF ABOVE l.

5. MOBILITY APPLIANCES/DEVICES — *(Check all that apply during last 7 days)*

Cane/walker	a.	Other person wheeled d. X
Brace/prosthesis	b.	Lifted (manually/mechanically) e. X
Wheeled self	c.	NONE OF ABOVE f.

6.	TASK SEG-MENTATION	Resident requires that some or all of ADL activities be broken into a series of subtasks so that resident can perform them	0
		0. No 1. Yes	
7.	ADL FUNC-TIONAL REHABILI-TATION POTENTIAL	Resident believes he/she capable of increased independence in at least some ADLs	a.
		Direct care staff believe resident capable of increased independence in at least some ADLs	b.
		Resident able to perform tasks/activity but is very slow	c.
		Major difference in ADL Self-Performance or ADL Support in mornings and evenings (at least a one category change in Self-Performance or Support in any ADL)	d.
		NONE OF ABOVE	e. X
8.	CHANGE IN ADL FUNCTION	Change in ADL self-performance in **last 90 days**	0
		0. No change 1. Improved 2. Deteriorated	

SECTION F. CONTINENCE IN LAST 14 DAYS

1. CONTINENCE SELF-CONTROL CATEGORIES *(Code for resident performance over all shifts)*

   0. CONTINENT — Complete control
   1. USUALLY CONTINENT — BLADDER, incontinent episodes once a week or less; BOWEL, less than weekly
   2. OCCASIONALLY INCONTINENT — BLADDER, 2+ times a week but not daily; BOWEL, once a week
   3. FREQUENTLY INCONTINENT — BLADDER, tended to be incontinent daily, but some control present (e.g., on day shift); BOWEL, 2-3 times a week
   4. INCONTINENT — Had inadequate control. BLADDER, multiple daily episodes; BOWEL, all (or almost all) of the time

a.	BOWEL CONTI-NENCE	Control of bowel movement, with appliance or bowel continence programs, if employed	4
b.	BLADDER CONTI-NENCE	Control of urinary bladder function (if dribbles, volume insufficient to soak through underpants), with appliances (e.g., foley) or continence programs, if employed	4

2. INCONTIN-ENCE RELATED TESTING — *(Skip if resident's bladder continence code equals 0 or 1 AND no catheter is used)*

Resident has been tested for a urinary tract infection	a. X
Resident has been checked for presence of a fecal impaction, or there is adequate bowel elimination	b. X
NONE OF ABOVE	c.

3. APPLIANCES AND PROGRAMS

Any scheduled toileting plan	a.	Pads/briefs used	f. X
External (condom) catheter	b.	Enemas/irrigation	g.
Indwelling catheter	c.	Ostomy	h.
Intermittent catheter	d.	NONE OF ABOVE	i.
Did not use toilet room/commode/urinal	e.		

4. CHANGE IN URINARY CONTINENCE — Change in urinary continence/appliances and programs in **last 90 days**   0. No change 1. Improved 2. Deteriorated   **0**

SECTION G. PSYCHOSOCIAL WELL-BEING

1. SENSE OF INITIATIVE/INVOLVEMENT

At ease interacting with others	a. X
At ease doing planned or structural activities	b.
At ease doing self-initiated activities	c.
Establishes own goals	d.
Pursues involvement in life of facility (e.g., makes/keeps friends; involved in group activities; responds positively to new activities; assists at religious services)	e.
Accepts invitations into most group activities	f. X
NONE OF ABOVE	

2. UNSETTLED RELATION-SHIPS

Covert/open conflict with and/or repeated criticism of staff	a.
Unhappy with roommate	b.
Unhappy with residents other than roommate	c.
Openly expresses conflict/anger with family or friends	d. X
Absence of personal contact with family/friends	e.
Recent loss of close family member/friend	f.
NONE OF ABOVE	g.

3. PAST ROLES

Strong identification with past roles and life status	a.
Expresses sadness/anger/empty feeling over lost roles/status	b. X
NONE OF ABOVE	c.

(continued)

Documenting health status for long-term care *(continued)*

SECTION H. MOOD AND BEHAVIOR PATTERNS

1.	SAD OR ANXIOUS MOOD	*(Check all that apply during last 30 days)*	
		VERBAL EXPRESSIONS of DISTRESS by resident (sadness, sense that nothing matters, hopelessness, worthlessness, unrealistic fears, vocal expressions of anxiety or grief)	a.
		DEMONSTRATED (OBSERVABLE) SIGNS of mental DISTRESS	
		— Tearfulness, emotional groaning, sighing, breathlessness	b.
		— Motor agitation such as pacing, handwringing or picking	c.
		— Failure to eat or take medications, withdrawal from self-care or leisure activities	d.
		— Pervasive concern with health	e.
		— Recurrent thoughts of death—e.g., believes he/she about to die, have a heart attack	f.
		— Suicidal thoughts/actions	g.
		NONE OF ABOVE	h. X

2.	MOOD PERSISTENCE	Sad or anxious mood intrudes on daily life over last 7 days — not easily altered, doesn't "cheer up"	
		0. No 1. Yes	0

3.	PROBLEM BEHAVIOR	*(Code for behavior in last 7 days)*	
		0. Behavior not exhibited in last 7 days 1. Behavior of this type occurred less than daily 2. Behavior of this type occurred daily or more frequently	
		WANDERING (moved with no rational purpose, seemingly oblivious to needs or safety)	a. 0
		VERBALLY ABUSIVE (others were threatened, screamed at, cursed at)	b. 0
		PHYSICALLY ABUSIVE (others were hit, shoved, scratched, sexually abused)	c. 0
		SOCIALLY INAPPROPRIATE/DISRUPTIVE BEHAVIOR (made disrupting sounds, noisy, screams, self-abusive acts, sexual behavior or disrobing in public, smeared/threw food/feces, hoarding, rummaged through others' belongings)	d. 0

4.	RESIDENT RESISTS CARE	*(Check all types of resistance that occurred in the last 7 days)*	
		Resisted taking medications/injection	a.
		Resisted ADL assistance	b.
		NONE OF ABOVE	c. X

5.	BEHAVIOR MANAGEMENT PROGRAM	Behavior problem has been addressed by clinically developed behavior management program. (Note: Do not include programs that involve only physical restraints or psychotropic medications in this category)	
		0. No behavior problem 1. Yes, addressed 2. No, not addressed	0

6.	CHANGE IN MOOD	Change in mood in last 90 days	
		0. No change 1. Improved 2. Deteriorated	0

7.	CHANGE IN PROBLEM BEHAVIOR	Change in problem behavioral signs in last 90 days	
		0. No change 1. Improved 2. Deteriorated	0

SECTION I. ACTIVITY PURSUIT PATTERNS

1.	TIME AWAKE	*(Check appropriate time periods over last 7 days)* Resident awake all or most of time (i.e., naps no more than one hour per time period) in the:			
		Morning	a. X	Evening	c.
		Afternoon	b. X	NONE OF ABOVE	d.

2.	AVERAGE TIME INVOLVED IN ACTIVITIES	0. Most—more than 2/3 of time 2. Little—less than 1/3 of time 1. Some—1/3 to 2/3 of time 3. None	2

3.	PREFERRED ACTIVITY SETTINGS	*(Check all settings in which activities are preferred)*			
		Own room	a. X	Outside facility	d.
		Day/activity room	b. X	NONE OF ABOVE	e.
		Inside NH/off unit	c.		

4.	GENERAL ACTIVITY PREFERENCES (adapted to resident's current abilities)	*(Check all PREFERENCES whether or not activity is currently available to resident)*				
		Cards/other games	a.	Spiritual/religious activities	f. X
		Crafts/arts	b.	Trips/shopping	g.
		Exercise/sports	c. X	Walking/wheeling outdoors	h.
		Music	d. X	Watch TV	i. X
		Read/write	e.	NONE OF ABOVE	j.

5.	PREFERS MORE OR DIFFERENT ACTIVITIES	Resident expresses/indicates preference for other activities/choices	
		0. No 1. Yes	1

SECTION J. DISEASE DIAGNOSES

Check only those diseases present that have a relationship to current ADL status, cognitive status, behavior status, medical treatments, or risk of death. (Do not list old/inactive diagnoses.)

1.	DISEASES	*(If none apply, CHECK the NONE OF ABOVE box)*

HEART/CIRCULATION		PSYCHIATRIC/MOOD	
Arteriosclerotic heart disease (ASHD)	a.	Anxiety disorder	p.
Cardiac dysrhythmias	b.	Depression	q. X
Congestive heart failure	c.	Manic depressive (bipolar disease)	r.
Hypertension	d.	**SENSORY**	
Hypotension	e.	Cataracts	s.
Peripheral vascular disease	f. X	Glaucoma	t.
Other cardiovascular disease	g.	**OTHER**	
NEUROLOGICAL		Allergies	u.
Alzheimer's	h.	Anemia	v. X
Dementia other than Alzheimer's	i. X	Arthritis	w.
Aphasia	j.	Cancer	x.
Cerebrovascular accident (stroke)	k.	Diabetes mellitus	y.
Multiple sclerosis	l.	Explicit terminal prognosis	z.
Parkinson's disease	m.	Hypothyroidism	aa. X
PULMONARY		Osteoporosis	bb.
Emphysema/Asthma/COPD	n.	Seizure disorder	cc.
Pneumonia	o.	Septicemia	dd.
		Urinary tract infection— in last 30 days	ee. X
		NONE OF ABOVE	ff.

2.	OTHER CURRENT DIAGNOSES AND ICD-9 CODES	a. *Hypertension*	4|0|2|.|1|1
		b. _____	
		c. _____	
		d. _____	
		e. _____	
		f. _____	

SECTION K. HEALTH CONDITIONS

1.	PROBLEM CONDITIONS	*(Check all problems that are present in last 7 days unless other time frame indicated)*			
		Constipation	a.	Pain—resident complains or shows evidence of pain daily or almost daily	j.
		Diarrhea	b. X		
		Dizziness/vertigo	c.	Recurrent lung aspirations in last 90 days	k.
		Edema	d. X	Shortness of breath	l.
		Fecal impaction	e.	Syncope (fainting)	m.
		Fever	f.	Vomiting	n.
		Hallucinations/delusions	g.	NONE OF ABOVE	o.
		Internal bleeding	h.		
		Joint pain	i.		

2.	ACCIDENTS	Fell in past 30 days	a.	Hip fracture in last 180 days	c.
		Fell in past 31-180 days	b. X	NONE OF ABOVE	d.

Documenting health status for long-term care *(continued)*

3.	STABILITY OF CONDITIONS	Conditions/diseases make resident's cognitive, ADL, or behavior status unstable—fluctuating, precarious, or deteriorating	a. X
		Resident experiencing an acute episode or a flare-up of a recurrent/chronic problem	b.
		NONE OF ABOVE	c.

SECTION L. ORAL/NUTRITIONAL STATUS

1.	ORAL PROBLEMS	Chewing problem	a.
		Swallowing problem	b.
		Mouth pain	c.
		NONE OF ABOVE	d. X

2.	HEIGHT AND WEIGHT	*Record height (a.) in inches and weight (b.) in pounds. Weight based on most recent status in last 30 days; measure weight consistently in accord with standard facility practice—e.g., in a.m. after voiding, before meal, with shoes off, and in nightclothes.* HT (in.) a. 7 0 WT (lb.) b. 1 8 0
		c. Weight loss (i.e., 5%+ in **last 30 days**; or 10% in **last 180 days**) 0. No 1. Yes c. 0

3.	NUTRITIONAL PROBLEMS	Complains about the taste of many foods	a.	Regular complaint of hunger	d.
		Insufficient fluid; dehydrated	b.	Leaves 25%+ food uneaten at most meals	e.
		Did **NOT** consume all/almost all liquids provided **during last 3 days**	c.	*NONE OF ABOVE*	f. X

4.	NUTRITIONAL APPROACHES	Parenteral/IV	a.	Dietary supplement between meals	f.
		Feeding tube	b.	Plate guard, stabilized built-up utensil, etc.	g.
		Mechanically altered diet	c.	*NONE OF ABOVE*	h.
		Syringe (oral feeding)	d.		
		Therapeutic diet	e. X		

SECTION M. ORAL/DENTAL STATUS

1.	ORAL STATUS AND DISEASE PREVENTION	Debris (soft, easily movable substances) present in mouth prior to going to bed at night	a.
		Has dentures and/or removable bridge	b. X
		Some/all natural teeth lost—does not have or does not use dentures (or partial plates)	c.
		Broken, loose, or carious teeth	d.
		Inflamed gums (gingiva); swollen or bleeding gums; oral abscesses, ulcers or rashes	e.
		Daily cleaning of teeth/dentures	f. X
		NONE OF ABOVE	g.

SECTION N. SKIN CONDITION

1.	STASIS ULCER	(open lesion caused by poor venous circulation to lower extremities) 0. No 1. Yes	0
2.	PRESSURE ULCERS	*(Code for highest stage of pressure ulcer)* 0. No pressure ulcers 1. Stage 1 A persistent area of skin redness (without a break in the skin) that does not disappear when pressure is relieved 2. Stage 2 A partial thickness loss of skin layers that presents clinically as an abrasion, blister, or shallow crater 3. Stage 3 A full thickness of skin is lost, exposing the subcutaneous tissues—presents as a deep crater with or without undermining adjacent tissue 4. Stage 4 A full thickness of skin and subcutaneous tissue is lost, exposing muscle and/or bone	1
3.	HISTORY OF RESOLVED/ CURED PRESSURE ULCERS	Resident has had a pressure ulcer that was resolved/cured in **last 90 days** 0. No 1. Yes	0

4.	SKIN PROBLEMS/ CARE	Open lesions other than statis or pressure ulcers (e.g., cuts)	a.
		Skin desensitized to pain, pressure, discomfort	b.
		Protective/preventive skin care	c. X
		Turning/repositioning program	d. X
		Pressure relieving beds, bed/chair pads (e.g., egg crate pads)	e. X
		Wound care/treatment (e.g., pressure ulcer care, surgical wound)	f. X
		Other skin care/treatment	g. X
		NONE OF ABOVE	h.

SECTION O. MEDICATION USE

1.	NUMBER OF MEDI- CATIONS	*(Record the number of different medications used in the last 7 days; enter "0" if none used)*	0 7
2.	NEW MEDI- CATIONS	Resident has received new medications during the **last 90 days** 0. No 1. Yes	0
3.	INJECTIONS	*(Record the number of days injections of any type received during the last 7 days)*	7
4.	DAYS RECEIVED THE FOLLOWING MEDICATION	*(Record the number of days during last 7 days; enter "0" if not used; enter "1" if long-acting meds. used less than weekly)*	
		Antipsychotics	a. 0
		Antianxiety/hypnotics	b. 0
		Antidepressants	c. 7
5.	PREVIOUS MEDICATION RESULTS	*(SKIP this question if resident currently receiving antipsychotics, antidepressants, or antianxiety/hypnotics—otherwise code correct response for last 90 days)* Resident has previously received psychoactive medications for a mood or behavior problem, and these medications were effective (without undue adverse consequences) 0. No, drugs not used 1. Drugs were effective 2. Drugs were not effective 3. Drug effectiveness unknown	

SECTION P. SPECIAL TREATMENT AND PROCEDURES

1.	SPECIAL TREATMENTS AND PROCE- DURES	SPECIAL CARE—*Check treatments received during the last 14 days*				
		Chemotherapy	a.	IV meds	f. X	
		Radiation	b.	Transfusions	g.	
		Dialysis	c.	O$_2$	h.	
		Suctioning	d.	Other _____	L	
		Trach. care	e.	*NONE OF ABOVE*	J.	
		THERAPIES—*Record the number of days each of the following therapies was administered (for at least 10 minutes during a day) in the last 7 days:*				
		Speech—language pathology and audiology services	a. 0			
		Occupational therapy	b. 0			
		Physical therapy	c. 0			
		Psychological therapy (any licensed professional)	d. 0			
		Respiratory therapy	e. 0			
2.	ABNORMAL LAB VALUES	Has the resident had any abnormal lab values during the **last 90 days**? 0. No 1. Yes 2. No tests performed	1
3.	DEVICES AND RESTRAINTS	*Use the following codes for last 7 days:* 0. Not used 1. Used less than daily 2. Used daily	
		Bed rails	a. 2
		Trunk restraint	b. 0
		Limb restraint	c. 0
		Chair prevents rising	d. 2

Identifying the patient's needs

What happens to the certification data compiled for a patient entering long-term care? It's analyzed to identify the primary problems and care needs. The result: a complementary form known as the "Resident Assessment Protocol" (RAP) summary. Completed, this form confirms a plan to meet the patient's health care needs. Directions for completing this document and an example appear below.

Resident's name: *Joseph McElroy*   Medical record no.: *000-926-705*

Signature of RN assessment coordinator: *Ann Jones, RN, BSN*

RESIDENT ASSESSMENT PROTOCOL SUMMARY

1. For each RAP area triggered, show whether you are proceeding with a care plan intervention.

2. Document problems, complications, and risk factors; the need for referral to appropriate health care professionals; and the reasons for deciding to proceed or not to proceed to care planning. Documentation may appear anywhere the facility routinely keeps such information, such as problem sheets or progress notes.

3. Identify the location of this information.

RAP problem area	Care planning decision		Location of information
	Proceed	Do not proceed	
Delirium	☑	☐	*Plan of Care #1*
Cognitive loss and dementia	☑	☐	*Plan of Care #1 and #3*
Visual function	☐	☐	
Communication	☑	☐	*Plan of Care #3*
ADL functional and rehabilitation potential	☑	☐	*Plan of Care #3*
Urinary incontinence and indwelling catheter	☑	☐	*Plan of Care #4*
Psychosocial well-being	☑	☐	*Plan of Care #2*
Mood state	☐	☐	
Behavior problem	☑	☐	*Plan of Care #2*
Activities	☑	☐	*Plan of Care #5*
Falls	☑	☐	*Plan of Care #7*
Nutritional status	☑	☐	*Plan of Care #6*
Feeding tubes	☐	☐	
Dehydration and fluid maintenance	☐	☑	*Not a valid problem. See dietary note 1/3/95*
Dental care	☐	☐	
Pressure ulcers	☑	☐	*Plan of Care #9*
Psychotroplc drug use	☑	☐	*Plan of Care #2*
Physical restraints	☑	☐	*Plan of Care #7*

BETTER CHARTING

Documenting mental status for long-term care

Before a patient covered by Medicare or Medicaid enters a long-term care facility, he must undergo various evaluations, one of which is known as the "Preadmission Screening Annual Resident Review" (PASARR).

PREADMISSION SCREENING ANNUAL RESIDENT REVIEW (PASARR)
IDENTIFICATION FORM PA-PASARR-ID

Applicant's/resident's name - Last, First	Social security number	Date
Perrone, Marie	*027-00-1111*	*1/10/95*

I. What are the applicant's/resident's current diagnoses? The individual named above is being considered for nursing facility services on the basis of the following medical diagnoses (Dx).

Primary Dx	*Fractured Ⓛ hip – Total Ⓛ hip replacement*
Secondary Dx	*NIDDM*
Target Dx	*Depression*

II. An individual is considered to have a serious mental illness (MI) if he/she meets all of the following requirements regarding diagnosis, level of impairment, and duration of illness.

   A. **Diagnosis:** The individual has a serious mental disorder diagnosable under the Diagnostic and Statistical Manual of Mental Disorders, 4th edition, revised in 1994.

   This mental disorder is:

   schizophrenia, delusional (paranoid) disorder, mood disorder, or psychotic disorder not otherwise specified; panic or other severe anxiety disorder; somatoform disorder; personality disorder; or another mental disorder that may lead to a chronic disability. Specify: *Depression*

   NOTE: For this purpose, individuals whose primary diagnosis is not considered a serious mental illness and who have a diagnosis of dementia (including Alzheimer's disease and other organic brain diseases) are to be excluded from PASARR evaluation and continue with regular admission.

   ☑ Yes   ☐ No

   B. **Level of impairment:** The mental disorder resulted in functional limitations in major life activities within the past 3 to 6 months that were not appropriate for the individual's developmental stage. An individual typically has at least one of the following characteristics on a continuing or intermittent basis. Check the appropriate box(es):

   ☑ 1. Interpersonal functioning. The individual has serious difficulty interacting appropriately and communicating effectively with other individuals, has a possible history of altercations, evictions, firing, fear of strangers, avoidance of interpersonal relationships, and social isolation.

   ☑ 2. Concentration, persistence, and pace. The individual has serious difficulty in sustaining focused attention for a long enough period to permit the completion of tasks commonly found in work settings or in worklike structured activities occurring in school or home settings. This manifests difficulties in concentration, inability to complete simple tasks within an established time period, making frequent errors, or requiring assistance in the completion of these tasks.

   ☑ 3. Adaptation to change. The individual has serious difficulty in adapting to typical changes in circumstances associated with work, school, family, or social interaction. This manifests in agitation, exacerbated signs and symptoms associated with the illness, or withdrawal from the situation, or requires intervention by the mental health or judicial system.

(continued)

Documenting mental status for long-term care *(continued)*

C. **Recent treatment:** The treatment history indicates that the individual has experienced at least one of the following (check the appropriate boxes):

☑ 1. Psychiatric treatment more intensive than outpatient psychiatric care more than once in the past 2 years (such as partial hospitalization or inpatient hospitalization). Name of inpatient facility partial program or other MH treatment: *Westover Hospital*

☑ 2. Within the last 2 years, due to his mental disorder, the individual experienced an episode of significant disruption to the normal living situation, for which supportive services were required to maintain functioning at home, or in a residential treatment environment, or which resulted in intervention by housing or law enforcement officials.

D. Does the applicant/resident meet all of the requirements of having a serious mental illness listed in Section II A-C?

☑ Yes   ☐ No

III. An applicant/resident is considered to be mentally retarded if all of the criteria listed below in A through C are met. If evidence is not present to at least suspect that the individual meets each of the three criteria, the individual should not be identified within the mental retardation target population. Documentation is not necessary to support each criterion as long as the individual is suspected to meet each criterion based on observations and knowledge about the individual. The individual completing this form is responsible for reporting the documentation used in making the identification and should complete the entire section, including "Related Questions."

A. The individual has significantly subaverage intellectual functioning (i.e., two standard deviations below the norm, an I.Q. of around 70 or below).

☐ Yes   ☐ No

Related Questions:

Is intellectual functioning documented on a standardized general intelligence test?

☐ Yes   ☐ No

If yes, what is the name and date of the test and the tester's professional qualifications?

_____

_____

_____

_____

If no, what is the basis of the reviewer's finding?

_____

_____

_____

_____

B. The individual has impairments in adaptive behavior that show (check all that apply):

☐ 1. Significant limitation in meeting the standards of maturation, learning, personal independence, and/or social responsibility of his/her age and cultural group.

Documenting mental status for long-term care *(continued)*

☐ 2. Substantial functional limitation in three or more of the following areas of major life activity which is not related to the normal aging process (check all that apply):

☐ a. Self-care ☐ b. Receptive and expressive language ☐ c. Learning

☐ d. Mobility ☐ e. Self-direction ☐ f. Capacity for independent living

☐ g. Economic self-sufficiency

Related Questions:

Are impairments in adaptive behavior documented by a standardized test?

☐ Yes ☐ No

If yes, what is the name and date of the test and the tester's professional qualifications?

_____

_____

If no, what is the basis for the reviewer's finding?

_____

_____

C. Is there documentation to substantiate that these conditions occurred between the individual's birth and 22nd birthday?

☐ Yes ☐ No

Related Questions:

What documentation substantiates that these conditions occurred between the individual's birth and 22nd birthday?

_____

_____

_____

D. Does the applicant/resident have presenting evidence to indicate mental retardation based on the criteria listed in A through C above?

☐ Yes ☑ No

E. Has the applicant/resident received mental retardation services from an MR agency in the past?

☐ Yes Identify agency: _____

☑ No

IV. "Other related condition" (ORC) includes physical, sensory, or neurologic disabilities that manifested before age 22, are likely to continue indefinitely, and result in substantial functional limitations in three or more of the following areas of major life activity: economic self-sufficiency, capacity for independent living, mobility, self-direction, learning, understanding and use of language, and self-care. Examples of individuals with other related conditions include individuals with paraplegia or quadriplegia (due to spinal cord injuries), spina bifida, cerebral palsy, blindness/deafness, epilepsy, head injuries or other injuries (such as gunshot wounds), so long as the injuries were sustained before age 22. It is important to note that an individual can have an ORC regardless of whether the ORC impairs his intellectual abilities.

(continued)

Documentation Methods

Documenting mental status for long-term care *(continued)*

The key to determining whether an individual has an ORC is the age of onset of the disability. It's the obligation of the nursing facility to determine age of onset. If the clinical record does not clearly eliminate the possibility that the individual's physical disability occurred before the age of 22, the nursing facility must ask the individual (or the individual's family if necessary), document the response, and target the individual accordingly. This information must be available upon request to representatives of the Department, which include the Community Services Program for Persons with Physical Disabilities (CSPPPD) contractors who serve individuals with other related conditions.

A. An individual is considered to have an ORC, which is a severe chronic developmental disability, if he meets all of the conditions in 1 through 4 below.

   1. The ORC is attributable to:

      a. Cerebral palsy, autism, epilepsy, Tourette syndrome, meningitis, encephalitis, hydrocephalus, multiple sclerosis, polio, anoxic brain damage, paraplegia or quadriplegia (due to spinal cord injuries), spina bifida, blindness or deafness, head injuries, or other injuries (such as gunshot wounds), as long as the injuries were sustained before age 22. Circle applicable condition(s).

      b. Any other condition, other than a serious mental illness, found to be closely related to mental retardation because this condition has resulted in impairment of general intellectual functioning or adaptive behavior similar to that of individuals with mental retardation, and requires treatment or services similar to those required for individuals with mental retardation.

   2. The ORC is manifested before the individual reaches age 22.

   3. The ORC is likely to continue indefinitely.

   4. The ORC results in substantial functional limitations in three or more of the following areas of major life activity. Check all areas of substantial functional limitation that were present prior to age 22 and were directly the result of the other related condition:

      ☐ a. Self-care   ☐ b. Understanding and use of language   ☐ c. Learning

      ☐ d. Mobility   ☐ e. Self-direction   ☐ f. Capacity for independent living

      ☐ g. Economic self-sufficiency

B. Does the applicant/resident meet the criteria of an ORC as defined in IV-A?

      ☐ Yes   ☑ No

C. Is there documentation that indicates the presence of an ORC as defined in IV-A?

      ☐ Yes   ☑ No

D. Was the individual referred for care by an agency that serves individuals with developmental disabilities or is the applicant/resident eligible for that agency's services?

      ☐ Yes   ☑ No

IF YOU ANSWER "YES" IN SECTIONS II-D (MH), III-D (MR), OR IV-B (ORC) - GO TO SECTION V.

IF YOU ANSWER "NO" IN SECTIONS II-D (MH), III-D (MR) AND IV-B (ORC) - GO TO SECTION VI-A-B.

Documenting mental status for long-term care *(continued)*

V. Does the applicant/resident meet the criteria for exceptional admission to a facility without PAS evaluation?

Criteria defined in A, B, and C of this section apply to applicants/residents who answered "Yes" in Sections II-D, III-D, or IV-B.

A. Is person an exempted hospital discharge?

☑ Yes   ☐ No

Although identified as an individual with a serious mental illness, mental retardation, or an ORC, an applicant/resident who is not dangerous to himself and/or others may be directly admitted for nursing facility services from an acute care hospital for a period up to 30 days without further evaluation if such admission is based on a written, medically prescribed period of recovery for the conditions requiring hospitalization.

If the individual is admitted under this criteria and continues in residence for more than 30 days, a new PA-PASARR-ID form must be completed. The Department must be notified on the MA 408, and an evaluation must be completed within 40 calendar days of admission to the nursing facility. Failure to report these changes in condition in a timely manner may result in financial sanctions against the nursing facility.

B. Does person require respite care?

☐ Yes   ☐ No

Although identified as an individual with a serious* mental illness, mental retardation, or other related condition, an applicant/resident who is not dangerous to self or others may be admitted for respite care for a period up to 14 days without further evaluation if he or she is certified by a referring or attending physician to require 24-hour nursing facility services and supervision.

If the individual's condition changes from respite to long-term and he/she is going to stay in the nursing facility, the department must be notified on the MA 408, and an evaluation must be completed within 24 days of admission to the nursing facility. Failure to report these changes in condition in a timely manner may result in financial sanctions against the nursing facility.

C. Is person in a coma or functioning at brain stem level?

☐ Yes   ☐ No

Although identified as an individual with a serious* mental illness, mental retardation, or other related condition, an applicant/resident who is not dangerous to himself and/or others may receive nursing facility services without further evaluation if certified by the referring or attending physician to be in a coma or functioning at brain stem level. The condition must require intense 24-hour nursing facility services and supervision and is so extreme that the individual cannot focus upon, participate in, or benefit from specialized services.

If there is a "No" response in Sections II-D, III-D, and IV-B, complete Section VI A-B.

If there is a "Yes" response in Sections II-D (MH), III-D (MR), or IV-B(ORC), and if all answers to Section V (Exceptional criteria) are "No," complete Sections VI-A and VI-C.

If there is a "Yes" response to any question in Section V (Exceptional criteria), complete Sections VI-A and VI-D.

*Serious only applies to mental illness

VI. Certifications

A. Individual Completing Form:

Jean Krenshaw, MSW   (615) 222-8100   1/11/95
SIGNATURE   TELEPHONE NUMBER   DATE

(continued)

Documenting mental status for long-term care *(continued)*

GO TO APPROPRIATE BLOCK: B, C, OR D.

B. Regular Admission - No further PASARR evaluation is needed. (Answers in Sections II-D, III-D, AND IV-B are all "No".) This is to certify that the applicant does not need to have a PASARR evaluation completed.

_____
SIGNATURE   TELEPHONE NUMBER   DATE

GO TO SECTION VII

C. Target Group - PASARR evaluation is required. (Answers in Sections II-D, III-D, or IV-B are "Yes" and answers to Section V are "No".) This is to certify that the applicant meets criteria for referral to the designated Area Agency on Aging for PAS evaluation or if a resident will be referred to the Department's Utilization Management Review Team for PASARR evaluation.

_____
SIGNATURE   TELEPHONE NUMBER   DATE

GO TO SECTION VII

D. Exceptional Admission (when answers in Sections II-D, III-D, or IV-B are "Yes" and one or more answers in Section V is "Yes"). This is to certify that the applicant/resident was targeted for evaluation but has a condition that meets the criteria for exceptional admission indicated in Section V.

Dr. James P. Spencer   *(615) 222-8888*
PRINT PHYSICIAN'S NAME   TELEPHONE NUMBER

James P. Spencer, MD   *1/11/95*
PHYSICIAN'S SIGNATURE   DATE

Medical Director Confirmation (must be completed for all exceptional admissions)

This is to confirm that I have reviewed the diagnosis and medical need of the applicant for the level of nursing services and medical services to be provided by the facility.

Dr. Susan Brown   *(615) 222-7177*
PRINT MEDICAL DIRECTOR'S NAME   TELEPHONE NUMBER

Susan Brown, MD   *1/12/95*
MEDICAL DIRECTOR'S SIGNATURE   DATE

GO TO SECTION VII

VII. Does the applicant/resident need an interpreter or other assistance to participate in or understand the PASARR evaluation process?

         ☐ Yes   Describe: _____

         ☐ No

GO TO SECTION VIII

VIII. Type of Admission

         ☐ Target group   ☑ Exceptional admission   ☐ Regular

            1. Report on MA 408   1. Report on MA 408 admission

            2. Refer to OPTIONS/UMR team

bladder function, skin care, and ambulation.

When the long-term care facility discharges a patient—for example, to a hospital or to his home—documented information should include the reason for discharge, the patient's destination at discharge, his mode of transportation, and the person or health care facility representative accompanying the patient (if applicable). Additional required data focus on the patient's medications, skin assessment findings, the overall condition of the patient, and the disposition of his personal belongings.

Documents that satisfy internal policies and procedures

Like government agencies, long-term care facilities have their own strict and comprehensive protocols (for bowel and bladder monitoring, physical and chemical restraints, safety, and infection control, for example).

Documentation related to these care categories should reflect the nursing process, especially in the areas of assessment and intervention.

Plans of care

Usual standards for plans of care developed for residents of long-term care facilities require that they be completed by the nurse within 7 days of the patient's admission. Usual standards also require documented review of the plan of care to be completed every 3 months or when a patient's status changes.

The plans of care themselves emerge from the patient's health problems, the nursing diagnoses, and the expected treatment outcomes.

Typically, plans of care for patients in long-term care facilities develop from an interdisciplinary approach to care. Ideally, the patient, his family, and each involved department—nursing, dietary, physical therapy, and social services, for example—contribute to the plan.

Documentation guidelines

Consider the following points when updating your records:
• When writing nursing summaries, be sure to address any specific patient problems noted in the plan of care.
• When writing progress notes, confirm that the patient's progress is being evaluated and reevaluated continually in relation to the goals or outcomes defined in the plan of care. If goals aren't met, this also needs to be addressed. Any additional actions should be described and documented.
• Record transfers and discharges according to institutional protocol.
• Be sure to report and document any change in the patient's condition (for example, a change resulting from an accident or a treatment) to the doctor and the patient's family—or others—within 24 hours.
• Document any follow-up interventions or other measures implemented in response to a reported change in the patient's condition.
• Keep a record of any visits (from family or friends) and phone calls regarding the resident in your notes. An institution may be fined by state or federal regulators if omissions like these occur.
• If an incident involving the patient occurs, such as a fall or a treatment error, be sure to maintain follow-up documenta-

tion for at least 48 hours after the event.
• Ensure that records for newly admitted patients are maintained in a thorough and detailed manner by the nursing staff on each shift during the patient's first week of residence.

Like patients affected by an incident and patients that need special monitoring, new patients should become well known to all staff members. Some long-term care facilities use a flagging system (such as a red dot on the patient's chart, bed, or door).
• When documenting, never lose sight of funding. To qualify for reimbursement, the records must reflect the level of care given to the patient. If you're providing care for your patient's pressure ulcer, for example, Medicare requires documentation that describes daily activity; skin condition; turning and positioning measures; the ulcer's location, size, and degree of healing; the patient's nutritional status and dietary intake; and so forth.
• Be certain that your records accurately reflect any skilled service that the patient receives.
• Always record a doctor's verbal and telephone orders. Then make sure that the doctor countersigns these orders within 48 hours.
• If appropriate, record when the doctor sees the patient because standards require that the doctor see each patient in a long-term care facility at least once every 60 days.

Selected references

Cordell, B., and Smith-Blair, N. "Streamlined Charting for Patient Education," *Nursing94* 24(1):57-59, January 1994.

Edelstein, J. "A Study of Nursing Documentation," *Nursing Management* 21(11):43, 46, November 1990.

Iyer, P.W. "New Trends in Charting," *Nursing91* 21(1):48-50, January 1991.

Iyer, P.W., and Camp, N.H. *Nursing Documentation: A Nursing Process Approach*, 2nd ed., St. Louis: Mosby–Year Book, Inc., 1995.

Patient Teaching Loose-leaf Library. Springhouse, Pa.: Springhouse Corp., 1990.

Rasmussen, N., and Gengler, T. "Clinical Pathways of Care: The Route to Better Communication," *Nursing94* 24(2):47-49, February 1994.

CHAPTER SIX

Documentation of the Nursing Process

Whether you document according to the source-oriented or the problem-oriented medical record system, your documentation must reflect the nursing process. In the current accreditation manual of the Joint Commission on Accreditation of Healthcare Organizations (JCAHO), the updated charting guidelines reaffirm this emphasis.

Based on theories of nursing and other disciplines, the nursing process follows the scientific method. This problem-solving process systematically organizes nursing activities to ensure the highest quality of care. It allows you to determine which problems you can help alleviate and which potential problems you can help prevent. The nursing process also helps you identify what kind of and how much assistance a patient requires, who can best provide that assistance, which desired outcomes the patient can achieve, and whether he achieves them.

To get such a complete picture of the patient's situation, you'll need to systematically follow the five steps of the nursing process — assessment, nursing diagnosis, planning, intervention, and evaluation — and document them effectively. (See *Five-step nursing process.*)

Fundamentals of nursing documentation

To ensure clear communication and complete, accurate documentation of your nursing care, you must keep in mind the fundamentals of documentation. Follow these guidelines.

Write neatly and legibly

One important reason to document your nursing care is to communicate with other members of the health care team. Sloppy or illegible handwriting confuses people and wastes their time as they try to decipher it. More seriously, the patient might be injured if other caregivers can't understand crucial information.

If you don't have room to chart something legibly, leave that section blank, put a bracket around it, and write, "See progress notes." Then record the information fully and legibly in the notes.

Write in ink

Because it's a permanent document, the clinical record should be completed in ink or printed out from a computer. Use only black or blue ink, if possible; green and red ink (traditionally used on evening and night shifts) don't photocopy well. Also, don't use felt-tipped pens on forms with carbons; the pens may not produce sufficient pressure for copies.

Use correct spelling and grammar

Notes filled with misspelled words and incorrect grammar create the same negative impression as illegible handwriting. To avoid spelling and grammatical errors:
• Keep a dictionary in charting areas.
• Post a list of commonly misspelled words, especially terms and medications regularly used on the unit.

Five-step nursing process

This flowchart shows the steps of the nursing process and lists the forms you should use to document them.

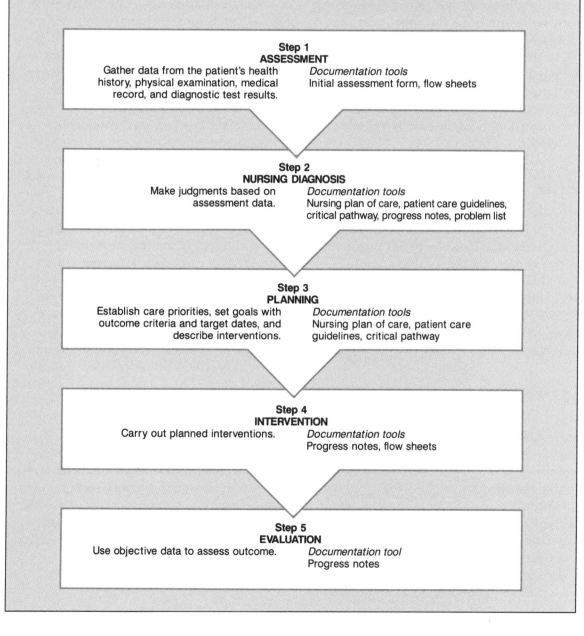

Step 1
ASSESSMENT
Gather data from the patient's health history, physical examination, medical record, and diagnostic test results.

Documentation tools
Initial assessment form, flow sheets

Step 2
NURSING DIAGNOSIS
Make judgments based on assessment data.

Documentation tools
Nursing plan of care, patient care guidelines, critical pathway, progress notes, problem list

Step 3
PLANNING
Establish care priorities, set goals with outcome criteria and target dates, and describe interventions.

Documentation tools
Nursing plan of care, patient care guidelines, critical pathway

Step 4
INTERVENTION
Carry out planned interventions.

Documentation tools
Progress notes, flow sheets

Step 5
EVALUATION
Use objective data to assess outcome.

Documentation tool
Progress notes

Use standard abbreviations

The JCAHO standards and many state regulations require health care facilities to use an approved abbreviations list to prevent confusion. Make sure that you know and use your facility's approved abbreviations. Using unapproved abbreviations can result in ambiguity, which may endanger a patient's health. (See the appendix Commonly Accepted Abbreviations.)

For example, if you use "o.d." for "once a day," another nurse may misinterpret it as "oculus dexter" (right eye) and mistakenly instill medication into the patient's eye instead of giving it once a day. (See *Abbreviations to avoid.*)

Write clear, concise sentences

Avoid using a long word when a short word will do. Clearly identify the subject of the sentence. Don't be afraid to use "I," as in "I contacted the patient's family at 1300 hours, and I explained the change in his condition."

This differentiates your actions from those of the patient, doctor, or another staff member.

Say what you mean

Many nurses were taught that nurses don't make diagnoses, so you may sometimes qualify your observations with such words as "appears" or "apparently" when describing symptoms.

However, if you use these inexact qualifiers, anyone reading the patient's chart may conclude that you weren't sure what you were describing or doing. Your best approach is to state clearly and succinctly what you see, hear, and do. Don't sound tentative.

Chart promptly

Do your charting as soon as possible after you make an observation or provide care because that's when you'll recollect the circumstances most clearly. If you leave your charting until the end of the shift, you may forget important details.

Bedside flow sheets make charting throughout the shift much easier. Some hospitals also place progress notes at the bedside. And, of course, bedside computers allow you to document promptly too.

But some nurses are uncomfortable about leaving written flow sheets or notes at the bedside — and understandably so. Although flow sheets don't usually contain confidential information, progress notes do. Unless the records can be kept in a secure place, confidentiality could be breached. Fold-down desks outside the patient's room are one solution: Besides giving you a handy writing surface, they provide a secure place for keeping the chart.

If bedside flow sheets or computers aren't available, consider making notes on worksheets or pads that you keep in your pocket. Jot down key phrases and times; then transcribe the information into the chart later.

Note the time

Be specific about times in the chart. In particular, note the exact time of all sudden changes in the patient's condition, significant events, and nursing actions. Avoid block charting such as "0700 to 1500." This sounds vague and implies inattention to the patient.

Abbreviations to avoid

The Joint Commission on Accreditation of Healthcare Organizations requires every health care facility to develop a list of approved abbreviations for staff use. But certain abbreviations should be avoided, if possible, because they're easily misunderstood, especially when handwritten. Here's a list of abbreviations to avoid.

ABBREVIATION	INTENDED MEANING	MISINTERPRETATION	CORRECTION
Apothecaries' symbols			
℥	fluidounce	Frequently misinterpreted	Use the metric equivalents.
ʒ	fluidram	Frequently misinterpreted	Use the metric equivalents.
♏	minim	Frequently misinterpreted	Use the metric equivalents.
Ɔ	scruple	Frequently misinterpreted	Use the metric equivalents.
Drug names			
MTX	methotrexate	mustargen (mechlorethamine hydrochloride)	Use the complete spelling for drug names.
CPZ	Compazine (prochlorperazine)	chlorpromazine	Use the complete spelling for drug names.
HCl	hydrochloric acid	potassium chloride ("H" is misinterpreted as "K")	Use the complete spelling for drug names.
DIG	digoxin	digitoxin	Use the complete spelling for drug names.
MVI	multivitamins *without* fat-soluble vitamins	multivitamins *with* fat-soluble vitamins	Use the complete spelling for drug names.
HCTZ	hydrochlorothiazide	hydrocortisone (HCT)	Use the complete spelling for drug names.
ara-a	vidarabine	cytarabine (ara-C)	Use the complete spelling for drug names.

(continued)

Abbreviations to avoid *(continued)*

ABBREVIATION	INTENDED MEANING	MISINTERPRETATION	CORRECTION
Dosage directions			
au	*auris uterque* each ear	Frequently misinterpreted as "OU" (*oculus uterque*— each eye)	Write it out.
Mg	microgram	Frequently misinterpreted as "mg"	Use "mcg."
OD	once daily	Frequently misinterpreted as "OD" (*oculus dexter*—right eye)	Don't abbreviate "daily." Write it out.
OJ	orange juice	Frequently misinterpreted as "OD" (*oculus dexter*—right eye) or "OS" (*oculus sinister*—left eye). Medications that were meant to be diluted in orange juice and given orally have been given in a patient's right or left eye.	Write it out.
ŤID	once daily	Misinterpreted as "t.i.d." (three times daily).	Write it out.
Per os	orally	The "os" is frequently misinterpreted as "OS" (*oculus sinister*—left eye).	Use "P.O." or "by mouth" or "orally."
q.d.	every day	The period after the "q" has sometimes been misinterpreted as "i," and the drug has been given q.i.d. rather than daily.	Write it out.
qn	nightly or at bedtime	Misinterpreted as "qh" (every hour)	Use "h.s." or "nightly."
qod	every other day	Misinterpreted as "q.d." (daily) or "q.i.d."	Use "q other day" or "every other day."
subq	subcutaneous	The "q" has been misinterpreted as "every." For example, a prophylactic heparin dose meant to be given 2 hours before surgery may be given *every* 2 hours before surgery.	Use "subcut," or write out "subcutaneous."
u u	unit	Misinterpreted as a "0" or a "4," causing a tenfold or greater overdose.	Write it out.

Chart in chronological order

Most of our assessments and observations are useful only as part of a pattern of assessments and observations. Isolated, most assessments tell us very little; in chronological order, they reveal a pattern of improvement or deterioration.

If you take the time to note your observations and assessments when you make them, they'll be recorded in chronological order. Too often, nurses wait until the end of the shift, then record groups of assessments that omit important variations.

Document accurately and completely

Record the facts, not opinions or assumptions. Although you don't need to chart routine tasks, such as changing bed linens, you do need to chart all relevant information relating to patient care and reflecting the nursing process.

Document objectively

Record exactly what you see, hear, and do. When you record a patient's statement, use his exact words. Avoid making subjective statements such as "Patient's level of cooperation has deteriorated since yesterday." Instead, include the facts that led you to this conclusion. For example, write "The patient stated, 'I don't want to learn how to inject insulin. I tried yesterday, but I'm not going to do it today.' " In some cases, you may include your conclusion, as long as you record the objective assessment data that supports it.

Remember to document only data you witness yourself or data from a reliable source—such as the patient or another nurse. When you include information reported by someone else, cite your source. (See *Watch your charting language,* page 184.)

Sign each entry

Sign each entry you make in your progress notes with your first name or initial, full last name, and professional licensure (such as RN or LPN). If you find the last entry unsigned, immediately contact the nurse who made the entry and have her sign her name. If you can't locate her, simply write and sign your progress notes. The different times and handwriting on the chart should dispel confusion as to the author. (See *Signing nurses' notes,* page 185.)

Assessment

Your assessment of a patient begins when you first encounter him. It continues throughout his hospitalization as you obtain more information about his changing condition. The initial step of the nursing process, assessment includes collecting relevant information from various sources and analyzing it to form a complete picture of your patient.

As you obtain assessment information, you need to document it accurately for several reasons. First of all, accurately recorded assessment information helps guide you through the rest of the nursing process. Using reliable assessment documentation, you can formulate nursing diagnoses, create patient problem lists, and write nursing plans of care. Properly documented assessment information also serves as a vital communication tool for

Watch your charting language

At times, some of us may speak and write in a vague or judgmental manner without being aware of it. However, when you're charting, you should conscientiously avoid ambiguous statements and inclusion of personal judgments.

Undefined time periods

"Mrs. Brown asks for pain medication *every so often*." How would you interpret "every so often"—once an hour, once a shift, or once a day? Although you can't time each and every interaction or occurrence precisely, you should document time relationships when appropriate. In this case, for example, you might chart, "Mrs. Brown asked for pain medication at 0800 and again at 1300."

Of course, such precision isn't always necessary. If you write "The patient was quiet for most of the shift," for example, the exact number of minutes she was quiet isn't necessary to communicate clearly.

Undefined quantities

"A *large amount* of bloody drainage drained from the nasogastric tube." That could mean 75 ml of fluid to you, 150 ml to the next nurse. Chart a specific measurement.

Interpretations of behavior without an objective basis

"Mr. Russo has a *good attitude*." How do you know? Support your judgment with an objective rationale. For example, "Mr. Russo states that he intends to learn insulin injection techniques before discharge."

Don't be afraid to give your impressions of the patient; just make sure that you support your observations. For example, "Leslie was frustrated, voicing dismay at being unable to walk around the room without help." Avoid using words such as "seems" or "appears"—they make you sound unsure of your observations.

---

other health care team members, forming a baseline from which to evaluate a patient's progress.

You also need to document your assessments accurately to meet the requirements of the JCAHO and various regulatory agencies. And good documentation provides a means of indicating that quality care has been given. Peer review organizations and other quality assurance reviewers often look to the nursing assessment data as proof of quality care. Finally, in case of litigation, your record of your assessments can be used as evidence in court.

Initial assessment

You'll perform your initial assessment when you first meet a patient. But before getting started, consider two questions:
• Which information will be most relevant for this patient?
• How much time do I have to gather the information? Your answers will help you collect meaningful information during your assessment. This in turn makes comprehensive, goal-directed nursing interventions possible.

Signing nurses' notes

To discourage others from adding information to the nurses' notes, draw a line through any blank spaces and sign your name at the far right of the column.

1/5/95	1200	P: Will continue plan and request enterostomal therapist to assess patient's knowledge and acceptance of colostomy on the 2nd postop day.————— *Nora Martin, RN*

If you don't have enough room to sign your name after the last word of your entry, draw a line from the last word to the end of the line. Then, drop down to the next line and draw a line from the left margin toward the right margin, leaving room to sign your name on the far right side.

1/5/95	0900	A: Pt.'s respiratory status markedly improved after diuretic and O₂ therapy. P: Continue to monitor ABGs, urine output, weight, and breath sounds. Continue diuretic therapy as prescribed. ————— ————— ————— *Nora Martin, RN*

If you want to record a lot of information but think you'll run out of room on the page, leave space at the bottom of the page to write "Continued on next page," and add your signature. Start the next page with "Continued from previous page." Then finish your notes and sign the second page as usual.

		Medication effective. Patient drowsy, (continued on next page) — *Nora Martin, RN*

1/5/95	1500	(continued from previous page) relaxed. States that pain is now 2 on a scale of 1 to 10.————— *Nora Martin, RN*

Collecting relevant information

Your initial assessment of a patient may begin with his signs and symptoms, chief complaint, or medical diagnosis. It also may center on the type of care he received in another unit, such as the critical care unit (CCU) or the emergency department (ED).

Start by finding out some basic information: Why has the patient sought health care? What are his immediate problems? Are these problems life-threatening? Does a potential for injury exist? What other influences — advanced age, fear, cultural differences, or lack of understanding, for instance — will affect treatment outcomes?

Complying with the time frame

Your time limit for completing the initial assessment depends on the policy of your health care facility. The JCAHO requires facilities to establish an assessment time frame for each type of patient they serve. Thus, depending on the unit where you work, the time frame for initiating the first assessment may range from 15 minutes to 8 hours.

On medical-surgical units, the initial assessment should usually be completed within 1 hour of the patient's arrival on the unit. Because many facilities offer a wide variety of care, they must establish individual assessment time frames for units or groups of units that share similar patient populations.

Thus, a nurse on a CCU or a trauma emergency unit would have a much shorter time frame for completing an initial assessment than a nurse on an elective surgical unit would have.

Categorizing assessment data

When you collect and analyze assessment information, you need to distinguish between two types — subjective and objective. Subjective information represents the patient's perception of his problem. A patient's complaint of chest pain, for example, would be subjective information. Objective information, on the other hand, is something you can observe and verify. A patient's blood pressure reading would be objective information. During your assessment, you'll gather both types of information from primary and secondary sources.

Subjective data

Subjective data collected during the patient history generally include the patient's chief complaint or concern, current health status, health history, family history, psychosocial history, activities of daily living (ADLs), and a review of body systems.

The patient's history, embodying his perception of his problems, is your most important source of assessment information. But it's also subjective, so you must interpret it carefully.

Suppose, for instance, that a patient complains of frequent stomach pain. To find out what he considers "frequent," ask if the pain occurs once a week, once a day, twice a day, or all day. To find out what he means by "stomach," have him point to the specific area affected. This also tells you if the pain is localized or generalized. To find out how he defines "pain," have him describe the sensation. Is it stabbing or dull, twisting or nagging? How does he rate its severity on a scale of 1 to 10?

When documenting subjective data, be sure to record it as such. Whenever possible, write the patient's own words in quo-

Nursing Process

tation marks. And introduce patient statements with a phrase such as "Pt. states...." For instance, you would document the previous example like this: "Pt. states that he has frequent stomach pain. He describes pain as dull and nagging. Patient rates pain as a 4 on a scale of 1 to 10. The pain occurs after eating, is relieved by antacids, and is located in the left lower quadrant."

If the patient uses unfamiliar words or phrases, such as slang words, ask him to define them. For clarity, record both the phrase and the patient's definition of it.

Objective data
Unlike subjective data, objective data involve no interpretation. If another practitioner were to make the same observations under the same circumstances, she'd obtain the same information. That's why it's important to be specific and avoid using subjective descriptions, such as "large," "small," or "moderate," when documenting your findings. Whenever possible, use measurements to record data clearly. Specify color, size, and location when appropriate. For instance, "small amount of abdominal wound drainage" could be more clearly described as "serosanguineous nonodorous abdominal wound drainage that completely saturated three 4″ × 4″s."

Also, avoid interpreting the data and reflecting your opinion. For example, don't write "patient is in shock." Instead, document the findings: "pale skin, pulse rate of 140, blood pressure of 90/60 mm Hg."

Sources of data
Usually, information gathered directly from the patient—known as primary source data—is the most valuable because it reflects his situation most accurately. Ad-

ditional data about a patient can be obtained from secondary sources, including family members, friends, and other members of the health care team. Written records—past clinical records, transfer summaries, and personal documents, such as a living will—also provide important information about the patient.

Information from secondary sources often gives you alternative viewpoints to the patient's. And sometimes, because of a patient's condition or age, secondary sources may be essential to establish a complete profile. For example, a child or a patient who's profoundly confused may be able to answer only the simplest questions.

Besides providing essential data, family members and friends give important indications of family dynamics, educational needs, and available support systems. Also, including persons close to the patient helps alleviate their feelings of helplessness during the hospitalization.

Performing the initial assessment
An initial assessment consists of your general observations, the health history, and the physical examination.

General observations
You can obtain a wealth of information simply by observing the patient. These observations can begin as soon as you meet him. You may, for instance, observe him while taking him to his room or helping him change into a hospital gown.

Continue to make general observations during the interview and physical examination, as well as throughout the patient's hospitalization. By looking critically at the patient, you can collect valuable information about his emotional state, immediate comfort level, and general physical condition. (See *Making general observations.*)

Keep your observations objective and don't draw conclusions. Just document the facts. Remember, initial conclusions are frequently wrong because they're based on too little evidence.

Suppose, for example, that your patient is a middle-aged man who's brought to the ED by ambulance after being found lying in a deserted alley. His clothes are soiled and torn and he smells of urine and feces. He babbles incoherently, although obscenities are clearly discernible.

To document properly, you should record these facts, but you shouldn't conclude that the patient is drunk. He may have diabetes mellitus and be suffering from acute hypoglycemia.

Health history

A guide to subsequent physical assessment, the health history organizes pertinent physiologic, psychological, cultural, and psychosocial information. It consists of subjective data about the patient's current health status and provides clues that point to actual or potential health problems. It also reveals the patient's ability to comply with health care interventions and his expectations for treatment outcomes. Finally, the health history yields details about the patient's lifestyle, family relationships, and cultural influences—all of which may affect his health care needs.

Use the health history to identify patient problems that your nursing interventions can help resolve. You'll then formulate your nursing diagnoses and subsequent plan of care based on these problems.

Preparing to take the health history

Obtain the patient's health history by interviewing him in a comfortable environment and recording his answers to your questions. If appropriate, also interview the patient's family members and close friends.

Before the interview, consider the patient's ability and readiness to participate. For example, if he's sedated or confused, hostile or angry, or experiencing pain or dyspnea, ask only the most essential questions. You can perform a more in-depth interview later, when his condition improves. In the meantime, secondary sources can often provide much of the needed information.

Try to alleviate as much of the patient's discomfort and anxiety as possible. Also attempt to create a quiet, private environment for your talk. Avoid interruptions by arranging for another nurse to cover your other patients during the interview. Your efforts let your patient know that you're interested in what he tells you and that you respect the confidentiality of the information he shares.

Tell the patient how long the interview will last—usually from 15 to 30 minutes for a medical-surgical patient. Explain the purpose of the history so he understands why you'll be asking him personal questions. Finally, be calm, relaxed, and unhurried. Your actions will convey to the patient the importance of the health history interview.

Conducting the interview

You need to show empathy, compassion, self-awareness, and objectivity to promote a trusting relationship with your patient—the first step toward a successful interview. To obtain a comprehensive health

Making general observations

Your general observations of the patient's appearance, mobility, communication ability, and cognitive functions form an important part of your initial assessment. To save you time, here are some specific characteristics to look for and to document.

Appearance

Age
- Appears to be stated age
- Appears older or younger than stated age

Physical condition
- Physically fit, strong, and appropriate weight for height
- Deconditioned, weak, and either underweight or overweight
- Apparent limitations, such as an amputation or paralysis
- Obvious scars, rash

Dress
- Dressed appropriately or inappropriately for season
- Clean and well-kept clothes
- Clothes soiled or torn; smell of alcohol, urine, or feces

Personal hygiene
- Clean and well-groomed
- Unkempt; dirty skin, hair, and nails; unshaved
- Body odor or unusual breath odor

Skin color
- Pale, ruddy, cyanotic, jaundiced, or tanned

Mobility

Ambulation
- Walks independently; steady gait
- Uses a cane, crutches, walker
- Unsteady, slow, hesitant, or shuffling gait; leans toward one side; can't support own weight

- Transfers from chair to bed independently
- Needs assistance (from one, two, or three people) to transfer from chair to bed

Movement
- Moves all extremities
- Has right- or left-sided weakness; paralysis
- Can't turn in bed independently
- Has jerky or spastic movements of body parts (specify)

Communication

Speech
- Speaks clearly in English or other language
- Speaks only with one-word responses; doesn't respond to verbal stimuli
- Speech seems slurred, hoarse, loud, soft, incoherent, hesitant, slow, fast, or nonsensical
- Has difficulty completing sentences because of shortness of breath or pain

Hearing
- Hears well enough to respond to questions
- Hard of hearing; wears hearing aid; must speak loudly into left or right ear
- Deaf; reads lips or uses sign language

Vision
- Sees well enough to read instructions in English or other language
- Wears glasses to see or to read
- Can't read
- Blind

(continued)

Making general observations   *(continued)*

Cognitive functions
Awareness
- Oriented; aware of surroundings
- Disoriented; unaware of person, place, time

Mood
- Responds appropriately; talkative
- Answers in one-word responses; offers information only in response to direct questions
- Hesitant to answer questions; looks to family member before answering

- Angry; states "Leave me alone" (or similar response); speaks loudly and abruptly to family members
- Maintains, or avoids, eye contact

Thought processes
- Maintains a conversation; makes relevant statements; follows commands appropriately
- Mind wanders; makes irrelevant statements; follows commands inappropriately

---

history, you'll also need to use a variety of interviewing techniques. Here are some examples.

Using general leads. Broad opening questions allow the patient to relate information that he deems essential. Asking something such as "What brought you to the hospital?" or "What concerns do you have?" encourages the patient to discuss what's most important to him.

Restating (summarizing) information. To help clarify the patient's meaning, restate the essence of his comments. For instance, suppose a patient says, "I have pain after I eat" and you respond, "So, you have pain about three times a day." This might prompt the patient to reply, "Oh no, I only eat breakfast and then the pain is so severe that I don't eat for the rest of the day."

Using reflection. Asking a question in a different way offers the patient an opportunity to reconsider his response. A patient

might state, "I've told you everything about my home life." Using reflection, you might respond, "Do you have any other concerns about your situation after you leave the hospital?"

Stating the implied meaning. A patient may hint at difficulties or problems. By stating what has been unspoken, you give him an opportunity to clarify his thoughts and accurately interpret the meaning of his statements. A patient who remarks, "I'm sure my wife is glad that I'm in the hospital" may be implying several things. To clarify this statement, you might respond, "By saying your wife is glad, do you mean she's been concerned about your condition, or do you feel you've been a burden to her at home?"

Focusing the discussion. Patients often stray from the topic at hand to relate other information they feel you should know. You need to get the conversation back on track without insulting the patient or making him feel that the information isn't important. To help him refocus the conversation, you might say, "That's very interesting, but first I'd like to get back to our discussion about your last hospitalization."

Asking open-ended questions. Questions that encourage the patient to express himself elicit more information than questions that call for a one-word response. If you ask, "Do you take your medications?" the patient may respond with a simple "Yes." But if you ask, "How do you take your medications?" you might discover that the patient takes his antihypertensive pills sporadically because they make him feel dizzy.

To avoid alienating the patient during the interview and thus hindering communication, don't use the techniques that follow.

Judgmental or threatening questions. A patient shouldn't have to justify his feelings or actions. Questions such as "Why did you do that?" or demanding statements such as "Explain your behavior" may be perceived as a threat or challenge. They force the patient to defend himself. What's more, when a patient doesn't have a specific answer to this type of question, he may invent an appropriate response merely to satisfy you.

Probing and persistent questions. This style of questioning can make the patient feel manipulated and defensive. Make only one or two attempts to obtain information about a particular subject. If the patient seems to be avoiding the topic or is hesitant to answer, reevaluate the rele-

vance of the information. Respect his right to privacy.

Inappropriate language. Don't use technical terms or jargon when interviewing the patient. Questions such as "Do you take that med q.i.d. or p.r.n.?" can intimidate or alienate the patient and his family. Using unfamiliar language can make the patient feel you're unwilling to share information about his condition or to converse on his level.

Advice. Giving advice implies that you know what's best for the patient. Instead, you should encourage the patient and family members to participate in health care decisions. If the patient asks for advice, help him explore his own opinions about the available options.

False reassurances. Statements such as "You'll be all right" or "Everything will work out fine" tend to devalue a person's feelings. By recognizing those feelings, you can open communication channels. Saying something such as "You seem worried or frightened" encourages the patient to speak candidly. Always try to be honest and sensitive. Even when a patient asks, "Am I going to die?" you can honestly state, "I don't know. Tell me what makes you ask that."

Timesaving measures
Increased patient acuity and staff shortages sometimes make conducting a thorough patient interview difficult. But certain strategies can help you make the most of the time you have without compromising quality.

In certain circumstances, you may not have to conduct a patient interview. In-

CHARTING TIMESAVER

When interview time is limited

When you're pressed for time, the following tips will help you obtain a health history more quickly.

• Before the interview, fill in as much of the health history information as you can from secondary sources, such as admission forms, transfer summaries, and the medical history. This avoids duplication of effort and reduces interview time. If some of this information needs clarification, you can ask the patient to give you a fuller explanation. For instance, you might say something such as "You told Dr. Smith that you have periodic dizzy spells. Do you think you could tell me more about those spells?"

• Check your facility's policy regarding who can gather assessment data. You may be able to have a nursing assistant collect routine information, such as allergies and past hospitalizations. Remember, however, you must review the information and verify it as necessary.

• Begin by asking about the patient's chief complaint and the reason for his hospitalization. Then, if the interview is interrupted, you'll have some initial information on which to base a plan of care.

• Use your facility's nursing assessment documentation form only as a guide to organize information. Ask your patient only pertinent questions from the form.

• Take only brief notes during the interview. That way, your note taking won't interrupt the flow of conversation. Complete longer summations or expand on information as soon as possible after you complete the interview. You can always go back to the patient if you need to clarify or verify information.

• Record your findings in concise, specific phrases. Use approved abbreviations.

stead, you can ask the patient to complete a questionnaire about his past and present health status. Then you can quickly and easily document his health history by reviewing the information on the questionnaire. This method has been most successful in short procedure units and before admission for elective procedures. But although it saves time, this method doesn't give you an opportunity to develop a positive relationship with your patient. (See *When interview time is limited.*)

Physical examination

Perform the physical examination by using the assessment techniques of inspection, palpation, percussion, and auscultation. During this phase of the assessment, you'll obtain objective data that may confirm or rule out suspicions raised during the health history interview. Your findings will enable you to plan care and start teaching your patient about his condition. For example, an elevated blood pressure reading tells you that a patient may need a sodium-restricted diet and, possibly, patient teaching on how to control hypertension.

The scope of the physical examination depends on the patient's condition, the clinical setting, and the policies and procedures established by your health care facility. A routine neurologic examination on a medical-surgical unit, for example, may include assessing level of consciousness, orientation, muscle strength, and pupillary response. Abnormal findings would then call for you to perform a more in-depth assessment — an assessment that would be routine on a neurologic unit or CCU.

The major components of the physical examination include height, weight, vital signs, and a review of the major body systems. A routine review for an adult patient on a medical-surgical unit includes the body systems that follow.

Respiratory system

Note the rate and rhythm of respirations, and auscultate the lung fields. Inspect the lips, mucous membranes, and nail beds. Also inspect any sputum, noting color, consistency, and other characteristics.

Cardiovascular system

Note the color and temperature of the extremities and assess the peripheral pulses. Also check for edema and note hair growth on the extremities. Inspect the neck veins and auscultate heart sounds.

Neurologic system

Inspect the patient's head for evidence of trauma. Then assess his level of consciousness, noting his orientation to time, place, and person and his ability to follow commands. Also assess his pupillary reactions. Check his extremities for movement and sensation.

Eyes, ears, nose, and throat

Assess the patient's ability to see objects with or without corrective lenses as appropriate. Also assess his ability to hear spoken words clearly. Inspect the eyes and ears for discharge; the nasal mucous membranes for dryness, irritation, and the presence of blood; and the teeth for cleanliness.

If appropriate, note how well the patient's dentures fit. Observe the condition of the oral mucous membranes, and palpate the lymph nodes in the neck.

GI system

Auscultate for bowel sounds in all quadrants. Note any abdominal distention or ascites, and assess the condition of mucous membranes around the anus.

Musculoskeletal system

Assess the range of motion of major joints. Look for any swelling at the joints, as well as for any contractures, muscular atrophy, or obvious deformity.

Genitourinary system

Note any bladder distention or incontinence. If indicated, inspect the genitalia for rashes, edema, or deformity. (Inspection of the genitalia may be waived at the patient's request or if no dysfunction was reported during the interview.)

Reproductive system

If indicated, inspect the genitalia for sexual maturity. Also examine the breasts, noting any abnormalities.

Integumentary system

Note any sores, lesions, scars, pressure ulcers, rashes, bruises, or petechiae. Also note the patient's skin turgor.

Meeting JCAHO requirements

The JCAHO requires that health care professionals in accredited facilities meet certain standards for performing patient assessments. By reviewing the documentation of patient assessments, the JCAHO determines whether these standards have been met. (See Chapter 3, Quality Improvement and Reimbursement, for more information on JCAHO requirements.)

One key JCAHO requirement is that you obtain assessment information from the patient's family or friends, when appropriate. When you interview someone close to the patient who isn't part of his family, make sure that you note the nature of the relationship and the length of time the person has known the patient. For instance, in your documentation, you might write something such as "Information supplied by Daniel Rosenberger, a friend who has lived with the patient for 3 years."

Assessment requirements

Current JCAHO standards mandate that each patient's initial assessment include six elements: biophysical factors, psychosocial factors, environmental factors, self-care capabilities, learning needs, and discharge planning needs.

Biophysical factors

These include physical examination findings from your review of the major body systems.

Psychosocial factors

These include the patient's fears, anxieties, and other concerns related to his hospitalization. To find out what support systems the patient has, you might ask something such as "How does being in the hospital affect your home situation?" or "How is your family coping while you're hospitalized?" A patient's concerns about these matters may impair his willingness or ability to comply with health care interventions.

Environmental factors

The patient's home environment affects his need for care both during hospitalization and after discharge. Ask where he lives and whether he lives in a house or an apartment. Does his home have adequate heat, ventilation, hot water, and bathroom facilities? How many flights of stairs does he have to climb? Does the layout of the home pose any hazards?

Ask if his home is near a shopping area. How far does he have to travel to visit a doctor or health care facility? When performing ADLs at home, does he use special equipment that isn't available in the hospital? Tailor your questions to the patient's condition and the geographic setting of his current residence.

Self-care capabilities

A patient's ability to perform ADLs affects how well he complies with his therapy both before and after discharge. So you must assess your patient's ability to eat, wash, dress, use the bathroom, turn in bed, get out of bed, and get around. At some health care facilities, you'll use a checklist to indicate if a patient can perform these tasks independently or if he needs partial or total assistance.

Learning needs

An early assessment of what the patient needs to know about his condition leads to effective patient teaching. During the initial assessment, you should evaluate your patient's knowledge of the disease process, self-care, diet, medications, lifestyle changes, treatment measures, and any limitations resulting from the disease or its treatment.

One way to evaluate your patient's educational needs is to ask open-ended questions, such as "What do you know about the medicine you take?" His response will tell you if he understands and complies with his medication regimen or if he needs more teaching.

You should also assess factors that may hinder learning. These include the nature of the patient's illness or injury, as well as his health beliefs, religious beliefs, educational level, sensory deficits (such as hearing difficulties), language barriers, stress level, age, and any pain or discomfort he may be experiencing.

Discharge planning needs
As with patient teaching, discharge planning should begin as soon as possible. You must identify the discharge planning needs of every patient—especially those who are most likely to require help after discharge.

Find out where the patient will go after discharge. Will follow-up care be accessible? Are community resources, such as visiting nurse services and Meals on Wheels, available where the patient lives? Answers to such questions help you to plan effectively for your patient's discharge.

Documenting the initial assessment
Depending on where you work, you may hear the initial assessment information referred to by any of several names, including the "nursing admission assessment" and the "nursing data base." Documentation styles and formats also vary, depend-ing on the facility's policy and the patient population. What's more, health care facilities have different policies for documenting learning needs, discharge planning, and incomplete initial assessment data. So you must be familiar with your facility's standards to document your initial assessment findings appropriately.

Documentation styles
Initial assessment findings are documented in one of three basic styles: narrative note, standardized open-ended style, and standardized closed-ended style. Many assessment forms use a combination of all three styles.

Narrative note
This consists of a handwritten account in paragraph form, summarizing information obtained by general observation, interview, and physical examination.

While narrative notes allow you to list your findings in order of importance, they also pose problems. Frequently, the notes mimic the medical model by focusing on a review of body systems. They're also time-consuming—both to write and to read. Plus, narrative notes require you to remember and record all significant information in a detailed, logical sequence—often an unrealistic goal in today's hectic world of health care. Finally, difficulty in interpreting handwriting can easily lead to a misinterpretation of findings.

Narrative notes are most practical for independent practitioners. Within health care institutions, however, exclusive use of narrative notes wastes time and may jeopardize quality monitoring.

BETTER CHARTING

Documenting assessment on an open-ended form

At some health care facilities, you may use a standardized open-ended form to document initial assessment information. Below you'll find a portion of such a form.

Reason for hospitalization *"My blood sugar is very high."*
Expected outcomes *By discharge, pt. and his family will verbalize an understanding of the disease process of diabetes mellitus, demonstrate correct insulin administration techniques, and identify signs and symptoms of hyperglycemia and hypoglycemia.*

Last hospitalization
Date *1/94*   Reason *high BP*

Medical history *hypertension, diabetes mellitus*

Medications and allergies

Drug	Dose	Time of last dose	Patient's statement of drug's purpose
Humulin N	*30 units*	*0730*	*for sugar*
Humulin R	*5 units*	*0730*	*for sugar*
furosemide	*20 mg*	*1000*	*water pill*
atenolol	*50 mg*	*0800*	*for BP*

Allergy	Reaction
shellfish	*hives*

Standardized open-ended style

The typical "fill-in-the blanks" assessment form comes with preprinted headings and questions. This form saves you time in a couple of ways. Information is categorized under specific headings, so you can easily record and retrieve it. And the form can be completed using partial phrases and approved abbreviations. (See *Documenting assessment on an open-ended form.*)

Unfortunately, however, open-ended forms don't always provide the space or the instructions to encourage thorough descriptions. Thus, following the heading *type of dwelling,* one nurse may write "apartment" whereas another may write

BETTER CHARTING

Documenting assessment on a closed-ended form

At some health care facilities, you may use a standardized closed-ended form to document initial assessment information. Below you'll find a portion of such a form.

SELF-CARE ABILITY

Activity	1	2	3	4	5	6
Bathing			✓			
Cleaning			✓			
Climbing stairs			✓			
Cooking			✓			
Dressing and grooming			✓			
Eating and drinking	✓					
Moving in bed	✓					
Shopping					✓	
Toileting			✓			
Transferring			✓			
Walking		✓				
Other home functions			✓			

KEY
1 = Independent
2 = Requires assistive device
3 = Requires personal assistance
4 = Requires personal assistance and assistive device
5 = Dependent
6 = Experienced change in last week

ASSISTIVE DEVICES
☐ Bedside commode
☐ Brace or splint
☑ Cane
☐ Crutches
☐ Feeding device
☐ Trapeze
☐ Walker
☐ Wheelchair
☐ Other
☐ None

ACTIVITY TOLERANCE
☐ Normal
☑ Weakness
☐ Dizziness
☑ Exertional dyspnea
☐ Dyspnea at rest
☐ Angina
☐ Pain at rest
☐ Oxygen needed
☐ Intermittent claudication
☑ Unsteady gait
☐ Other

REST PATTERN
Sleep habits
☑ Less than 8 hours
☐ 8 hours
☐ More than 8 hours
☑ Morning or afternoon nap

Sleep difficulties
☐ Insomnia
☑ Early awakening
☐ Unrefreshing sleep
☐ Nightmares
☐ None

"apartment with four-flight walk-up, without heat or hot water."

Nonspecific responses can lead to misinterpretation. For instance, a nurse may write that a patient performs a task "within normal limits." But unless normal limits have been defined, this notation is neither clear nor legally sound.

Standardized closed-ended style

This type of assessment form provides preprinted headings, checklists, and questions with specific responses. You simply check off the appropriate response. (See *Documenting assessment on a closed-ended form.*)

Besides saving time, the closed-ended form eliminates the problem of illegible handwriting and makes checking documented information easy. In addition, the form can be easily incorporated into most computerized systems.

This kind of form also clearly establishes the type and amount of information required by the health care facility. And even though the closed-ended forms usually use nonspecific terminology, such as "within normal limits" or "no alteration," guidelines clearly define these responses.

The closed-ended form also creates some problems. For instance, many of these forms provide no place to record relevant information that doesn't fit the pre-printed choices. And the forms tend to be lengthy, especially when a hospital's policy calls for recording in-depth physical assessment data.

Documentation formats

Historically, nursing assessment has followed a medical format, emphasizing the patient's initial symptoms and a comprehensive review of body systems. Although many health care facilities still use a medical format to organize their nursing assessment forms, some facilities have adopted formats that more readily reflect the nursing process.

Most facilities that use a nursing format for assessment base it on either human response patterns or functional health care patterns. Other documentation formats are modeled on specific conceptual frameworks based on published nursing theories.

Human response patterns

As you know, the North American Nursing Diagnosis Association (NANDA) has developed a classification system for nursing diagnoses based on human response patterns. These patterns relate directly to actual or potential health problems as indicated by assessment data.

Thus, when you use an assessment form organized by these patterns, you can easily establish appropriate diagnoses while you record assessment data—especially if a listing of diagnoses is included with the form. The main drawback is that these forms tend to be lengthy.

Functional health care patterns

Some health care facilities organize their assessment data according to functional health care patterns. Developed by Marjory Gordon, this system classifies nursing data according to the patient's ability to function independently. Many nurses consider functional health care patterns easier to understand and remember than human response patterns.

Conceptual frameworks

At some health care facilities, assessment forms have been modeled on the nursing philosophies that the nursing departments follow. Some examples include Dorothea Orem's self-care model, Imogene King's theory of goal attainment, and Sister Callista Roy's adaptation model. Assessment forms based on these nursing philosophies reflect the individual theory's approach to nursing care.

Documenting learning needs

Most initial assessment forms have a separate section for documenting a patient's learning needs. When you reassess your patient's learning needs, you can document your findings in the progress notes, on an open-ended patient education flow sheet, or on a structured patient education flow sheet designed for a specific problem such as diabetes mellitus.

Documenting discharge planning needs

Effective discharge planning begins when you identify and document the patient's needs during the initial assessment. Depending on the policy at your health care facility, you'll record the patient's discharge needs on the initial assessment form (in a designated section), on a specially designed discharge planning form, in a separate section on the patient care card file, in the progress notes, or on a discharge planning flow sheet. (See *Documenting discharge planning needs,* page 200.)

Documenting incomplete initial data

No matter which assessment tool you use, you may not always be able to obtain a complete health history during the initial assessment. For instance, the patient may be too ill to participate, and secondary sources may be unavailable.

When this occurs, base your initial assessment on your observations and physical examination of the patient. When documenting your findings, be sure to write something such as "Unable to obtain complete data at this time." Otherwise, it might appear that you failed to perform a complete assessment.

Try to obtain missing information as soon as possible, when the patient's condition improves or family members or other secondary sources are available. Be sure to record how and when you obtained the

missing data. Depending on your facility's policy, you may record the information on the progress notes, or you may return to the initial assessment form and add the new information along with the date and your signature. Both methods have advantages and disadvantages.

Adding to the initial assessment form makes it easy to retrieve the data when it's needed—either during the patient's hospitalization or after discharge for quality assurance. Putting the information into the nursing progress notes aids in the day-to-day communication with others who read the notes but makes it difficult to retrieve the data later.

Remember, when you add information to complete an initial assessment, be sure to revise your nursing plan of care accordingly. (See *Adding to the initial assessment,* pages 201 to 204.)

Ongoing assessment

Your assessment of a patient, of course, is a continuous process. Reassessment lets you evaluate the effectiveness of your nursing interventions and determine your patient's progress toward the desired outcomes. Effective documentation of your assessment findings facilitates communication with other health care practitioners, allowing you to plan the most appropriate patient care.

How often should you reassess a patient? That depends primarily on his condition. However, the JCAHO has a list of suggestions you can use as a basis for reassessing certain types of patients. Your health care facility's policy should also define specific conditions under which you must reassess—for instance, when a patient is trans-

(Text continues on page 205.)

BETTER CHARTING

Documenting discharge planning needs

How and where you document your discharge planning will depend on the policy at the health care facility where you work. Here's one of the more common ways of documenting this information.

DISCHARGE PLANNING NEEDS

Occupation *Retired college professor*   **Language spoken** *English*

Patient lives with *Wife*

Self-care capabilities *Needs extensive assistance*

Assistance available
- ☑ Cooking
- ☑ Dressing changes/treatments *Irrigate ⓛ lower leg wound b.i.d. with ½ strength H₂O₂, followed by rinse with normal saline solution. Pack with ½" iodoform gauze. Apply dry sterile dressing.*
- ☐ Cleaning
- ☑ Shopping

Medication administration routes
- ☑ P.O.
- ☐ I.V.
- ☐ I.M.
- ☐ S.C.
- ☐ Other:

Dwelling
- ☐ Apartment
- ☑ Private home
- ☐ Single room
- ☐ Institution
- ☐ Elevator
- ☑ Outside steps (number) *6*

- ☑ Inside steps (number) *12*
- ☑ Kitchen
  - gas stove
  - electric stove
  - wood stove
- ☐ Other

- ☑ Bathrooms (number) *2* (location) *1 upstairs   1 downstairs*
- ☑ Telephones (number) *1* (location) *kitchen*

Transportation
- ☐ Drives own car
- ☐ Takes public transportation
- ☑ Relies on family member or friend

After discharge, patient will be:
- ☐ Home alone
- ☑ Home with family
- ☐ Other:

Patient has had help from:
- ☑ Visiting nurse
- ☑ Housekeeper
- ☑ Other: *Social worker*

Anticipated needs *Nurse for dressing changes, transportation for groceries, etc.*

Social service requests *VNA*

Date contacted *1/10/95*   **Reason** *Contacted VNA for dressing changes and transportation needs.*

BETTER CHARTING

Adding to the initial assessment

The sample below shows you how to complete an initial assessment form. You can add information to the form where it will be easy to retrieve when you need it later.

INITIAL ASSESSMENT

GENERAL INFORMATION

Age _44_ Sex _F_ Height _5' 1"_ Weight _137 lb_
T _99_ P _74_ R _18_ B/P(R) _124/64_ (L) _122/64_
Room _408B_ Admission time _1400_
Admission date _1/6/95_ Doctor _R. Wright_
Admitting diagnosis _cholecystitis_
Patient's stated reason for
hospitalization _"To have my gallbladder removed."_

Allergies
PCN

Current medications

Name	Dosage	Last taken
none		

Medical history
appendectomy, age 12

Orientation
☑ Identification band ☑ Bed position and side rails ☑ Television
☑ Visiting policy ☑ Call light ☑ Telephone
☑ Smoking policy ☑ Intercom ☑ Bathroom
                                              ☑ Signed consent

I understand the explanations I've received during orientation.
Patient's signature _Julie Stephan_

Personal possessions
☑ Money _$20_
☑ Clothing _One knee-length, yellow nightgown,_
pink robe, one pair pink slip-on slippers

☑ Jewelry _One white metal wedding ring, yellow_
metal lady's watch.

☑ Glasses _Red wire-rim_
☑ Contact lenses _R and L soft_
☑ Dentures _Partial, upper_
☐ Hearing aid
☐ Other

VALUING

Religion _Lutheran_

☑ Request for clerical visit
☐ Request for religious rites

SUBJECTIVE DATA

☑ From patient   ☐ From other

OBJECTIVE DATA

RELATING, CHOOSING

☐ Single   ☑ Divorced
☐ Married   ☐ Widowed
Most supportive person _sister_
☑ Alcohol use
How much? _4 cans lt. beer_ How often? _every weekend_
☐ Substance abuse
Type _none_

Pertinent nonverbal behavior _____

Describe patient's ability to comply with therapy for long-term health problems.
_N/A_

Date _1/6/95_   Signature _Theresa Doria, RN_

(continued)

Adding to the initial assessment *(continued)*

INITIAL ASSESSMENT	**page 2**

SUBJECTIVE DATA	**OBJECTIVE DATA**

☑ From patient   ☐ From other

EXCHANGING

Oxygenation

Yes	No	
☐	☑ Dyspnea	
☐	☑ Painful breathing	
☐	☑ Cough	
☐	☑ Sputum	
☐	☑ Use of oxygen at home	

Smoking history *Quit 17 years ago*

☑ Regular respirations
☐ Irregular respirations
☑ Normal breath sounds
☐ Abnormal breath sounds

Circulation

Yes	No	
☐	☑ Chest pain	
☐	☑ Palpitations	
☐	☑ Leg pain	
☐	☑ Limbs numb	
☐	☑ Limbs cold	

☑ Regular heart rhythm
☐ Irregular heart rhythm
☑ Normal heart sounds
☐ Abnormal heart sounds
☑ Adequate capillary refill
☐ Edema

Apical rate _74_   Radial rate _74_
Carotid pulse R   Radial pulse R
Femoral pulse R   Pedal pulse R
Comments *All pulses palpable*

Reproduction
☐ Menarche
Last menstrual period *2½ weeks ago*
Last Pap smear *Oct. 1993*

Tissue, skin integrity

Yes	No	
☐	☑ Dry	
☐	☑ Pale	
☐	☑ Itchy	
☐	☑ Bruised	
☐	☐ Other	

☐ Flushed
☐ Pale
☐ Cyanotic
☑ Pink
☐ Dry
☑ Moist
☐ Cool
☑ Warm

Mark illustrations, using key.

1 Blister	6 Rash
2 Bruise	7 Scar *Appendectomy 6 cm*
3 Burn	8 Ulcer
4 Pressure ulcer	9 Wound
5 Nevi *℗ lower leg 4 mm*	10 Other

Date _1/6/95_   Signature *Theresa Doria, RN*

Adding to the initial assessment *(continued)*

INITIAL ASSESSMENT   page 3

SUBJECTIVE DATA   **OBJECTIVE DATA**

☑ From patient   ☐ From other

NUTRITION

Yes	No						

Yes		**No**		**Breath**	**Teeth**	**Gums**

Yes **No**

☐   ☑ Recent weight gain
☑   ☐ Recent weight loss
☐   ☑ Recent increase in appetite
☑   ☐ Recent decrease in appetite
☑   ☐ Food intolerance
☑   ☐ Nausea
☐   ☑ Vomiting
☐   ☑ Heartburn
☐   ☑ Swallowing problems

Diet   *Low-fat diet*
Comments *Intolerant of fat in diet. Nausea,*
decrease in appetite and recent 5-lb weight loss
related to gallbladder

Breath
☑ Normal
☐ Fruity
☐ Halitosis
☐ Other _____

Teeth
☑ Normal
☐ Caries
☐ Loose
☐ Broken
☐ Missing

Gums
☑ Moist
☑ Pink
☐ Pale
☐ Bleeding

Tongue
☑ Moist
☐ Dry
☐ Pink
☐ Other _____

Body type
☑ Normal
☐ Thin
☐ Emaciated
☐ Obese

Elimination

Yes **No**

☑   ☐ Continent (urine) _____
☑   ☐ Continent (stool) _____
☐   ☑ Urinary problems _____
☑   ☐ Constipation *occasionally*
☐   ☑ Hemorrhoids _____
☐   ☑ Rectal bleeding _____

Date of last bowel movement _1/5/95_
Patient's constipation remedy _milk of magnesia_
_____

☑ Bowel sounds
☐ Abdominal distention
☐ Ostomy _____
☐ Urinary catheter _____
Appearance of urine _____
Appearance of diarrheic stool _____
Comments _____

MOVING

Rest, activity, self-care

Yes **No**

☑   ☐ Ambulates _____
☑   ☐ Bathes self _____
☐   ☑ Paralysis _____
☐   ☑ Seizures _____
☐   ☑ Sleeping problems _____

Activities _Step aerobics, reading_
_____
_____

☑ Steady gait
☐ Unsteady gait
☐ Cane
☐ Walker
☑ Moves limbs *normal ROM*
☐ Has stiffness _____
☐ Contractures _____
☐ Deformities _____
☐ Amputation _____

Date _1/6/95_   Signature _Theresa Doris, RN_ _____

(continued)

Adding to the initial assessment *(continued)*

INITIAL ASSESSMENT   page 4

SUBJECTIVE DATA   **OBJECTIVE DATA**

☑ From patient   ☐ From other

PERCEIVING, COMMUNICATING

Yes   **No**
☑   ☐ Visual impairment *Contacts during*   ☑ Alert
                    day. Glasses in evening.   ☐ Lethargic
☐   ☑ Hearing impairment _____   ☐ Semicomatose
☐ Other sensory impairment _____   ☐ Unconscious

_____   ☐ Ocular drainage _____
_____   ☐ Ear drainage _____
                                                                 ☑ Normal speech _____
                                                                 ☐ Abnormal speech _____
                                                                 ☐ Language barrier _____

FEELING

Yes   **No**
☑   ☐ Pain not noted elsewhere *occasional*   ☑ Calm
RUQ abdominal ache   ☐ Apprehensive
☐   ☐ Recent sensory loss _____   ☐ Grimaces
                                                                 ☐ Guarding _____
_____   ☐ Other signs of pain _____
_____

KNOWING

Highest grade completed *16* _____   ☑ Answers questions appropriately
☑ Reads English   ☑ Follows directions
☑ Reads other language *Spanish* _____   ☑ Teaching needs *Preoperative teaching. Care*
☑ Understanding of illness *Able to accurately state*   *required postoperatively including nutrition.*
knowledge of cholecystitis and related
treatments.

DISCHARGE PLANNING

Patient and family postdischarge intentions *Pt. states that sister will help her at home and that no*

further assistance will be necessary.

_____

_____

Date *1/6/95* _____   Signature *Theresa Doni, RN* _____

ferred to another unit. (See *When to reassess.*)

Planned reassessment

A planned reassessment provides the routine data you must obtain to evaluate a patient on a daily basis. On a medical-surgical unit, this may include reviewing the patient's mental status, respiratory status, vital signs, skin integrity, self-care capabilities, appetite, and fluid balance, as well as psychosocial factors. You'll also need to regularly reassess environmental factors and his learning and discharge needs. Based on the patient's condition, your nursing plan of care may specify other reassessments as well.

At some facilities, health care team members must meet every 2 or 3 days during a patient's hospital stay to discuss and update discharge plans. At these meetings, staff representatives from various departments—including nursing, medicine, social services, physical therapy, and dietary—evaluate the patient's progress toward established goals and revise the plan of care as needed. Records of these meetings are maintained in the clinical record to ensure communication with other team members.

Unplanned reassessment

An unplanned reassessment occurs whenever the patient's condition or circumstances change unexpectedly. For example, suppose a patient with no previous cardiac dysfunction suddenly develops severe chest pain and shortness of breath. You'd perform a complete assessment and schedule future cardiac reassessments according to the revised plan of care.

Or suppose you're caring for an elderly patient whose wife is his primary home

When to reassess

The Joint Commission on Accreditation of Healthcare Organizations suggests the following time intervals for patient reassessment. Keep in mind that these are minimum standards; some patients may need more frequent assessment.

TYPE OF PATIENT	WHEN TO REASSESS
Stable medical-surgical patient	Every 24 hours
Long-term care patient	Monthly
Patient in rehabilitation	Every 1 to 2 weeks
Same-day surgery patient	On return from post-anesthesia care unit and immediately before discharge
Patient in labor	Every 15 minutes
Patient with decreasing neurologic status	Every 15 minutes
Suicidal patient	Continuously on a one-to-one basis
Patient with active GI bleeding	Continuously on a one-to-one basis

caregiver. If his wife suddenly becomes incapacitated, you'd need to perform an unplanned reassessment of the patient's discharge needs to accommodate this change.

Documenting ongoing assessment

You'll usually document ongoing assessment data on flow sheets or in narrative notes on the patient's progress report. Ideally, you should use flow sheets to document all routine assessment data and nursing interventions. That way, you can shorten the narrative notes to include only information regarding the patient's progress toward achieving desired outcomes and any unplanned assessments.

Flow sheets come in many varieties, including temperature graphs and intake and output forms. When used to record routine assessment data, flow sheets can be a quick and consistent way to highlight trends in the patient's condition. A flow sheet for documenting information about a patient's skin integrity, for instance, will clearly show the progression of any pressure ulcers or reddened areas.

Because flow sheets are legally accepted components of the patient's clinical record, they must be documented correctly. Give yourself enough time to evaluate each piece of information on the flow sheet. And keep in mind that it must accurately reflect the patient's current clinical status.

In some cases, you'll find that recording only the information requested on a flow sheet won't be sufficient to give a complete picture of the patient's status. When this occurs, record additional information in the space provided on the flow sheet. If additional information isn't necessary, draw a line through the space. Doing so indicates that, in your judgment, further information isn't required. If your flow sheet doesn't have additional space and you need to record more information, use the progress notes.

Nursing diagnosis and plan of care

When you formulate nursing diagnoses and write a plan of care for a patient, you're playing a key role in his recovery. To build a solid foundation for your plan of care, you need to identify nursing diagnoses carefully. Then you must write a plan that not only fits your nursing diagnoses, but also fits your patient—taking into account his needs, age, developmental level, culture, strengths and weaknesses, and willingness and ability to take part in his care.

Your plan should help him reach his highest functional level with minimal risk and without new problems. If he can't recover completely, your plan should help him cope physically and emotionally with his impaired or declining health. And, of course, you need to document all of this—carefully and completely.

That's a tall order. But this section will help you fill it by explaining the nursing diagnosis and planning processes and showing you how to document them most effectively. The first section covers how to formulate nursing diagnoses. Next comes a section on how to rank these diagnoses so you treat your patient's most urgent problems first.

The third section reviews how to develop realistic expected outcomes—goals your patient should reach by or before discharge so he can function as effectively as possible. In the fourth section, you'll read about choosing the nursing interventions that will help your patient reach those expected outcomes.

Nursing diagnoses: Avoiding the pitfalls

To avoid making common mistakes when formulating your nursing diagnoses, follow these guidelines.

Use nursing diagnoses
Don't use medical diagnoses or interventions. Terms such as *angioplasty* and *coronary artery disease* belong in a medical diagnosis—not in a nursing diagnosis.

Use all relevant assessment data
If you just focus on the physical assessment, for instance, you might miss psychosocial or cultural information relevant to your diagnoses.

Take enough time
Take enough time to analyze the assessment data. If you rush, you might easily miss something important.

Interpret the assessment data accurately
Make sure that you follow established norms, professional standards, and interdisciplinary expectations. In addition, don't permit your biases to interfere with your interpretation of information.

For instance, don't assume your patient is exaggerating if he states that he feels pain during what you would consider a painless procedure. If possible, have the patient verify your interpretation.

Keep data up-to-date
Don't stop assessing and updating your diagnoses after the initial examination. As the patient's condition changes, so should your evaluation.

The next section explains how to write plans of care. As you'll see, the discussion includes how to use practice guidelines to make planning and documentation more efficient and how to document your patient teaching and discharge planning. The final section looks at case management, a comprehensive way of caring for a patient that attempts to meet both clinical and financial goals.

Formulating nursing diagnoses

Unlike a medical diagnosis, which focuses on the patient's pathophysiology or illness, a nursing diagnosis focuses on the pa-

tient's responses to illness. (See *Nursing diagnoses: Avoiding the pitfalls.*)

Types of nursing diagnoses
Depending on the policy of your health care facility, you'll either use standardized diagnoses or formulate your own diagnoses.

Using standardized diagnoses
To make nursing diagnoses consistent, several organizations have developed standardized lists, which are used by a growing number of health care facilities. The North American Nursing Diagnosis Association (NANDA) has developed the

CHARTING TIMESAVER

Evaluating assessment data

To formulate your nursing diagnoses, you must evaluate the essential assessment information. These questions will help you quickly zero in on the appropriate data.
• Which signs and symptoms does the patient have?
• Which assessment findings are abnormal for this patient?
• How do particular behaviors affect the patient's well-being?
• What strengths or weaknesses does the patient have that affect his health status?
• Does he understand his illness and treatment?
• How does the patient's environment affect his health?
• Does he want to change his state of health?
• Do I need to gather any further information for my diagnoses?

most widely accepted taxonomy of nursing diagnoses. (See the appendix NANDA Taxonomy I, Revised, for a complete list.) NANDA categorizes nursing diagnoses according to the human response patterns of exchanging, communicating, relating, valuing, choosing, moving, perceiving, knowing, and feeling. The association meets every 2 years to consider new diagnoses.

Diagnoses can also be categorized according to nursing models, such as the one developed by Marjory Gordon. In this model, nursing diagnoses correspond to functional health patterns. Other ways of categorizing diagnoses—for instance, ac-

cording to Orem's universal self-care demands—may also be used. Or your health care facility or unit can establish its own list of nursing diagnoses, categorizing them according to medical diagnoses and surgical procedures, for example.

No accrediting organization requires the use of standardized diagnoses. But by using nationally accepted nursing diagnoses like the NANDA taxonomy, health care facilities help establish a common language for nursing diagnoses—making communication easier and diagnoses more precise.

Formulating your own nursing diagnoses

Developing your own diagnoses takes more effort than using standardized ones. But some nurses prefer this approach because they find the standardized diagnoses incomplete or their language overly formal or abstract. Such an approach can also help you characterize a problem that standardized diagnoses don't readily address.

Deciding on a diagnosis

Before using or developing nursing diagnoses, you must evaluate relevant assessment data. You'll usually find this data on a standardized assessment form that groups related information into categories. Looking at the data in these groupings lets you determine which patient needs require nursing intervention. (See *Evaluating assessment data.*)

Components of the diagnosis

Once you've examined the assessment data, you're ready to devise your nursing diagnoses. A diagnosis usually has three components: the human response or problem, related factors, and signs and symptoms.

Human response or problem. The first part of a diagnosis, the human response, identifies an actual or a potential problem that can be affected by nursing care. For instance, if assessment information on a patient with osteoarthritis shows that he has trouble moving, you might turn to the NANDA taxonomy, look under the human response pattern of moving, and identify the problem as impaired physical mobility. If the NANDA taxonomy doesn't provide a label that fits a patient's problem or if your facility doesn't use standardized diagnoses, create your own label for the patient's condition.

Related factors. The second part of the nursing diagnosis identifies related factors. Such factors may precede, contribute to, or simply be associated with the human response. But no matter how they relate, these factors make your diagnosis more closely fit the particular patient and help you choose the most effective interventions.

For example, for your patient with osteoarthritis you may write "Impaired physical mobility related to pain" or "Impaired physical mobility related to depression." Based on these related factors, you'd intervene differently.

When you can't determine the related factors, write "related to unknown etiology" and modify your diagnosis as you obtain more information. To save charting time, use the standard abbreviation "R/T" for "related to" when writing your nursing diagnoses.

Signs and symptoms. Finally, a complete nursing diagnosis includes the signs and symptoms — or defining characteristics, as NANDA calls them — that led you to the diagnosis. You'll draw these from the assessment data. Not all nurses include signs and symptoms in their diagnoses but, like related factors, they help tailor the nursing diagnosis to the particular patient.

To help keep the nursing diagnosis brief, choose only the key characteristics. You can list them after the human response and related factors. For instance, you might write "Impaired thought processes R/T uncompensated perceptual or cognitive impairment. Defining characteristics: short attention span during conversation; minimal speech; confused, oriented to person."

Alternatively, you can join the signs and symptoms to the first part of the nursing diagnosis with the words "as evidenced by," abbreviated AEB. For example, you'd write "Fluid volume excess R/T increased sodium intake AEB edema, weight gain, shortness of breath, and S_3 heart sounds."

Setting priorities

Once you've made your nursing diagnoses, you'll need to rank them based on which problems require more immediate attention. Whenever possible, you should include the patient in this process. Maslow's hierarchy of needs is generally accepted as the basis for setting priorities. (See *Relating assessment to nursing diagnoses,* page 210.)

Typically, the first nursing diagnosis will stem from the primary medical diagnosis or from the patient's chief complaint. This nursing diagnosis points out a threat to the patient's physical well-being — some-

Relating assessment to nursing diagnoses

Some assessment forms group assessment information and relevant nursing diagnoses together so that you can immediately relate one to the other. This saves you from looking back through the form for assessment data when determining the nursing diagnosis. Here's a section of this type of form.

Patient _John Ramsey_   **Age** _72_

Medical diagnosis _CHF_

ASSESSMENT FINDINGS   **NURSING DIAGNOSES**

Cardiopulmonary

Breath sounds _crackles bilat. bases_

Breathing pattern ☑ cough _dry_   ☐ smoker

Dyspnea   ☑ on exertion   ☑ nocturnal

Sputum   color _____

        consistency _____

Heart sounds _S3 and S4 present_

Peripheral pulses _All peripheral pulses +1_

Edema   ☑ extremities _ankles_

        ☐ other _____

Cyanosis   ☑ extremities _nail beds_

        ☑ other _lips_

☑ Impaired gas exchange

☐ Ineffective airway clearance

☐ Inability to sustain spontaneous ventilation

☑ Ineffective breathing pattern

☑ Decreased cardiac output

☐ Altered peripheral tissue perfusion

☐ Altered cardiopulmonary tissue perfusion

Nutrition

Diet   _2 G Na, low cholesterol_

Appetite

☐ normal   ☐ increased   ☑ decreased

☐ vomiting   ☐ nausea

☑ Altered nutrition: less than body requirements

☐ Altered nutrition: more than body requirements

☐ Altered nutrition: potential for more than body requirements

---

times to his life. For a patient who has a primary medical diagnosis of congestive heart failure (CHF), for instance, you'd give first priority to the nursing diagnosis of "Decreased cardiac output R/T de-creased contractility and altered heart rhythm."

Related nursing diagnoses come next. These define problems that pose less immediate threats to the patient's well-being. For instance, you may have also selected for the CHF patient the nursing diagnosis of "Fluid volume excess R/T compromised regulatory mechanism."

Then, you'll usually list nursing diagnoses that refer to the patient's psychosocial, emotional, or spiritual needs. For the CHF patient, a nursing diagnosis of "Anxiety R/T possible loss of employment" doesn't carry the same urgency as the previous two nursing diagnoses.

But just because a nursing diagnosis has a lower priority doesn't mean that you should wait to intervene until you've resolved all the higher-priority problems. By helping the CHF patient cope with anxiety about losing his job, for example, you may speed his recovery—helping to resolve problems related to his physical well-being.

Developing expected outcomes

After you've established and ranked nursing diagnoses, you're ready to develop relevant expected outcomes, an increasingly important planning step. Based on nursing diagnoses, expected outcomes are goals the patient should reach as a result of planned nursing interventions. (Once achieved, an expected outcome is called a patient outcome.) You may find that one nursing diagnosis requires more than one expected outcome.

An outcome can specify an improvement in the patient's ability to function—an increase in the distance he can walk, for example. Or an outcome can specify an amelioration of a problem, such as a reduction of pain. Each outcome should call for the maximum realistic improvement for a particular patient.

Writing outcome statements

Ideally, an outcome statement should include four components: the specific behavior that will demonstrate the patient has reached his goal, criteria for measuring the behavior, the conditions under which the behavior should occur, and the time by which the behavior should occur. (See *Writing an outcome statement*, page 212.)

When you're writing outcome statements, follow these guidelines: Make your statements specific, focus on the patient, let the patient help you, take medical orders into account, adapt the outcome to the circumstances, and change your statements as necessary.

Make your statements specific

If someone writes a statement such as "Understand relaxation techniques," you don't have much to go on. How do you observe a patient's understanding? A more specific statement such as "Practice progressive muscle relaxation techniques unassisted for 15 minutes daily by 10/9/94" tells you exactly what to look for when assessing the patient's progress. (See *Writing outcomes more efficiently*, page 213.)

Focus on the patient

Make sure that the outcome statement reflects the patient's behavior—not your intervention. The statements "Medication brings chest pain relief" and "Nurse to change pt.'s position every 2 hours to promote comfort" don't say anything about the patient's behavior. A proper statement would be "Express relief of chest pain within 1 hour of receiving medication."

Writing an outcome statement

An outcome statement should consist of four components.

B	M	C	T
Behavior A desired behavior for the patient. This behavior must be observable.	**Measure** Criteria for measuring the behavior. The criteria should specify how much, how long, how far, and so on.	**Condition** The conditions under which the behavior should occur.	**Time** The time by which the behavior should occur.

As indicated, the two outcome statements below have these four components.

Limit sodium intake	2 g/day	using hospital menu	by 1/10/95
Eat	50% of all meals	unassisted	by 1/10/95

Let the patient help you

If the patient has a part in developing outcome statements, he's more motivated to achieve his goals. And his input—and the input of family members—can help you set realistic goals.

Take medical orders into account

Make sure that you don't write outcome statements that ignore or contradict medical orders. For example, before writing the outcome statement "Ambulate 10′ unassisted twice a day by 12/5/94," you should make sure that the medical orders don't call for more restricted activity.

Adapt the outcome to the circumstances

Take into account the patient's coping ability, age, educational level, cultural influences, family support, living conditions, and socioeconomic situation. Also consider his anticipated length of stay when you're deciding on time limits for achieving goals. In some cases, you'll need to consider the health care setting itself. For instance, an outcome statement such as "Ambulate outdoors with assistance for 20 minutes t.i.d. by 12/14/94" may be unrealistic in a large city hospital.

Change your statements as necessary

Sometimes, you may need to revise even the most carefully written outcome statements. You may have to choose a later target date if the patient has trouble reaching his goal, for instance. Or you may need to change the goal to one the patient can reach more easily.

Selecting interventions

Now, you're ready to select interventions— nursing actions that you and your patient agree will help him reach the expected outcomes. Base these interventions on the second part of your nursing diagnosis, the related factors. With a nursing diagnosis of "Impaired physical mobility R/T arthritic morning stiffness," for example, you'd select interventions that reduce or eliminate the patient's stiffness, such as mild stretching exercises. You'll need to write at least one intervention for each outcome statement.

Considering potential interventions

You can come up with interventions in several ways. Start by considering ones that your patient or you have successfully tried before. Say your patient is having trouble sleeping. He knows he sleeps better at home if he has a glass of warm milk at bedtime. That could work as an intervention for the expected outcome "Sleep through the night without medication by 12/14/94."

You can also pick interventions from standardized plans of care, talk with your colleagues about interventions they've used successfully, or check nursing journals that discuss interventions for standardized nursing diagnoses. If these

CHARTING TIMESAVER

Writing outcomes more efficiently

Save yourself charting time by including only the essentials in your outcome statements. For example:

• Avoid unnecessary words. You don't need to refer to the patient as this statement does: "Pt. will demonstrate insulin self-administration, unassisted, by 12/5/94." Simply drop the first two words of the statement— the reader knows you're referring to the patient. You only need to specify the person if you're referring to someone else.

• Use accepted abbreviations wherever possible. If your health care facility uses relative dates, use abbreviations like HD2 for hospital day 2 or POD3 for postoperative day 3.

methods don't yield anything useful, try brainstorming.

Guidelines for writing interventions

When you write your interventions, be sure to follow these guidelines: Clearly state the action to be taken, make the intervention fit the patient, keep the patient's safety in mind, follow the rules of your health care facility, take other health care activities into account, and include the available resources.

Clearly state the necessary action

To ensure continuity of care, write your interventions with as much specific detail as possible. Note how and when to perform the intervention, and include any special instructions. An intervention such as "Promote comfort" doesn't tell another nurse what specific actions she should take. But "Administer ordered analgesic ½ hr before dressing change" lets her know exactly what to do and when to do it.

Make the intervention fit the patient

Keep in mind the patient's age, condition, developmental level, environment, and value system. For instance, if your patient is a vegetarian, you shouldn't write an intervention that requires him to eat lean meat to gain extra protein for healing. Instead, your intervention can call for him to eat legumes and dairy products.

Keep the patient's safety in mind

This means taking into account both the patient's physical and mental limitations. For instance, before teaching a patient to give himself medication, make sure that he's physically able to do so and that he can remember and follow the medication regimen.

Follow the rules of your health care facility

If your facility has a rule that only nurses may administer medications, you obviously wouldn't write an intervention calling for the patient to "Administer hemorrhoidal suppositories as needed."

Take other health care activities into account

Sometimes, other necessary activities may interfere with interventions you want to use. For example, you may want your patient to get plenty of rest on a day he has several diagnostic tests scheduled. In this case, you'd need to adjust your interventions.

Include the available resources

If your patient needs to learn about his cardiac problem, use your health care facility's education department, literature from the American Heart Association, local support groups—anything that might help you carry out the intervention effectively. Then write the intervention to reflect the use of these resources.

Writing your plan of care

A good plan of care is the blueprint for concise, meaningful charting. Write a good plan of care and your nurses' notes will practically write themselves. A good plan consists of the following:
• patient problems identified during the admission interview and hospitalization
• realistic, measurable expected outcomes and their target dates
• nursing interventions that will help the patient or his family achieve these outcomes.

To document your nursing diagnoses, expected outcomes, and interventions, you can use either a traditional or a standardized plan of care. You also may decide to use protocols along with one of these plans. In some cases, you can use protocols alone to demonstrate planned care. Your plan of care will also include your patient-teaching and discharge plans.

Types of nursing plans of care

Two basic types of plans of care exist: traditional and standardized. No matter which you use, your plan should cover all nursing care from admission to discharge and should be a permanent part of the patient's clinical record. Be sure to write the plan of care and put it into action as soon as possible after the initial assessment.

Then you can revise and update it throughout the patient's hospitalization.

Traditional plan of care
Also called the individually developed plan of care, the traditional plan of care is written from scratch for each patient. After analyzing the assessment data, you'll either write the plan or enter it into a computer.

The basic form can vary, depending on the needs of the health care facility or department. Most forms have three main columns: one for nursing diagnoses, another for expected outcomes, and a third for interventions. Other columns allow you to enter the date you initiated the plan of care, the target dates for expected outcomes, and the dates for review, revisions, and resolution. Most forms also have a place for you to sign or initial when you make an entry or a revision.

What you must include on these forms also varies. With shorter stays brought on by the advent of diagnosis-related groups (DRGs), most facilities require you to write only short-term outcomes that the patient should reach by or before discharge. But some facilities—particularly long-term care facilities—also want you to include long-term outcomes that reflect the maximum functional level the patient can reach. Such facilities frequently use forms that provide separate places for the two types of outcomes. (See *Using a traditional plan of care,* page 216.)

Standardized plan of care
Developed to save documentation time and improve the quality of care, standardized plans of care provide a series of interventions for patients with similar diagnoses. Most standardized plans also supply

root outcome statements. Some of these plans are classified by medical diagnoses or DRGs; others, by nursing diagnoses.

The early versions of standardized plans of care made no allowances for differences in patient needs. But current versions allow you to customize the plan to fit your patient's specific needs. In fact, they require you to explain how you've individualized the plan of care. To use such a plan, you'll usually fill in the following information:
• related factors and signs and symptoms for a nursing diagnosis. For instance, the form will provide a root diagnosis such as "Pain R/T...." You might fill in "inflammation as exhibited by grimacing, expressions of pain."
• the time limits for the outcomes. To a root statement of "Perform postural drainage without assistance," you might add "for 15 minutes immediately upon awakening in the morning by 12/11/94."
• frequency of interventions. You can complete an intervention such as "Perform passive range-of-motion exercises" with "twice a day: 1× each in the morning and evening."
• specific instructions for interventions. For a standard intervention of "Elevate patient's head," you might specify "Before sleep, elevate the patient's head on three pillows."

When a patient has more than one diagnosis, the resulting combination of standardized plans of care can be long and cumbersome. But computerized documentation can help. With computerized plans, you can pull only what you need from each one and combine them to make one manageable plan. Some computer programs simply provide a checklist of inter-

BETTER CHARTING

Using a traditional plan of care

This sample shows how a traditional plan of care organizes key information. Keep in mind that the plans of care you'll use will have wider columns to allow more room for your notes.

Date	Nursing diagnoses	Expected outcomes	Interventions	Revision (initials and date)	Resolution (initials and date)
1/8/95	Decreased cardiac output R/T reduced stroke volume secondary to fluid volume overload.	Lungs clear on auscultation by 1/10/95. BP will return to baseline by 1/10/95.	Monitor for signs and symptoms of hypoxemia, such as dyspnea, confusion, arrhythmias, restlessness, and cyanosis. Ensure adequate oxygenation by placing patient in semi-Fowler's position and administering supplemental O2 as ordered. Monitor breath sounds q4hr. Administer cardiac medications as ordered and document pt.'s response, their effectiveness, and any adverse reactions. Monitor and document heart rate and rhythm, heart sounds, and BP. Note the presence or absence of peripheral pulses. KK		

Review dates

Date	Signature	Initials
1/8/95	Karen Kubrak, RN	KK

ventions you can use to build your own plan.

Keep in mind that standardized plans usually include only essential information. But most provide space for you to add further nursing diagnoses, expected outcomes, and interventions. (See *Using a standardized plan of care,* page 218.)

Practice guidelines

A newer documentation tool, practice guidelines give specific sequential instructions for treating patients with particular problems. Developed to help nurses manage equipment and provide specific treatments, practice guidelines now are also used to manage patients with specific nursing diagnoses. (See *Practice guidelines for acute pulmonary edema,* pages 220 and 221, and *Managing ineffective breathing pattern,* page 222.)

Practice guidelines offer several advantages. Because they spell out the steps to follow for a patient with a particular nursing diagnosis, they can help you provide thorough care and ensure that the patient receives consistent care from all caregivers. Many detailed practice guidelines even specify what to teach the patient and what to document, and they include a reference section that lets you quickly determine how up-to-date they are.

Some practice guidelines also spell out the role of other health care professionals, helping all team members coordinate their efforts. And by supplying such comprehensive instruction, practice guidelines help teach inexperienced staff members. Used in conjunction with other plans of care or alone, practice guidelines can also save documentation time.

Using practice guidelines

Use the practice guidelines that best fit your patient. You'll use some practice guidelines, such as the generic one for pain, for several patients. You'll use others rarely. For example, the practice guideline — Potential for violence: self-directed — applies mainly to patients in psychiatric settings. If you find that a practice guideline doesn't exist for a patient problem, you can help develop a new one.

Once you've selected a practice guideline, make sure that you tailor it to fit your patient's needs. Record any modifications you made on the patient's plan of care.

Documenting practice guidelines

To document a practice guideline on a plan of care, note in the interventions section that you'll follow the guideline. Write, for instance, "Follow impaired gas exchange guideline." Or list the practice guidelines you plan to use on a flow sheet. Be sure to document any modifications you'll need to make.

After you intervene, simply write in your progress notes that you followed the practice guidelines, or check the practice guidelines off on your flow sheet and initial it. The guidelines themselves usually remain at the nurses' station.

Patient-teaching plan

You'll also need to include a patient-teaching plan as part of your plan of care. You may either include this on your main plan or write a separate plan. Today, many health care facilities require a separate plan because of the emphasis placed on patient teaching by accrediting and regulatory organizations. The need to control costs and the current practice of discharg-

Nursing Process

Using a standardized plan of care

The plan of care below is for a patient with a nursing diagnosis of decreased cardiac output. To customize it to your patient, you'd complete the diagnosis—including signs and symptoms—and fill in the expected outcome. You'd also modify, add, or delete interventions as necessary.

Date _1/8/95_

Nursing diagnosis
Decreased cardiac output R/T reduced stroke volume secondary to fluid volume overload.

Target date _1/9/95_

Expected outcome
Adequate cardiac output (AEB): _>4.0 L/min_
Heart rate: _Apical rate <90_
BP: _140/80 mm Hg_
Pedal pulse: _palpable and regular_
Radial pulse: _palpable and regular_
Cardiac rhythm: _normal sinus rhythm_
Cardiac index: _>3L/min/m²_
Pulmonary artery wedge pressure (PAWP): _10 mm Hg_
Pulmonary artery pressure (PAP) _20/12 mm Hg_
SvO_2: _Between 60% and 80%_
Urine output in ml/hr: _>30 ml/hr_

Date _1/8/95_

Interventions
- Monitor ECG for rate and rhythm; note ectopic beats. If arrhythmias occur, note patient's response. Document and report findings and follow appropriate arrhythmia protocol.
- Monitor SvO_2, T, R, and central pressures continuously.
- Monitor other hemodynamic pressures q _1_ hr and p.r.n.
- Auscultate heart sounds and palpate peripheral pulses q _2_ hr and p.r.n.
- Monitor I & O q _1_ hr. Notify doctor if output <30 ml/hr x 2 hr.
- Administer medications and fluids as ordered, noting effectiveness and adverse reactions. Titrate vasoactive drugs p.r.n. Follow appropriate vasoactive drug protocol to wean pt. as tolerated.
- Monitor O_2 therapy or other ventilatory assistance.
- Decrease patient's activity to reduce O_2 demands. Increase as tolerated.
- Assess and document LOC. Assess for changes q _1_ hr and p.r.n.
- Additional interventions:
Inspect for pedal and sacral edema q 2 hr.

ing patients earlier also calls for more extensive teaching plans.

Purpose of the teaching plan
Besides identifying what the patient needs to learn and how he'll be taught, a teaching plan sets criteria for evaluating how well he learns. The plan also helps all the patient's educators coordinate their teach-

ing. Plus, it serves as legal proof that the patient received appropriate instruction and satisfies the requirements of regulatory agencies such as the JCAHO.

To make sure that your teaching plan does all that it should, you must carefully organize what the patient needs to learn and how you'll provide the instruction and measure the results. Work closely with other health care team members as well as with the patient and his family to make the plan's content realistic and attainable during his stay. And include provisions for follow-up teaching at home.

Also, keep your patient-teaching plan flexible. Take into account such variables as the patient being unreceptive because of a poor night's sleep as well as your own daily time limits.

Components of the plan

Although the scope of each teaching plan differs, all should contain the same elements:
• patient-learning needs
• expected learning outcomes
• teaching content, organized from the simplest concepts to the most complex
• teaching methods and tools.

Patient-learning needs. Identifying learning needs helps you decide which outcomes you should establish for your patient. Be sure to take into account not only what you, the doctor, and other health care team members want the patient to learn, but also what he wants to learn.

Expected learning outcomes. As with your other patient care outcomes, expected learning outcomes should focus on the patient and be readily measurable.

Your patient's learning behaviors and the outcomes you develop fall into three categories:
• cognitive, relating to understanding
• psychomotor, covering manual skills
• affective, dealing with attitudes.

For a patient learning to give himself subcutaneous injections, identifying an injection site would be the cognitive outcome; giving the injection, the psychomotor outcome; and coping with the need for injections, the affective outcome. (See *Writing clear learning outcomes,* page 223.)

To help formulate precise, measurable outcomes, decide which evaluation techniques will best reveal the patient's progress. For cognitive learning, you might use questions and answers; for psychomotor learning, you might use return demonstration. To measure affective learning, which can be difficult because changes in attitudes develop slowly, you can use several evaluation techniques. To determine whether a patient has overcome his anxiety about giving himself an injection, you can ask him if he still feels anxious. You can also assess his willingness to perform the procedure. And you can observe whether he hesitates or shows other signs of stress while doing it.

Teaching content. Next, you'll need to select what to teach the patient to help him achieve the expected outcomes. As you make these decisions, be sure to include family members and other caregivers in your plan. Even if a patient will learn to care for himself, you can teach a family member how to provide physical and emotional support. You can also teach a family member to serve as a source of informa-

(Text continues on page 223.)

Practice guidelines for acute pulmonary edema

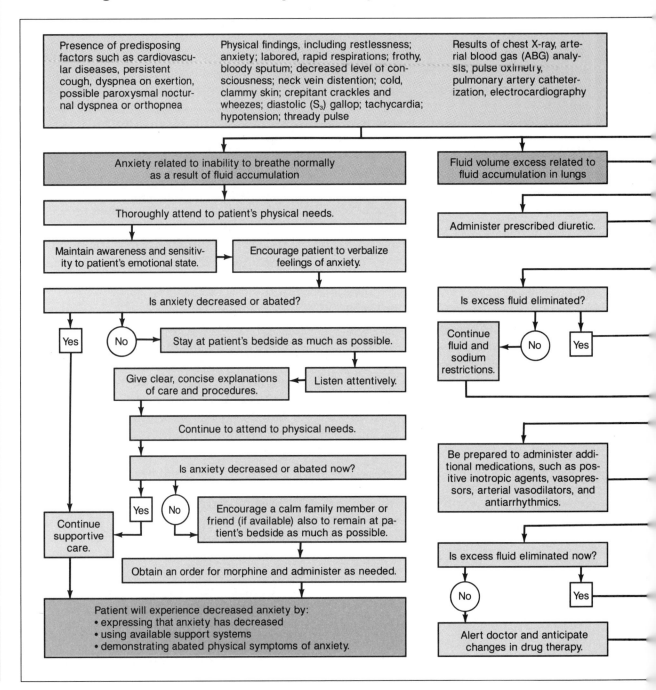

Nursing Process

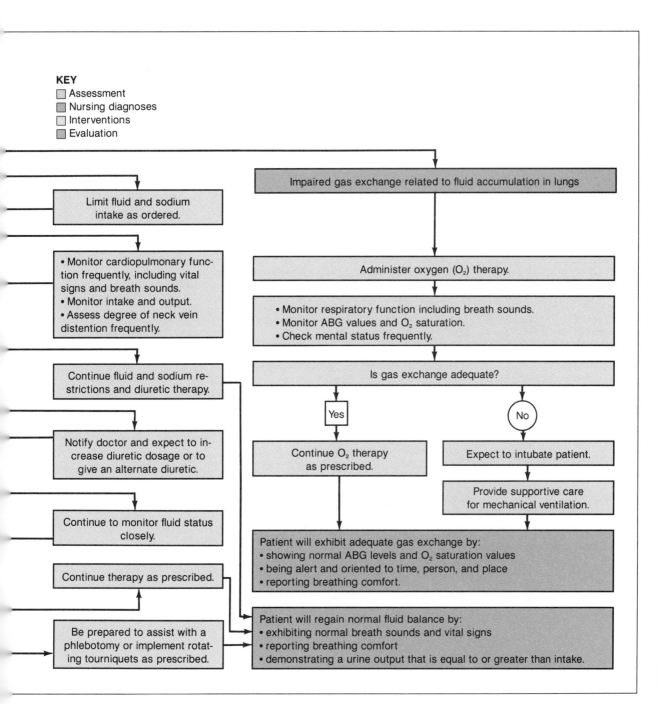

KEY
☐ Assessment
▨ Nursing diagnoses
☐ Interventions
▨ Evaluation

Impaired gas exchange related to fluid accumulation in lungs

Limit fluid and sodium intake as ordered.

Administer oxygen (O_2) therapy.

• Monitor cardiopulmonary function frequently, including vital signs and breath sounds.
• Monitor intake and output.
• Assess degree of neck vein distention frequently.

• Monitor respiratory function including breath sounds.
• Monitor ABG values and O_2 saturation.
• Check mental status frequently.

Continue fluid and sodium restrictions and diuretic therapy.

Is gas exchange adequate?

Yes

No

Notify doctor and expect to increase diuretic dosage or to give an alternate diuretic.

Continue O_2 therapy as prescribed.

Expect to intubate patient.

Continue to monitor fluid status closely.

Provide supportive care for mechanical ventilation.

Patient will exhibit adequate gas exchange by:
• showing normal ABG levels and O_2 saturation values
• being alert and oriented to time, person, and place
• reporting breathing comfort.

Continue therapy as prescribed.

Be prepared to assist with a phlebotomy or implement rotating tourniquets as prescribed.

Patient will regain normal fluid balance by:
• exhibiting normal breath sounds and vital signs
• reporting breathing comfort
• demonstrating a urine output that is equal to or greater than intake.

Managing ineffective breathing pattern

A portion of a practice guideline appears below for a patient who has chronic obstructive pulmonary disease (COPD) with the nursing diagnosis of ineffective breathing pattern.

NURSING DIAGNOSIS AND PATIENT OUTCOMES	IMPLEMENTATION	EVALUATION
Ineffective breathing pattern related to decreased lung compliance and air trapping By _____ , the patient will: • demonstrate a respiratory rate within ±5 of baseline • maintain ABG levels within acceptable ranges • verbalize his understanding of the disease process, including its causes and risk factors • demonstrate diaphragmatic pursed-lip breathing • take all medication as prescribed • use oxygen as prescribed.	• Monitor respiratory function. Auscultate breath sounds, noting improvement or deterioration. Obtain arterial blood gas (ABG) levels and pulmonary function tests as ordered. • Explain lung anatomy and physiology, using illustrated teaching materials if possible. • Explain COPD, its physiologic effects, and its complications. • Review the most common signs and symptoms associated with the disease: dyspnea, especially with exertion; fatigue; cough; occasional mucus production; weight loss; rapid heart rate; irregular pulse; and use of accessory muscles to help with breathing because of limited diaphragm function. • Explain the purpose of diaphragmatic pursed-lip breathing for patients with COPD; demonstrate the correct technique and have the patient perform a return demonstration. • If the patient smokes, provide information about smoking cessation groups in the community. • Explain the importance of avoiding fumes, respiratory irritants, temperature extremes, and exposure to upper respiratory tract infections. • Review the patient's medications and explain the rationale for their use, their dosages, and possible adverse effects. Advise him to report any adverse reactions to the doctor immediately. • For the patient receiving oxygen, explain the rationale for therapy and the safe use of equipment. Explain that the oxygen flow rate should never be increased above the prescribed target.	• The patient's respiratory rate remains within ±5 of baseline. • ABG levels return to established limits and remain within them. • Patient verbalizes an understanding of his disease. • Patient properly demonstrates diaphragmatic pursed-lip breathing. • Patient takes all medication as prescribed. • Patient demonstrates the appropriate use of oxygen as prescribed.

Writing clear learning outcomes

The patient's learning behaviors fall into three categories: cognitive, psychomotor, and affective. With these categories in mind, you can write clear, concise, expected learning outcomes. Remember, your outcomes should clarify what you're going to teach, indicate the behavior you expect to see, and set criteria for evaluating what the patient has learned.

Review the two sets of sample learning outcomes for a patient with chronic renal failure. Notice that the outcomes in the well-phrased set start with a precise action verb, confine themselves to one task, and describe measurable and observable learning. In contrast, the poorly phrased outcomes may encompass many tasks and describe learning that's difficult or even impossible to measure.

WELL-PHRASED LEARNING OUTCOMES	POORLY PHRASED LEARNING OUTCOMES
Cognitive domain	
The patient with chronic renal failure will be able to:	
• state when to take each prescribed drug	• know his medication schedule
• describe symptoms of elevated blood pressure	• know when his blood pressure is elevated
• list permitted and prohibited foods on his diet.	• realize his dietary restrictions.
Psychomotor domain	
The patient with chronic renal failure will be able to:	
• take his blood pressure accurately, using a stethoscope and a sphygmomanometer	• take his blood pressure
• read a thermometer correctly	• use a thermometer
• collect a urine specimen, using sterile technique.	• bring in a urine specimen for laboratory studies.
Affective domain	
The patient with chronic renal failure will be able to:	
• comply with dietary restrictions to maintain normal electrolyte values	• appreciate the relationship of diet to renal failure
• verbally express his feelings about adjustments to be made in the home environment	• adjust successfully to limitations imposed by chronic renal failure
• keep scheduled doctors' appointments.	• realize the importance of seeing his doctor.

tion in case the patient forgets some aspect of his care.

Once you've decided what to teach, carefully organize it. Start with the simplest concepts and work toward the more complex ones. You'll find this especially helpful for teaching a patient with little education or one who doesn't learn well by listening.

Teaching methods. You'll also need to select the appropriate teaching method for your patient. You can probably plan to do most of your teaching on a one-on-one basis. This method gives you a chance to learn about your patient, build a relationship with him, and tailor your teaching to his learning needs.

But you can use other methods too—either in place of or in conjunction with one-on-one teaching. For instance, you may want to incorporate demonstration, practice, and return demonstration in your teaching plan. Role playing can help involve your patient in learning, as can case studies, which call for him to evaluate how someone else with his disorder responds to different situations. Self-monitoring also involves the patient because he must assess his situation and determine which aspects of his environment or behavior need correction. If you have several patients who need similar instruction, you can also try group teaching or lecturing.

Teaching tools. Finally, you must include the teaching tools you intend to use. These tools—ranging from printed pamphlets to closed-circuit television programs—can help familiarize the patient with a topic.

When choosing your tools, focus on what will work best for the particular patient. For instance, if your patient likes to watch how something is done, he may respond best to a videotape of a procedure, a closed-circuit television demonstration, or a slide show. For a patient who prefers a hands-on approach, you might use a working model or let him handle the equipment he'll use. A computerized patient-teaching program may be best for a patient who likes to work interactively at his own pace. And some patients may simply want to read about their disorders.

Keep the abilities and limitations of your patient in mind as you choose. For instance, if you plan to provide him with written materials to reinforce your instructions, make sure that he can understand them. (The average adult has only a seventh-grade reading level.)

To get the tools you need, consult the staff-development instructors on your unit, the health care facility's librarian, or staff specialists. If your facility doesn't have what you need, you might try the pharmaceutical and medical supply companies in your community. And don't overlook national associations and foundations such as the American Cancer Society. These organizations usually have large supplies of patient-education materials written with the layperson in mind.

Documenting the patient-teaching plan

Several forms are available for documenting your patient-teaching plan. Many of them include the phases of the nursing process as they relate to patient education. (See *Documenting patient teaching*.)

Patient-teaching plans come in two basic types. Like the traditional plan of care, one type provides only the format and calls for you to come up with the plan. When a patient requires extensive teaching, you may be able to use a standardized plan instead, checking off or dating steps as you complete them and adding or deleting information to individualize the plan.

Depending on the plan's format, it may include space for problems that may hinder learning, comments and evaluations, and dates and signatures. Or you may be instructed to include this information in the progress notes. No matter

BETTER CHARTING

Documenting patient teaching

Below you'll find the first page of a patient-teaching flow sheet. Such flow sheets let you quickly and easily tailor your teaching plan to fit your patient's needs.

PATIENT-TEACHING FLOW SHEET

DIABETES MELLITUS

Problems affecting learning

☐ None
☑ Fatigue or pain
☐ Communication problem

☐ Cognitive or sensory impairment
☐ Physical disability

☐ Lack of motivation
☐ Other _____

LEARNING OUTCOMES	INITIAL TEACHING						REINFORCEMENT					
	Date	Time	Learner	Techniques and tools	Evaluation	Initials	Date	Time	Learner	Techniques and tools	Evaluation	Initials
Basic knowledge • Define diabetes mellitus (DM).	1/11/95	1000	P	E,W	S	JM	1/11/95	1100	P	E,W	S	JM
• List four symptoms of DM.	1/11/95	1000	P	E,W	S	JM	1/11/95	1100	P	E,W	S	JM
Medication • State the action of insulin and its effects on the body.	1/11/95	1000	P	E,W	S	JM						
• List the three major classifications of insulin. Give their onsets, peaks, and durations.	1/11/95	1000	P	E,W,V	Dv	JM						
• Demonstrate the ability to draw up insulin in a syringe and mix the correct amount.	1/11/95	1000	P	D	S	JM						

KEY

Learner
P = patient
S = spouse
M = mother
F = father
D1 = daughter 1
D2 = daughter 2
S1 = son 1
S2 = son 2
O = other

Teaching techniques
D = demonstration
E = explanation
R = role-playing

Teaching tools
F = filmstrip
P = physical model
S = slide
V = videotape
W = written material

Evaluation
S = states understanding
D = demonstrates understanding
Dp = demonstrates understanding with physical coaching
Dv = demonstrates understanding with verbal coaching
T = passes written test
N = no indication of learning
NE = not evaluated

which plan you use, it becomes a permanent part of the medical record.

Discharge planning
The final part of the planning process, the discharge plan has become more important in recent years because of the trend toward shorter hospital stays. You'll need to start your discharge planning the day your patient is admitted—or sooner for a planned admission. Such early planning can help avert problems.

Responsibility for discharge planning
In some health care facilities, the social services department carries the major responsibility for discharge planning. Larger organizations may hire a nurse discharge planner to facilitate home care planning. But staff nurses still play the major role in preparing patients and caregivers to assume responsibility for ongoing care.

Even if you don't have the primary responsibility for discharge planning, you still play an important part. You and other health care team members need to coordinate your efforts with the discharge planners or social services department. Typically, you'll do this at a multidisciplinary discharge conference, in which team members evaluate the patient's discharge needs, discuss appropriate plans, and evaluate his progress.

Components of the plan
A discharge plan should note the anticipated length of stay and specify what the patient needs to learn, including:
• diet
• medications
• treatments
• physical activity limitations

• signs and symptoms to report to the doctor
• follow-up medical care
• equipment
• appropriate community resources and support groups.

As part of your plan, make sure that the patient receives an instruction sheet to reinforce what he learns during patient teaching and what he needs to remember about follow-up care.

The discharge plan should also spell out future care, including the setting for it, the patient's intended caregiver and support systems, actual or potential barriers to care, and any referrals.

Documenting the discharge plan
How you document the discharge plan will depend on the policy at your health care facility. Some policies require you to include your assessment of discharge needs on the initial assessment form, then document the discharge plan itself on a separate form. At many facilities, you must include the discharge plan as a component of the discharge summary. Some forms used for discharge planning allow several members of the health care team to include information.

Case management
A method of delivering health care that controls costs while still ensuring quality care, case management goes a step beyond planned care to managed care. It came into being after the government introduced the prospective payment system in 1983. Under this system Medicare pays the facility based on the patient's diagnosis—not on his length of stay or the number or types of services he receives. Thus, the fa-

cility loses money if the patient has a lengthy stay or develops complications.

Such a system forces health care facilities to deliver cost-effective care—without compromising the quality of care. And the case management system proposes to help them do that by managing each patient's care to meet both clinical and financial goals.

Your role in case management

If you become a case manager, your role will expand beyond giving nursing care. You'll learn to manage a closely monitored and controlled system of multidisciplinary care. And you'll take on responsibility for outcomes, length of stay, and use of resources throughout the patient's illness—not just during your shift.

How the system works

When a patient is assigned a particular DRG, he's also assigned a case manager. (In some facilities, a patient isn't assigned a DRG until after discharge—in which case, you'll need to make an educated guess about which DRG he'll be assigned to.) Each DRG case management plan has standard outcome criteria and includes medical and nursing interventions as well as interventions from other disciplines.

As the case manager for a patient, you'll discuss the outcomes with the patient and his family, using the established time line for the patient's DRG. This time line should cover all the processes that must occur for the patient to reach the expected outcome, including tests, procedures, and patient teaching, and the resources such as social services the patient will need. If it doesn't, you'll adapt it as necessary to fit the patient's needs. If possible, you should do all this before the

patient is even admitted, but you must complete these steps within the time limit set by your facility—usually 24 hours.

Once the patient is admitted, the multidisciplinary team evaluates his progress and suggests any necessary revisions, keeping in mind the need for continuity of care and the best use of resources. You'll document any variations in the time line, processes, or outcomes, along with the reasons for the changes. Plus, you'll keep a lookout for duplication of services and medical orders.

You must also start discharge planning, beginning an assessment of the patient's discharge needs at or before admission. And you're responsible for activating home health care services—including obtaining personnel and equipment—well before discharge.

Case management systems

Several case management systems and various adaptations exist. And health care facilities continue to create new systems. But most facilities pattern their systems after the one developed at the New England Medical Center (NEMC), one of the first centers to use case management in an acute care setting. Facilities typically adapt this system to meet their own needs and philosophy of care.

Tools for case management

Most facilities also pattern their case management tools after those used in the NEMC system. Called the case management plan and the critical pathway or health care map, these tools allow you to direct, evaluate, and revise patient progress and outcomes.

Case management plan

The basic tool of case management systems, the case management plan spells out the standardized care a patient with a specific DRG should receive. The plan covers:
• nursing-related problems
• patient outcomes
• intermediate patient outcomes
• nursing interventions
• medical interventions
• target times.

Each subsection of the plan covers a care unit the patient may be admitted to during his illness. For instance, a patient with a myocardial infarction may go to both the critical care and medical-surgical units.

Critical pathway

Because of the length of case management plans, you probably won't use them on a daily basis. Instead, you'll turn to an abbreviated form of the plan: the critical pathway. The pathway covers only the key events that must occur for the patient to be discharged by the target date. Such events include consultations, diagnostic tests, physical activities the patient must perform, treatments, diet, medications, discharge planning, and patient teaching. (See *Following a critical pathway for congestive heart failure.*)

Once you've established a pathway, you must note any variances from it, grouping them by cause. Variances may result from the system, the caregivers, or a problem the patient develops, and they can be justifiable or not. For instance, you may have a patient who doesn't walk in the hall as scheduled. If he has a secondary infection that prevents him from walking, you'll list the variance as justifiable. But if the patient simply prefers to stay in bed watching television, you'll need to list the variance as unjustifiable and take steps to correct the problem.

At shift report each day, you should review the critical pathways with the other nurses. Before you go off duty, note any changes in the expected length of stay and point out critical events scheduled for the next shift to the nurses coming on duty. Also, discuss any variances that may have occurred during your shift.

Drawbacks of case management

The case management system usually works well for a patient with one primary diagnosis, no secondary diagnoses, and few complications. But for some patients, you'll have trouble even establishing a time line. For instance, you can't easily predict when treatment will succeed for a patient with a seizure disorder. And for a patient with several variances, the expected course of treatment and length of stay will likely change, and documentation can become lengthy and complicated.

Nursing interventions

Documenting nursing interventions has long been standard practice. But documentation methods have changed dramatically over the years, mainly because of frustration with tedious traditional methods and the urgent economic need to streamline hospital operations. No longer must you always write lengthy narrative notes. In many cases, you can use flow sheets or refer to practice guidelines instead.

This section will help you keep pace with these changes by explaining how to perform and document your interventions.

Following a critical pathway for congestive heart failure

Below is a critical pathway for nursing care for 4 days—the estimated hospital stay for congestive heart failure. The patient's copy of the pathway may be followed by the nurse's copy or vice versa.

CRITICAL PATHWAY: Congestive heart failure PATIENT COPY
ESTIMATED LENGTH OF STAY: 4 Days

CARE CATEGORIES	Day of Admission	Day 2	Day 3	Day 4
ACTIVITY	• Walk around as you are able. Don't become overtired or short of breath. • Remain in bed for 30 minutes before and 60 minutes after meals.	• Increase your activity slowly. Start by sitting up in the chair for meals and walking short distances with the help of the nurses twice a day.	• You should start to feel better and be able to do mild activities without your O_2. If your doctor suggests using O_2 at home, a home health nurse will check on you for a few weeks.	• You should be able to walk in the halls and take your own bath without trouble breathing. • You'll go home today if your doctor feels you're ready.
NUTRITION	• You'll be on a no added salt diet. The dietitian will explain this. (Salt makes your swelling worse and causes your heart to work even harder.) A salt substitute is available if you need it.	• Low-salt diet	• Low-salt diet	• Low-salt diet. Ask your doctor or nurse if you should continue this diet at home.
TREATMENTS	• The nurse will check your vital signs. • The nurse will measure the amount of fluid you take in and put out. • The nurse will listen to your heart and lungs to see if they are getting better. • You may have to use O_2 for the first day or two to help you breathe easier. • You'll be weighed daily. • You'll have an I.V. catheter placed in your hand or arm. This will be used to give you medication. • You may be placed on a telemetry heart monitor. Nurses in the intensive care unit will monitor your heart's rhythm.	• Treatments will remain the same.	• Some treatments will remain the same. • You'll use O_2 only when you feel you need it. • The heart monitor will be discontinued if previously ordered.	• Some treatments will remain the same. • Your O_2 may be discontinued. • Your I.V. catheter will be removed if you're going home.
TEACHING	• The nurse will explain CHF and your medications. • Please ask questions about anything you don't understand.	• The nurse will give you information sheets that explain the medication you'll take at home. • The nurse will review the right foods to eat and which foods to avoid.	• Make sure you keep your follow-up appointment with your doctor and know which problems may require medical attention.	• Your doctor may order follow-up teaching and care by a home health nurse.

(continued)

Following a critical pathway for congestive heart failure *(continued)*

NURSE'S COPY

CRITICAL PATHWAY: Congestive heart failure
Supplies given: Adm. kit *PN2/1/95*   **Urinal** *PN2/1/95*   **Bedpan** *PN2/1/95*   **Air Mattress** *PN2/1/95*

CARE CATEGORIES	Day of admission	Day 2	Day 3	Day 4
ACTIVITY	**Nursing diagnosis** Activity intolerance related to dyspnea • Restrict activity 30 minutes before and 60 minutes after meals. **Expected outcome** • Activity as tolerated	• Restrict activity 30 minutes before and 60 minutes after meals. • Pt . should sit up in a chair 30 min t.i.d. for meals. • Pt . may ambulate 60′ in hall b.i.d. with assistance. • Pt . has bathroom privileges. **Expected outcome** • Able to tolerate activity without distress	• Pt . may ambulate 100′ t.i.d. **Expected outcome** • Able to perform ADLs and ambulation without O_2	• Prepare pt. for discharge home. **Expected outcome** • Able to tolerate activity without distress and without O_2
NUTRITION Needs assistance? *no* Consultation needed? *no*	• No added salt diet • Other _____ _____	• No added salt diet • Other _____	No added salt diet • Other _____	• No added salt diet • Other _____
TREATMENTS	**Nursing diagnosis** Fluid volume excess related to compromised regulatory mechanisms • Monitor VS every 4 hr. • Monitor I & O. • Weigh the pt. daily. • Institute telemetry monitoring if ordered. • Insert an intermittent infusion device for medication administration if necessary. • Administer O_2 at *3 L/min.* • Assess breath and heart sounds every 8 hr and p.r.n. • Assess peripheral pulses and edema q 8 hr. **Expected outcomes** • Pt.'s foot edema decreases or pt. loses weight (minimum 1 lb [0.5 kg]) by Day 2. • Pt.'s breath sounds improve by Day 2.	• Monitor VS every 4 hr. • Monitor I & O. • Weigh the pt. daily. • Perform telemetry monitoring if ordered. • Maintain pt.'s intermittent infusion device. • Administer O_2 at *3 L/min.* • Assess breath and heart sounds every 8 hr and p.r.n. • Assess peripheral edema and pulses every 8 hr. **Expected outcomes** • Pt.'s foot edema is decreased or pt. has lost weight (minimum 1 lb [0.5 kg]). • Pt. has improved breath sounds.	• Monitor the pt'.s VS every 8 hr. • Monitor I & O. • Weigh the pt. daily. • Discontinue telemetry monitoring if ordered. • Maintain the intermittent infusion device. • Administer O_2 p.r.n. (If still needed, consult cardiopulmonary services for need for home O_2.) • Assess breath and heart sounds every 8 hr. • Assess peripheral pulses and edema every 8 hr. **Expected outcomes** • Foot and ankle edema resolves by Day 4. • Unlabored respirations by Day 4	• Monitor VS every 8 hr. • Monitor I & O. • Weigh the pt. daily. • Remove the intermittent infusion device. • Discontinue O_2. • Assess breath and heart sounds every 8 hr. • Assess peripheral edema and pulses every 8 hr. **Expected outcomes** • Foot and ankle edema resolved • Unlabored respirations

Following a critical pathway for congestive heart failure   *(continued)*

CARE CATEGORIES	Day of admission	Day 2	Day 3	Day 4
Teaching	• Review plan of care with pt. and give him a copy. • Discuss the disorder and explain medications. • Is a home health care referral needed? *yes* • Is home O₂ needed? *possibly* **Expected outcome** • Pt. can verbalize understanding of present medications by Day 2.	• Reinforce teachings of admission day. **Expected outcome** • Pt. can verbalize understanding of present medications.	• Give pt. written instructions about his medication and home care. • Arrange home health care referral if needed. • Arrange home O₂ if needed. **Expected outcome** • Pt. can verbalize understanding of present medications, home care, and follow-up medical plans by Day 4.	• Reinforce teachings of Day 3. **Expected outcomes** • Pt. can verbalize understanding of present medications. • Review discharge instructions and medications, and make sure that patient can verbalize understanding. • Pt. can verbalize importance of follow-up visit and when to call doctor.
Nurse's signature and date	*Patricia Norris, RN* 2/1/95	*Patricia Norris, RN* 2/2/95	*Patricia Norris, RN* 2/3/95	*Patricia Norris, RN* 2/4/95

OTHER FOCAL AREAS
Durable power of attorney *yes PN 2/1/95*   Living will *yes PN 2/1/95*   Code status *full PN 2/1/95*

And you'll read how to document patient teaching and your patient's discharge summary.

Performing interventions

Nursing intervention represents a crucial step in the nursing process. When you carry out your interventions, you're putting your carefully constructed plan of care into action.

Once you've established and recorded your plan of care, you'll begin to implement it. You'll find that your interventions fall into two general categories: interdependent and independent. Before performing either type, you'll need to make a brief reassessment.

Need for reassessment

Just before performing a particular intervention, you should quickly reassess the patient to ensure that your plan of care remains appropriate. For example, what if the plan calls for helping the patient walk every 2 hours throughout the day, but your reassessment reveals that he recently returned from a physical therapy session and feels fatigued? In this case, making the patient walk would be inappropriate — despite the plan of care.

Types of interventions

Interdependent interventions include those you perform in collaboration with other health care professionals to help achieve a patient outcome. For example, if the outcome calls for the patient to walk independently on level surfaces, you'd support the physical therapist's regimen by reinforcing positioning and ambulation techniques between therapy sessions.

Interdependent interventions also include activities you perform at a doctor's request to help implement the medical regimen. These activities include administering medications and performing invasive procedures, such as indwelling urinary catheter insertion and venipuncture.

Independent interventions are measures you take at your own discretion, independent of other health care team members. Such interventions include instituting common comfort measures and teaching routine self-care techniques.

Documenting interventions

You need to record the fact that you performed an intervention, the time you performed it, the patient's response to it, and any other interventions that you took based on his response. You should also include your reasons for these additional interventions. Recording all this information makes your documentation outcome-oriented.

You can document interventions on graphic records, a patient care flow sheet that integrates all nurses' notes for a 1-day period, integrated or separate nurses' progress notes, and other specialized documentation forms, such as the medication administration record (MAR). Your facility's policies will dictate the exact style, format, and location of your documentation. You'll record interventions when you give routine care, observe changes in the patient's condition, give emergency care,

and administer medications. (See Chapter 7, Documentation of Everyday Events, and Chapter 8, Legally Perilous Charting Practices, for more information on charting specific interventions.)

Routine care
For years, the JCAHO has encouraged health care facilities to use flow sheets for documenting routine care measures. In response, many facilities have developed these forms for such measures as making basic assessments, giving wound care, and providing hygiene. In many facilities, you may also use flow sheets to document vital signs checks, I.V. monitoring, equipment checks, patient education, and discharge summaries. Some flow sheets are simple patient care checklists; others provide space for you to record specific care given. (See Chapter 5, Documentation Methods, for more information on flow sheets and samples of different types.)

Because of their brevity, flow sheets make documenting and reviewing documented material quick and easy. Specifically, they allow you to evaluate patient trends at a glance. But keep in mind that overusing flow sheets can lead to fragmented documentation that may obscure the patient's clinical picture.

Changes in condition
In your progress notes, you'll need to document any changes in your patient's condition. Suppose, for instance, that you observe a sudden increase in your patient's wound drainage. In a narrative format, your progress note describing this observation should look something like the sample note on page 233.

12/5/94	1100	℗ arm wound drainage has
		saturated six 4" x 4" gauze
		pads and one 4" x 8" dress-
		ing since last dressing check
		at 1000. Wound dimensions
		remain as on 12/4 note, but
		drainage now dark yellow and
		foul-smelling. Obtained speci-
		mens for culture and sensitivity
		testing and sent to the lab
		per impaired skin integrity
		practice guidelines. Cleaned
		wound with 0.9% sodium
		chloride solution. (See plan
		of care for dressing change
		orders.) Pt. states, "My arm
		is really throbbing." Adminis-
		tered Darvocet-N and repo-
		sitioned patient to semi-
		Fowler's position with ℗ arm
		supported on pillow. ————
		———————— Louise Davis, RN

This example refers to a practice guideline or standard of care for patients with a nursing diagnosis of impaired skin integrity. Because this protocol mandates cleaning with 0.9% sodium chloride solution and culture and sensitivity testing for a patient with purulent wound drainage, no further orders or clarification are required.

The note also directs readers to the patient's plan of care for specific dressing change methods. The reader would also know to check the MAR for specific information about the pain medication given.

The note goes on to specify information about the other pain-relief measure implemented as well as the patient's comments about the pain's characteristics. And it doesn't repeat information recorded elsewhere in the chart, so it's concise yet informative.

Patient teaching

With each patient, you'll need to implement the teaching plan you've created and evaluate its effectiveness. And, of course, you'll need to clearly and completely document your teaching sessions and the results. Doing so provides a permanent legal record of the extent and success of teaching. Thus, your documentation may serve as your defense against charges of insufficient patient care—even years later. Your clear documentation also helps administrators gauge the overall worth of a specific patient-education program. And your documentation can help you demonstrate cost-effectiveness or support your requests for improving patient care.

Direct benefits

Documenting exactly what you've taught the patient also saves time by preventing duplication of patient-teaching efforts by other staff members. By checking your notes, another nurse can determine precisely what's been covered and what she should teach next, without skipping essential information. This is important for patients with complicated needs who may receive care from several nurses.

Take the case of a hypertensive patient who requires instruction in several areas, including diet, medication, exercise, and self-care. Successful teaching hinges on a clear record of what's been taught by everyone involved in his care. When staff members communicate by documenting what they've taught and how well the patient has learned, the teaching plan can be evaluated and revised as needed. And the patient will get the care he needs.

You can also use your documentation to help motivate your patient. As appropriate, show him your record of his learning successes and encourage him to continue. Moreover, by recording the patient's response to your teaching and your assessment of his progress, you're gathering some of the data necessary to evaluate the effectiveness of your teaching, the patient's degree of knowledge or competency, and the appropriateness of his learning outcomes.

Documentation tools

In many facilities, you'll document patient teaching on preprinted forms that become part of the clinical record. Using these forms not only makes documentation quicker, but also ensures that it's complete.

If your facility doesn't have a preprinted form, you might talk to your supervisor about developing one. In the meantime, write accurate, detailed narrative notes to document your patient teaching.

Whether you use a preprinted form or narrative notes, keep these tips in mind:
• Check your facility's policies and procedures regarding when, where, and how to document your teaching.
• Each shift, ask yourself these questions: "What part of the teaching plan did I complete?" and "What other teaching have I given this patient or his significant other?" Then document your answers.
• Be sure that your documentation indicates that the patient's ongoing educational needs are being met.
• Before discharge, document the patient's remaining learning needs.

Patient discharge

JCAHO requirements specify that when preparing a patient for discharge, you must document your assessment of his continuing care needs as well as referrals for such care. To facilitate this documentation (and to save charting time), many facilities have developed combined discharge summaries and patient instructions. (See *Documenting discharge and patient instruction.*)

This documentation tool combines all the essential information required on a discharge summary as well as the instructions given to the patient. Typically, you'll keep one copy of the form in the clinical record and give one copy to the patient. The copy you keep can then provide useful information for further teaching and evaluation.

Of course, not all facilities use these forms. Some still require a narrative discharge summary. If you must use this type of documentation, be sure to include the following information:
• patient's status on admission and discharge
• significant highlights of the hospitalization
• outcomes of your interventions
• resolved and unresolved patient problems, continuing care needs for unresolved problems, and specific referrals for continuing care
• instructions given to the patient or significant other about medications, treatments, activity, diet, referrals, and follow-up appointments, as well as any other special instructions.

BETTER CHARTING

Documenting discharge and patient instruction

This sample combines your discharge summary with your postdischarge instructions for the patient. You'd give a copy of this form to the patient at discharge.

DISCHARGE SUMMARY

Date: _1/2/95_
Time: _1100_

Destination
☑ Home
☐ Nursing home
☐ Other

Mobility
☑ Ambulatory
☐ Wheelchair
☐ Stretcher

PATIENT STATUS
General
☑ TPR   _97.7 P.O. – 82 – 18_
☑ BP   _126/82_
☑ Eating regularly
☐ Comments _____

Skin
☑ Good condition
☐ Wound _____
☐ Other _____

Bowels
☑ Regular movement
☐ Irregular movement
☐ Ostomy

Bladder
☑ Continent
☐ Urinary frequency
☐ Incontinent
☐ Catheter
   Type _____
   Date changed _____

Compliance
☑ Understands physical condition
☑ Willing to comply with regimen
☑ States understanding of instructions
☐ Comments _____
_____

Medications
☐ Preadmission medications returned
_____
☑ Prescriptions given to patient
_____
☐ Medications given to patient
_____
☑ Patient or family knows of allergies
_____
Nurse's signature: _Helen P. Long, RN_

PATIENT INSTRUCTIONS

Diet
☑ Unrestricted
☐ Restricted _____
_____
_____
☐ Restricted low sodium _____
☐ Comments _____
_____

Activities
☑ Walking
☑ Climbing stairs
☑ Riding in car
☑ Driving car
☑ Showering

☐ Taking a tub bath
☑ Engaging in sexual intercourse
☑ Resuming regular activity
☑ Lifting
☑ Exercising

☐ Other _____
_____

(continued)

Documenting discharge and patient instruction (continued)

Medications

Tylenol #3

Dosage, route, and time

1 2 tablets orally every 8 hours as needed for headache

Special instructions

Referral

☑ Call Dr. Cook and schedule an appointment 1 week from today

☐ Home health care agency

☐ Other

If you have questions, call Dr. Cook at 555-1930.

I've read and understood these instructions, and I've received a copy of this form.

Date: 1/2/95

Patient or significant other

Grace Borden

Nurse and doctor

Helen P. Long, RN   Nathan J. Cook MD

Evaluation

The current emphasis on evaluating your interventions has changed documentation. Traditional documentation methods didn't always reflect the end results of nursing care. But today, your progress notes must include an assessment of your patient's progress toward the expected outcomes you've established in the plan of care.

This new method, called outcomes and evaluation documentation, focuses on the patient's response to nursing care and thus enables the nurse to provide high-quality, cost-effective care. It's now replacing narrative charting and lengthy, hand-written plans of care. (See *Writing clear evaluation statements.*)

The belief that hands-on care is more important than documentation is one reason why nurses often focus more on nursing interventions than on documenting patient responses. Outcomes and evaluation documentation force nurses to focus on patient responses. And when you evaluate the results of your interventions, you help ensure that your plan is working.

Evaluation of care gives the nurse a chance to:
• determine if her original assessment findings still apply
• uncover complications
• analyze patterns or trends in the patient's care and his responses to it
• assess the patient's response to all aspects of care, including medications, changes in diet or activity, procedures, unusual incidents or problems, and teaching
• determine how closely care conforms with established standards
• measure how well she has cared for the patient
• assess the performance of other members of the health care team
• identify opportunities to improve the quality of care.

When to perform evaluation

Evaluation itself is an ongoing process that takes place whenever you see your patient. But how often you're required to make evaluations will be influenced by several factors, including where you work. If you work in an acute care setting, your facility's policy may require you to review

Writing clear evaluation statements

Below you'll find examples of clear evaluation statements describing common outcomes. Note that they include specific details of care provided and objective evidence of the patient's response to care.

■ *Response to p.r.n. medication within 1 hour of administration*
"Pt. states pain decreased from 8 to 4 (on a scale of 1 to 10) 10 minutes after receiving I.V. morphine."
"Vomiting subsided 1 hr after 25 mg P.O. of prochlorperazine."

■ *Response to patient education*
"Able to describe the signs and symptoms of a postoperative wound infection."
"Despite repeated attempts, pt. couldn't identify signs of hypoglycemia."

■ *Tolerance of change or increase in activity*
"Able to walk across the room, approximately 15′, without dyspnea."

■ *Ability to perform activities of daily living, particularly those that may influence discharge planning*
"Unable to wash self independently because of left-sided weakness."
"Requires a walker to ambulate to bathroom."

■ *Tolerance of treatments*
"Consumed full liquid lunch; pt. stated she was hungry and wanted solid food."
"Skin became pink and less dusky 15 minutes after nasal O_2 was administered at 4 liters/min."
"Unable to tolerate having head of bed lowered from 90 degrees to 45 degrees; became dyspneic."

plans of care every 24 hours. But if you work in a long-term care facility, the required interval between evaluations may be up to 30 days. In either case, this doesn't mean that you shouldn't evaluate and revise the plan of care more often, if warranted.

Evaluating expected outcomes

Evaluation includes gathering reassessment data, comparing findings with the outcome criteria, determining the extent of outcome achievement (outcome met, partially met, or not met), writing evaluation statements, and revising the plan of care.

Revision starts with determining whether the patient has achieved the outcomes. If they have been fully met, and you decide that the problem is resolved, the plan can be discontinued. If the problem persists, the plan continues, with new target dates, until the desired status is achieved.

If outcomes are partially met or unmet, you must identify interfering factors, such as misinterpreted information, and revise the plan accordingly. This may involve the following:
• clarifying or amending the data base to reflect newly discovered information
• reexamining and correcting nursing diagnoses
• establishing outcome criteria that reflect new information and new or amended nursing strategies
• adding the revised nursing plan of care to the original document
• recording the rationale for the revisions in the nurse's progress notes.

Documenting evaluation

Evaluation statements should indicate whether expected outcomes were achieved and should list evidence supporting this conclusion. Base these statements on outcome criteria from the plan of care, and use active verbs, such as "demonstrate" or "ambulate." Include the patient's response to specific treatments (such as medication administration or physical therapy), and describe the conditions under which the response occurred or failed to occur. Document patient teaching and palliative or preventive care as well.

After evaluating the outcome, be sure to record it in the patient's chart with clear statements that demonstrate the patient's progress toward meeting the expected outcomes.

Selected references

Edelstein, J. "A Study of Nursing Documentation," *Nursing Management* 21(11):40-43, 46, November 1990.

Eggland, E.T. *Nursing Documentation Resource Guide.* Gaithersburg, Md.: Aspen Pubs., Inc., 1993.

Murray, R.B., and Zentner, J.P. *Nursing Assessment and Health Promotion Strategies Through the Lifespan,* 5th ed. Norwalk, Conn.: Appleton & Lange, 1993.

Rasmusen, N., and Gengler, T. "Clinical Pathways of Care: The Route to Better Communication," *Nursing94* 24(2):47-49, February 1994.

Nursing Process

CHAPTER SEVEN

Documentation of Everyday Events

Your patient's chart communicates important information about his condition and hospital course to other nurses and members of the health care team. Without this record, neither you nor other caregivers can do an appropriate job. That's why incomplete or improper charting has enormous implications.

Poor charting poses a threat to your patient's health and to your career as well. To avert serious problems, take the time to document not only accurately, objectively, and thoroughly but also consistently and legibly—in routine and exceptional situations.

In this chapter, you'll read about specific situations that you may encounter in your practice. A discussion of each is followed by a documentation example. Among the situations discussed are nursing procedures, common charting flaws, patient noncompliance, interdisciplinary communications, doctors' orders, and incidents.

Nursing procedures

Your notes about routine nursing procedures should appear in the patient's chart. Include information about the procedure, who performed it, how it was performed, how the patient tolerated it (if applicable), and any subsequent adverse effects (if applicable).

Typically, your documentation will include drug administration, I.V. therapy, supportive care, assistive procedures, infection control, diagnostic tests, pain control, codes, intake and output monitoring, skin and wound care, patient's belongings, and shift reports.

Drug administration

Your employer probably includes a medication administration record (MAR) in your documentation system. Commonly included in a card file (a medication Kardex) or on a separate medication administration sheet, the MAR serves as the central record of medication orders and their execution. The MAR is part of the patient's permanent record.

When using the MAR, consider these guidelines:
• Know and follow your hospital's policies and procedures for recording drug orders and charting drug administration.
• Make sure that all drug orders include the patient's full name, the date, the drug's name, dose, administration route or method, and frequency. When appropriate, include the specific number of doses given or the stop date. When administering a drug dose immediately—or stat—make sure to record the time. Also be certain to include drug allergy information.
• Write legibly.
• Use only standard abbreviations approved by the hospital. When doubtful about an abbreviation, write out the word or phrase.
• After administering the first dose, sign your full name, licensure status, and your initials in the appropriate space on the MAR.
• Record drugs immediately after administration so that another nurse doesn't give the drug again. (See *Using a medication administration record.*)

If you document medication administration by computer, chart your information

Using a medication administration record

This sample shows how to chart the administration of drugs, including those given as needed (p.r.n.)

MEDICATION ADMINISTRATION RECORD

ALLERGIES — (use red)

Penicillin

PLATE: James Row

00012345

Diagnosis: HTN, TIAs

Order date	Expiration date	Discontinued date	Drug and dosage	Refrigeration necessary	Time given	Date given					
						1/20	1/21	1/22			
1/20/95	1/27		hydralazine 50 mg		0600	DG	AO	AO			
			↑ P.O. q.i.d.		1200	RM	CB	CB			
					1800	GF	MD	GF			
					2400	GF	MD	GF			
1/20/95	1/27		Dyazide 25 mg		0900	RM	CB	CB			
			↑ P.O. q.d. in a.m.								
1/20/95	1/23		warfarin 2.5 mg		1400	RM	CB	CB			
			P.O. q.d. @ 1400 hr.								
			(Call H.O. c̄ PT q.d.)								
1/20/95	1/27		ferrous sulfate		0900	RM	CB	CB			
			325 mg ↑ P.O. t.i.d.		1300	RM	CB	CB			
			c̄ meals		1800	GF	MD	GF			

Initials	Signature	Initials	Signature
DG	Diane Holmen, RN		
RM	Rose Malecki RN		
GF	Grace Fedor, RN		
AO	Andrew Ortiz, RN		
CB	Carl Barton, RN		

(continued)

Using a medication administration record *(continued)*

_314A_	_Langley_	_Stephen_		_Dr. Murphy_	_HTN_
BED NO.	NAME-LAST	FIRST		PHYSICIAN	DIAGNOSIS

P.R.N. MEDICATIONS, SINGLE ORDERS, PREOPERATIVE ORDERS

Drug and dosage	Order date	Expiration date	Discontinued date	Refrigeration necessary					
acetaminophen gr X P.O. _94° p.r.n. headache_	_1/20/95_	_1/27_			Date	_1/20_			
					Time given	_0700_			
					Initials	_RM_			
flurazepam 15 mg _ẗ P.O. qhs p.r.n._	_1/20/95_	_1/23_			Date				
					Time given				
					Initials				
mom 30 ml P.O. qhs _p.r.n. constipation_	_1/20/95_	_1/27_			Date				
					Time given				
					Initials				
Mylanta 30 ml P.O. _q 4 hr p.r.n._ _indigestion_					Date				
					Time given				
					Initials				

Initials	Signature	Initials	Signature
_RM_	_Rosi Malecki RN_		

for each drug right after you give it. This is particularly important if you don't use printouts as a backup. By keying in information immediately, you ensure that all health care team members have access to the latest drug administration data for the patient.

Document the reason a drug was not given (for example, if the patient is having a test, which requires him not to take the drug). Many nurses leave out this important step.

Occasionally, you may suspect a connection between a patient's medication and an adverse event such as illness, injury, or even death. In such a case, report this information to the Food and Drug Administration (FDA) on a MedWatch form issued by the FDA. (See *Reporting adverse events and product problems to the FDA.*)

Reporting adverse events and product problems to the FDA

Even large, well-designed clinical trials can't guarantee that adverse reactions will never arise once a drug or medical device is approved for use. If a drug causes an adverse reaction in only 1 in 5,000 patients, such a reaction could easily be missed in clinical trials. Or the drug could interact with other drugs in ways unrevealed during clinical trials.

As a nurse, you play a key role in reporting adverse events and product problems. Reporting such problems helps ensure the safety of products that the Food and Drug Administration (FDA) regulates.

What to report

Complete a MedWatch form when you suspect that a drug, a medical device, a special nutritional product, or other products regulated by the FDA are responsible for:
• death
• life-threatening illness
• initial or prolonged hospitalization
• disability
• congenital anomaly
• the need for any medical or surgical intervention to prevent a permanent impairment or an injury.

Also inform the FDA promptly of product quality problems, such as:
• defective devices
• inaccurate or unreadable product labels
• packaging or product mix-ups
• contamination or stability problems
• particulates in injectable drugs.

Your responsibility in reporting

When filing a MedWatch form, keep in mind that you're not expected to establish a connection between the product and the problem. You don't have to include a lot of details; you only have to report the adverse event or the problem with the drug or the product.

What's more, you don't even have to wait until the evidence seems compelling. FDA regulations protect your identity and the identities of your patient and employer.

Further guidelines

The MedWatch form merges the individual forms used in the past to report adverse drug reactions, drug quality product problems, device quality product problems, and adverse reactions to medical devices. Send completed forms to the FDA by using the fax number or mailing address on the form.

File a separate MedWatch form for each patient, and attach additional pages if needed. If appropriate, report product problems to the manufacturer as well as to the FDA. Also remember to comply with your health care facility's protocols for reporting adverse events associated with drugs and medical devices.

FDA response

The FDA will report back to you on the actions it takes and will continue to work to instruct health care professionals about adverse events.

(continued)

Reporting adverse events and product problems to the FDA *(continued)*

Form Approved: OMB No. 0910-0291 Expires: 12/31/94
See OMB statement on reverse

MEDWATCH
THE FDA MEDICAL PRODUCTS REPORTING PROGRAM

For **VOLUNTARY** reporting
by health professionals of adverse
events and product problems

Page ___ of ___

FDA Use Only (NUR 93)

Triage unit
sequence #

A. Patient information

1. Patient identifier

In confidence

2. Age at time of event:
or ___
Date of birth:

3. Sex
☒ female
☐ male

4. Weight
___ lbs
or
59 kgs

B. Adverse event or product problem

1. ☒ Adverse event and/or ☐ Product problem (e.g., defects/malfunctions)

2. Outcomes attributed to adverse event (check all that apply)
☐ death ___ (mo/day/yr)
☐ life-threatening
☐ hospitalization – initial or prolonged
☐ disability
☐ congenital anomaly
☐ required intervention to prevent permanent impairment/damage
☐ other: ___

3. Date of event (mo/day/yr) 3/8/94

4. Date of this report (mo/day/yr) 3/8/94

5. Describe event or problem

After Reconstituting 100 mg
Vial with 10 ml. of
bacteriostatic water, the
drug crystallized and
turned yellow.
Drug was Not given.

6. Relevant tests/laboratory data, including dates

7. Other relevant history, including preexisting medical conditions (e.g., allergies, race, pregnancy, smoking and alcohol use, hepatic/renal dysfunction, etc.)

C. Suspect medication(s)

1. Name (give labeled strength & mfr/labeler, if known)
#1 Leucovorin Calcium for
#2 Injection – 100 mg vial

2. Dose, frequency & route used
#1 100 mg IV x1
#2

3. Therapy dates (if unknown, give duration) from/to (or best estimate)
#1 3/8/94
#2

4. Diagnosis for use (indication)
#1 Megaloblastic Anemia
#2

5. Event abated after use stopped or dose reduced
#1 ☐ yes ☐ no ☐ doesn't apply
#2 ☐ yes ☐ no ☐ doesn't apply

6. Lot # (if known)
#1 # 891
#2

7. Exp. date (if known)
#1
#2

8. Event reappeared after reintroduction
#1 ☐ yes ☐ no ☐ doesn't apply
#2 ☐ yes ☐ no ☐ doesn't apply

9. NDC # (for product problems only)
— — —

10. Concomitant medical products and therapy dates (exclude treatment of event)

D. Suspect medical device

1. Brand name

2. Type of device

3. Manufacturer name & address

4. Operator of device
☐ health professional
☐ lay user/patient
☐ other:

5. Expiration date (mo/day/yr)

6.
model # ___
catalog # ___
serial # ___
lot # ___
other # ___

7. If implanted, give date (mo/day/yr)

8. If explanted, give date (mo/day/yr)

9. Device available for evaluation? (Do not send to FDA)
☒ yes ☐ no ☐ returned to manufacturer on ___ (mo/day/yr)

10. Concomitant medical products and therapy dates (exclude treatment of event)

E. Reporter (see confidentiality section on back)

1. Name, address & phone #
Patricia Cohen
987 Elm Ave
Cincinatti, Ohio

2. Health professional? ☒ yes ☐ no

3. Occupation R.N.

4. Also reported to
☐ manufacturer
☐ user facility
☒ distributor

5. If you do NOT want your identity disclosed to the manufacturer, place an "X" in this box. ☐

Mail to: MEDWATCH
5600 Fishers Lane
Rockville, MD 20852-9787
or **FAX to:** 1-800-FDA-0178

FDA

Drugs given p.r.n.

Chart all drugs administered as needed (p.r.n.). For eye, ear, or nose drops, for example, chart the number of drops and where they were inserted. For suppositories, chart the type of suppository (rectal, vaginal, or urethral) and how it was tolerated by the patient. For dermal drugs, chart the size and location of the area to which you applied the drug. Also describe the condition of the skin or wound. For dermal patches, chart the location of the patch.

If you administer all drugs according to the accepted standards, you don't need to include more specific information in the chart. However, if the MAR doesn't include space to document exceptional data (such as the patient's response to drugs given p.r.n. or deviations from the drug order, such as patient refusal), document the information as narrative in the chart.

12/8/94	0900	Pt. refused KCL elixir, stating
		that it makes her feel nause-
		ated and she can't stand the
		taste. Dr. Miller notified .
		K-Dur tabs ordered and
		given. Pt. tolerated K-Dur well.
		—————— Betty Griffin, RN

Narcotic drugs

When you administer a narcotic, you must give the drug and document administration according to federal, state, and institutional regulations. These regulations require narcotic drugs to be counted after each nursing shift to ensure an accurate drug count. Before administering a narcotic, verify the amount of drug in the container, and sign out the medication on the appropriate form.

Another regulation requires that a second nurse document your activity and observe you if a narcotic or part of a dose must be wasted.

If you discover a discrepancy in the narcotic count, follow your employer's policy for reporting this. You'll need to file an incident report as well. An investigation will follow.

I.V. therapy

Currently, more than 80% of hospitalized patients receive some form of I.V. therapy. Whether providing fluid or electrolyte replacement, total parenteral nutrition (TPN), drugs, or blood products, you'll need to document all facets of I.V. therapy carefully—including not only administration but also subsequent complications of I.V. therapy.

Keep in mind that an accurate description of your care provides a clear record of treatments and drugs received by your patient. This record provides legal protection for you and your employer and furnishes health care insurers with the data they need to approve and provide reimbursement for equipment and supplies.

Depending on your facility's policy, document I.V. therapy in your progress notes or on a special I.V. therapy sheet or flowchart or in another format. (See *Using a flow sheet to document I.V. therapy,* pages 246 and 247.)

If venipuncture requires more than one attempt, document the number of attempts made and the type of assistance required.

Once you establish an I.V. route, remember to document the date, time, and venipuncture site together with the equipment

(Text continues on page 248.)

Using a flow sheet to document I.V. therapy

This sample shows the typical features of an I.V. therapy flow sheet.

I.V. THERAPY FLOW SHEET

Diagnosis: ℞ mastectomy
Venipuncture limitations: Ⓛ arm only
Permanent access: None

Date and time	1/14/95 1400	1/15 0800					
Patient visit	2	1					
Site status	1	1					
Procedure	R	C					
Gauge I.V. device	20	✓					
Catheter type	J	J					
Location	LPF	LPF					
Date of insertion	1/14	1/15					
Routine site rotation	—	—					
Phlebitis	1+	1					
Infiltration	1	O					
Other	1	—					
No. of failed attempts	O	—					
Lock status	—	—					
Flush	—	—					
Tubing: Macrodrip	✓	✓					
Minidrip							
Valleylab							
Filter							
Extension	✓	✓					
Dressing change	✓	—					
Blood sample drawn	—	—					
Subcutaneous access port	—	—					
Patient response	1	1					
Patient teaching	1	1					
Nurse's initials	BG	KC					

Initials	Signature		Initials	Signature
BG	Betty Griffin, RN			
KC	Kathy Collins, RN			

Using a flow sheet to document I.V. therapy *(continued)*

Date	Time	Patient care notes
1/14/95	1400	IV D5½NSS c̄ 40 meq KCL infusing @ 125 ml/hr. ——Patricia Quinn

KEY

Patient visit
1 Routine rounds
2 Unit request
3 Patient not available for rounds

Site status
1 Within normal limits
2 Dressing intact

Procedure
S Start
R Restart
C Check
D Discontinue

Catheter Type
J Jelco
P Protective Cath
H Huber
I Intima
TC Twin Cath

Location
RH right hand
RW right wrist
RA right arm
RPF right posterior forearm
RC right antecubital
RU right upper arm
LH left hand
LW left wrist
LA left arm
LPF left posterior forearm
LC left antecubital
LU left upper arm
RF right foot
LF left foot
RJ right jugular
LJ left jugular

AB abdomen
BR Broviac
CD cutdown
IP introducer port
PRT subq port
GR Groshong catheter
DD double lumen dialysis catheter
PICC peripherally inserted central catheter
TL triple lumen catheter
HI Hickman catheter
SC subclavian catheter
SG Swan-Ganz catheter
TE Tenckhoff catheter

Phlebitis
1 No pain to slight pain at site; erythema; edema; no streak; no palpable cord
1 + Pain at site; erythema or edema; no streak, no palpable cord
2 + Pain at site; erythema or edema streak formation; nonpalpable cord
3 + Pain at site; erythema or edema; streak formation; palpable cord

Infiltration
0 + Slight edema - no infiltration
1 + Slight puffiness at site
2 + Swelling above or below site
3 + Skin cool and pale; large area of swelling above or below site

Other
1 Leaking
2 Occluded
3 Patient removed catheter
4 Other (see patient care notes)

Lock status
1 Site locked
2 Site unlocked
3 Caps changed

Flush
1 Heparin
2 Saline

Patient response
1 Patient tolerated
2 Unresponsive
3 Patient agitated or combative
4 Other (see patient care notes)

Patient teaching
1 Patient or family member indicates understanding of procedure
2 Instructed to call nurse for signs of redness, swelling, leaking, pain, or problem
3 Patient unable to comprehend
* Further documentation in patient care notes

used, such as the type and gauge of catheter or needle. You'll need to update your records each time you change the insertion site and change the venipuncture device or the I.V. tubing. Also document any reason for changing the I.V. site, such as extravasation, phlebitis, occlusion, patient removal, or a routine change according to hospital policy.

1/6/95	0200	A #20 Fr. angiocath inserted in the anterior portion of the right hand. Good blood return noted. I.V. of 1,000 ml D5½NSS with 20 mEq KCL running at 125 ml/hr. On Imed. I.V. tolerated well. Taught pt. about the need for I.V. therapy, its complications, and how to ambulate with I.V. Pt. stated that he understood. ———— *Kathy Collins, RN*

On each shift, be sure to document the type, amount, and flow rate of I.V. fluid, along with the condition of the I.V. site. Document each time that you flush the I.V. line, and identify any medication used to flush the line as well.

Take the time to document any complication precisely. For example, if extravasation occurs, stop the I.V. Then assess the amount of fluid infiltrated and notify the doctor.

If a chemotherapeutic drug extravasates, follow the procedure specified by your health care facility. In the chart, document the appearance of the I.V. site, the type of treatment given (especially any medication used as an antidote), and the kind of dressing applied to the site. Also

be sure to record every time that you flush this kind of I.V. line and the type and amount of fluid used.

If an allergic reaction occurs while the patient is receiving I.V. therapy, notify the doctor immediately. Document all pertinent information about the reaction in addition to your nursing interventions and the patient's response to them.

Record any patient teaching that you perform with the patient and his family, such as explaining the purpose of I.V. therapy, describing the procedure itself, and discussing any possible complications.

Total parenteral nutrition

If a patient is receiving TPN, document the type and location of the central line, the condition of the insertion site, and the volume and rate of the solution infused. Monitor any patient receiving TPN for adverse reactions and document your observations and interventions.

When you discontinue a central or peripheral I.V. line for TPN, record the date and time and the type of dressing applied. Also describe the appearance of the administration site.

Blood transfusions

Whether you administer blood or blood components, such as packed cells, plasma, platelets, or cryoprecipitates, you must use proper identification and cross-matching procedures to ensure that the patient receives the correct blood product for transfusion. After matching the patient's name, medical record number, blood group (or type) and Rh factor (both the patient's and the donor's), the cross-match data, and the blood bank identification number with the label on the blood bag, you'll need to clearly document that you did so.

The blood or blood component must be identified and documented properly by two health care professionals as well.

Once you have determined that all the information is correct and matches, you may administer the transfusion. On the transfusion record, document the date and time the transfusion was started and completed, the name of the health care professional that verified the information, the type and gauge of the catheter, and the total amount of the transfusion. Also record the patient's vital signs before and after the transfusion as well as any infusion device used, the flow rate, and any blood warming unit that was used.

If the patient receives his own blood, document the amount of autologous blood retrieved and reinfused in the intake and output records. Also monitor and document laboratory data during and after the autotransfusion as well as the patient's pre- and post-transfusion vital signs.

Pay particular attention to the patient's coagulation profile, hemoglobin and hematocrit values, and arterial blood gas and calcium levels.

Transfusion reaction

During a blood transfusion, the patient is at risk for developing a transfusion reaction. If he develops a reaction, stop the transfusion immediately and notify the doctor. Be sure to document the time and date of the reaction, the type and amount of infused blood or blood products, the time you started the transfusion, and the time you stopped it. Also record the clinical signs of the reaction in order of occurrence, the patient's vital signs, any urine specimen and blood samples sent to the laboratory for analysis, any treatment given, and the patient's response to the treatment. If required by the health care facility, complete a transfusion reaction form.

1/13/95	1400	Pt. reports chills. Cyanosis of the lips noted at 1350 hours, with PRBCs transfusing. Stopped infusion. Tubing changed. I.V. of 1,000 ml D₅NSS infusing at KVO rate in ®. Notified Dr. Evans. BP, 168/88; P, 104; R, 25; T, 97.6R. Blood sample taken from PRBCs. Two red-top tubes of blood drawn from pt. and sent to the laboratory. Urine specimen obtained from catheter. Urine specimen to lab for UA. Gave pt. diphenhydramine 50 mg I.M. Two blankets placed on pt.
	1415	Pt. reports he's getting warmer. BP, 148/80; P, 96; R, 20; T, 97.6 R.
	1430	Pt. no longer complaining of chills. I.V. of 1,000 ml D₅NSS infusing at 125 ml/hr. in ®. BP, 138/76; P, 80; R, 18; T, 98.4 R. ———— ——— Mary Jane Belinsky, RN

Supportive care procedures

Your daily nursing interventions constitute supportive care measures. Many can be documented on graphic forms and flow charts. Others must be described in progress notes or other forms. Among commonly documented nursing interventions are those that are provided after a major or minor surgical procedure (for example, pacemaker insertion, paracentesis, peritoneal dialysis, peritoneal lavage, or thoracic drainage) and those provided to support the patient throughout treatment (for example, cardiac monitoring, chest physiotherapy, mechanical ventilation, nasogastric [NG] tube insertion and removal, seizure management, tube feedings, and withdrawing arterial blood for analysis).

Surgical incision care

Besides documenting vital signs and level of consciousness (LOC) when the patient returns from surgery, pay particular attention to maintaining records pertaining to the surgical incision and drains and the care you provide.

11/10/94	0830	Dressing removed from midline abd. incision; no drainage noted on dressing. Incision well approximated and intact with staples. Margins ecchymotic; small amt. of serosanguineous drainage noted from distal portion of wound. Dry 4" x 4" sterile gauze pad applied. JP in LLQ draining serosanguineous fluid. Emptied 40 ml. JP drain intact. Insertion site without redness or drainage. Split 4" x 4" gauze applied to site and taped securely.————— Grace Fedor, RN

Also read the records that travel with the patient from the postanesthesia care unit. (See *Documenting postsurgical status.*) Look for a doctor's order directing whether you or the doctor will perform the first dressing change. The following features of documenting surgical wound care are important:

• the date, time, and type of wound care performed
• the wound's appearance (size, condition of margins, necrotic tissue if any), odor (if any), location of any drains, and drainage characteristics (type, color, consistency, and amount)
• dressing information, such as type and amount of new dressing or pouch applied
• additional wound care procedures provided, such as drain management, irrigation, packing, or application of a topical medication
• the patient's tolerance of the procedure.

Record special or detailed wound care instructions and pain management measures on the nursing plan of care. Document the color and amount of measurable drainage on the intake and output form.

If the patient will need wound care after discharge, provide and document appropriate instruction. The record should show that you explained aseptic technique, described how to examine the wound for signs of infection and other complications, demonstrated how to change the dressing, and provided written instructions for home care.

Pacemaker care

Record the date and time of temporary pacemaker placement, the reason for placement, the pacemaker settings, and the patient's response.

Document the patient's LOC and vital signs, noting which arm you used to obtain the blood pressure reading. Also note any complications (such as infection or chest pain) and interventions taken (such as X-ray studies to verify correct electrode placement).

Document the information obtained from a 12-lead electrocardiogram (ECG).

CHARTING GUIDELINES

Documenting postsurgical status

When your patient recovers sufficiently from the effects of anesthesia, he can be transferred from the operating room-postanesthesia care unit (OR-PACU) to his assigned unit for ongoing recovery and care. As the nurse on this service, you're responsible for the four-part documentation that travels with the patient. Here are some tips for making sure that all parts of the record are present and complete.

Part 1: History
Make sure this section of the OR-PACU report includes the patient's pertinent medical and surgical history (information that might affect the patient's response to anesthesia and his postoperative course).

Include drug allergies, medication history, chronic illnesses (coronary artery disease or chronic obstructive pulmonary disease, for example), significant surgical history and hospitalizations, and smoking history.

Part 2: Operation
Check that the following information is recorded in this section of the report, describing the surgery itself:
• the procedure performed
• the type and dosage of anesthetics administered
• the length of time the patient was anesthetized
• the patient's vital signs throughout surgery
• the volume of fluid lost and replaced
• drugs administered
• surgical complications
• tourniquet time

• any drains, tubes, implants, or dressings used in surgery and removed or still in place.

Part 3: Postanesthesia period
Be certain that this part of the record includes information about:
• pain medications and pain control devices that the patient received and how he responded to them.
• interventions that should continue on the unit. For example, if the patient underwent leg surgery and had a tourniquet on for a long time, he will need more frequent circulatory, motor, and neurologic checks. Or, if the anesthesiologist inserted an epidural catheter, the record should note any doctor's orders regarding medication administration or special care procedures.
• a flow sheet showing the patient's postanesthesia recovery scores on arrival and discharge in these areas: activity level, respiration, circulation, level of consciousness (LOC), and color.
• an account of unusual events or complications that occurred on the PACU—for instance, nausea or vomiting, shivering, hypothermia, arrhythmias, central anticholinergic syndrome, sore throat, back or neck pain, corneal abrasion, tooth loss during intubation, swollen lips or tongue, pharyngeal or laryngeal abrasion, and postspinal headache.

Part 4: Current status
Expect this section to describe the patient's status at the time of transfer. Information should include the patient's vital signs, LOC, and sensorium.

Obtain and include rhythm strips in the medical record at these times: before, during, and after pacemaker placement; anytime pacemaker settings change; and anytime the patient receives treatment resulting from a pacemaker complication.

1/9/95	0920	Pt. c̄ temporary transvenous
		pacer in Ⓛ subclavian vein.
		Rate 70, mA2, mV full
		demand. 100% ventricular
		paced rhythm noted on moni-
		tor. ECG obtained. Pacer sens-
		ing & capturing correctly. Site
		w/o redness or swelling.
		Dressing D&I.————
		———— John Mora, RN

As ECG monitoring continues, note capture, sensing rate, intrinsic beats, and competition of paced and intrinsic rhythms.

If the patient has a transcutaneous pacemaker, document the reason for this kind of pacing, the time pacing started, and the locations of the electrodes.

Paracentesis

When caring for a patient during and after paracentesis, be sure to document the date and time of the procedure, the puncture site, and whether or not the site was sutured. Also record the amount, color, viscosity, and odor of the initially aspirated fluid in your notes and in the fluid intake and output record.

If you're responsible for ongoing patient care, be sure to keep a running record of the patient's vital signs and nursing activities related to drainage and to dressing changes.

The record should indicate the frequency of drainage checks (typically, every 15 minutes for the first hour, every 30 minutes for the next 2 hours, every hour for the next 4 hours, then every 4 hours for the next 24 hours) and the patient's response to the procedure. Continue to document drainage characteristics, including color, amount, odor, and viscosity.

If peritoneal fluid leakage occurs, notify the doctor and document that you did so. Be sure to include the time and the date.

Also document daily patient weight and abdominal girth measurements and the number of fluid specimens sent to the laboratory for analysis.

1/10/95	1100	After procedure explained
		to pt. and consent obtained,
		Dr. Mayberry performed para-
		centesis in RLQ as per proto-
		col. 1,500 ml cloudy, pale-
		yellow fluid drained and
		sent to lab as ordered. Site
		sutured with one 3-0 silk
		suture. Sterile 4" x 4" gauze
		pad applied. No leakage noted
		at site. Abd. girth 44" pre-
		procedure and 42³/₄" post-
		procedure. Pt. tolerated pro-
		cedure w/o difficulty. VSS be-
		fore and after procedure as
		per flow sheet. Emotional
		support given to pt. ————
		———— Carol Barton, RN

Peritoneal dialysis

During and after dialysis, monitor and document the patient's response to treatment. Record his vital signs every 10 to 15 minutes for the first 1 to 2 hours of exchanges, then every 2 to 4 hours or as often as necessary. Also document any abrupt changes in the patient's condition, notify the doctor, and document doing so.

Document the amount of dialysate infused and drained and any medications added. Be sure to complete a peritoneal dialysis flowchart every 24 hours. Keep a record of the effluent's characteristics and the assessed negative or positive fluid balance at the end of each infusion-dwell-drain cycle. Also record each time that you notify the doctor of an abnormality.

Chart the patient's daily weight (immediately after the drain phase) and abdominal girth. Note the time of day and any variations in the weighing-measuring technique. Also daily, document physical assessment findings and fluid status.

Keep a record of equipment problems, such as kinked tubing or mechanical malfunction, and your interventions. Also note the condition of the patient's skin at the dialysis catheter site, the patient's reports of unusual discomfort or pain, and your interventions.

1/15/95	0700	Pt. receiving exchanges q̄ 2 hr
		of 1,500 cc 4.25 dialysate with
		500 units heparin and 2
		mEq KCL. Dialysate infused
		over 15 min. Dwell time 75
		min. Drain time 30 min.
		Drainage clear, pale-yellow
		fluid. (See flow sheet for
		fluid balance.) VSS. Pt.
		tolerates procedure. No
		cramping or discomfort.
		Skin warm, dry at RLQ cathe-
		ter site and no redness. Dry
		split 4" x 4" dressing applied
		p̄ site cleaned per protocol.
		———— Pamela Worth, RN

Peritoneal lavage

Frequently monitor and document the patient's vital signs and any signs or symptoms of shock—for example, tachycardia, decreased blood pressure, diaphoresis, dyspnea, or vertigo.

Keep a record of the incision site's condition and document the type and size of peritoneal dialysis catheter used, the type and amount of solution instilled and withdrawn from the peritoneal cavity, and the amount and color of fluid returned. Note whether the fluid flowed freely into and out of the abdomen. Record which specimens were obtained and sent to the laboratory.

Also note any complications that occurred and the nursing actions you took to manage them.

1/2/95	1500	NG tube inserted via L̇ nos-
		tril, to low Gomco suction. #16
		Fr. Foley catheter inserted to
		straight drainage. Dr. Mangle
		inserted #15 Fr. peritoneal
		catheter below umbilicus via
		trocar. Clear fluid withdrawn.
		700 ml warm NSS instilled
		as ordered and clamped. Pt.
		turned from side to side. NSS
		dwell time of 10 min. Then
		NSS drained freely from ab-
		domen. Fluid samples sent to
		lab. as ordered. Peritoneal
		catheter removed and incision
		closed by Dr. Mangle. 4" x 4"
		gauze pad c̄ povidone-iodine
		ointment applied to site. Pt.
		tolerated procedure well, VSS
		pre- and post-procedure.——
		———— Pamela Worth, RN

Thoracic drainage

Record the date and time thoracic drainage began, the type of system used, the amount of suction applied to the pleural cavity, and the initial presence or absence of bubbling or fluctuation in the water-seal chamber. Also record the initial amount and type of drainage and the patient's respiratory status.

At the end of each shift, record how frequently you inspected the drainage system and how frequently chest tubes were milked or stripped. Again, note the presence or absence of bubbling or fluctuation in the water-seal chamber, and enter the patient's respiratory status.

12/11/94	0900	ⓛ anterior CT intact to
		Pleurevac suction system to
		20 cm of suction. All connec-
		tions intact. 50 ml BRB drain-
		age noted since 0800. No air
		leak noted, + fluctuation. CT
		site dressing D&I, no crepitus
		palpated. Lungs clear bilater-
		ally. Chest expansion equal
		bilaterally. No SOB noted.
		RR 18-20 nonlabored. O₂ @
		2 L/min via NC.
		———— Andrew Ortiz, RN

Also record the condition of the chest dressings; the name, amount, and route of any pain medication you gave; complications that developed; and any subsequent interventions that you performed.

When documenting ongoing drainage characteristics, describe the color, consistency, and amount of thoracic drainage in the collection chamber. Be sure to include the time and date of each instance that you make such observations.

Keep a record of patient-teaching sessions and subsequent activities that the patient will perform, such as coughing and deep-breathing exercises, sitting upright, and splinting the insertion site to minimize pain.

Record the results of your respiratory assessments, including the rate and quality of the patient's respirations and auscultation findings. Also document the time and date when you notify the doctor of serious patient conditions, such as cyanosis, rapid or shallow breathing, subcutaneous emphysema, chest pain, or excessive bleeding.

Be sure to document each chest tube dressing change and findings related to the patient's skin condition at the chest tube site.

Cardiac monitoring

In your notes, document the date and time that monitoring begins and the monitoring leads used. Commit all rhythm strip readings to the record. Be sure to label the rhythm strip with the patient's name, his room number, and the date and time. Also document any changes in the patient's condition.

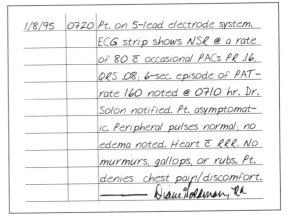

1/8/95	0720	Pt. on 5-lead electrode system.
		ECG strip shows NSR @ a rate
		of 80 c̄ occasional PACs PR .16,
		QRS .08; 6-sec. episode of PAT-
		rate 160 noted @ 0710 hr. Dr.
		Solon notified. Pt. asymptomat-
		ic. Peripheral pulses normal; no
		edema noted. Heart c̄ RRR. No
		murmurs, gallops, or rubs. Pt.
		denies chest pain/discomfort.
		———— Diane Holleman, RN

If cardiac monitoring will continue after the patient's discharge, document which caregivers can interpret dangerous rhythms and can perform cardiopulmonary resuscitation. Also teach troubleshooting techniques to use if the monitor malfunctions, and document your teaching efforts or referrals (for example, to equipment suppliers).

Chest physiotherapy

Whenever you perform chest physiotherapy, document the date and time of your interventions, the patient's positions for secretion drainage and length of time the patient remains in each position, the chest segments percussed or vibrated, and the characteristics of the secretion expelled (include color, amount, odor, viscosity, and the presence of blood). Also record indications of complications, the nursing actions taken, and the patient's tolerance of the treatment.

11/20/94	1415	Pt. placed on Ⓛ side c̄ foot of bed elevated. Chest PT and postural drainage performed for 10 min. from lower to middle then upper lobes as ordered. Pt. had productive cough and expelled large amt. of thick yellow sputum. Lungs clear p̄ chest PT. Procedure tolerated w/o difficulty. ————— Rose Malecki RN

Mechanical ventilation

Document the date and time that mechanical ventilation began. Note the type of ventilator used for the patient and its settings. Describe the patient's subjective and objective responses to mechanical ventilation (including vital signs, breath sounds, use of accessory muscles, intake and output, and weight).

12/6/94	1015	Pt. on Servo ventilator set at TV 750; F I O₂ 45%; 5 cm PEEP; AC of 12. RR 20 non-labored. #8 ETT in Ⓡ corner of mouth taped securely at 22-cm mark. Suctioned via ETT for large amt. of thick white secretions. Pulse oximeter reading 98%, Ⓛ lung clear. Ⓡ lung with basilar crackles and expiratory wheezes. No SOB noted. ————— Grace Fluharty, RN

Throughout mechanical ventilation, list any complications and subsequent interventions. Record all pertinent laboratory data, including results of any arterial blood gas (ABG) analyses and oxygen saturation findings.

If the patient is receiving pressure support ventilation or using a T-piece or tracheostomy collar, note the duration of spontaneous breathing and the patient's ability to maintain the weaning schedule. If the patient is receiving intermittent mandatory ventilation, with or without pressure-support ventilation, record the control breath rate, the time of each breath reduction, and the rate of spontaneous respirations.

Record any adjustments made in ventilator settings as a result of ABG levels, and document any adjustments of ventilator components, such as draining condensate into a collection trap and changing, cleaning, or discarding the tubing.

Note interventions implemented to promote mobility, to protect skin integrity, or to enhance ventilation. For example, record when and how you perform active or passive range-of-motion exercises, turn the patient, or position him upright for lung expansion.

Document assessment findings related to peripheral circulation, urine output, decreased cardiac output, fluid volume excess, or dehydration.

When possible, document sleep and wake periods, noting significant trends as appropriate.

Record any teaching efforts (involving the patient and appropriate caregivers) that you carried out in preparation for the patient's discharge. Take special care to record teaching associated with ventilator care and settings, artificial airway care, communication, nutrition, and therapeutic exercise.

Also indicate teaching discussions and demonstrations related to signs and symptoms of infection and equipment functioning. List any referrals you made to equipment vendors, home health agencies, and other community resources.

NG tube insertion and removal

Record the type and size of the NG tube that you insert and the date, time, and route of insertion as well. Describe the type and amount of suction (if used); drainage characteristics, such as amount, color, consistency, and odor; and the patient's tolerance of the insertion procedure.

1/15/95	1605	#12 Fr. NG tube placed in Ⓛ
		nostril. Placement verified and
		attached to low intermittent
		suction as ordered. Drainage
		pale green; heme −. Irrigated
		with 30 ml NSS q 2 hr. Pt. tol-
		erated procedure. Hypoactive
		b.s. in all 4 quadrants. ⸻
		⸻ MARL Roister, RN

Include in your notes any signs and symptoms signaling complications, such as nausea, vomiting, and abdominal distention. Document any subsequent irrigation procedures and continuing problems after irrigation.

Record the date and time of NG tube removal, the patient's tolerance of the procedure, and unusual events accompanying NG tube removal, such as nausea, vomiting, abdominal distention, and food intolerance.

Seizure management

Note in the medical record that the patient requires seizure precautions; also record all precautions taken. Record the date and time that a seizure began, as well as its duration and any precipitating factors. Identify any sensation that may be considered an aura. Describe any involuntary behavior occurring at onset, such as lip smacking, chewing movements, or hand and eye movements. Record any incontinence occurring during the seizure.

Document the patient's response to the seizure, the medications given, any complications resulting from the medications or the seizure, and any interventions performed. Finally, record your assessment of the patient's postseizure mental status.

1/10/94	1712	Pt. observed with generalized
		seizure activity lasting 2½
		min. Pt. sleeping at time
		of onset. Urinary inconti-
		nence during seizure. Seizure
		pads in place on bed before
		seizure. Pt. placed on Ⓛ side,
		airway patent, no N/V. Dr.
		Gordon notified of seizure.
		Diazepam 10 mg given I.V. as
		ordered. VS taken q 15 min.
		and p.r.n. (see flow sheet). Pt.
		currently obtunded (see neu-
		rologic flow sheet). No further
		seizure activity noted. ———
		——— Karen Huntsman, RN

1/8/95	0700	Full strength Pulmocare in-
		fusing via Flexiflow pump
		thru Dobhoff tube in Ⓡ nos-
		tril at 50 ml/hr. Tube place-
		ment checked and pt. main-
		tained with HOB raised about
		45°. 5 ml residual obtained.
		Pt. denies any N/V. normal
		active bowel sounds auscul-
		tated x 4 quad. Diphenoxylate
		elixir 2.5 mg given via f.t. for
		continuous diarrhea. Tube
		flushed with 30 ml H2O this
		shift as ordered. Pt. instructed
		to tell nurse of discomfort.
		——— Faye Gayle, RN

Tube feedings

Besides frequently assessing and documenting the patient's tolerance of the procedure and the feeding formula, keep careful records of the kind of tube feeding the patient is receiving (for example, duodenal or jejunal feedings or continuous drip or bolus), and the amount, rate, route, and method of feeding.

If you need to dilute a feeding formula, note the dilution strength for the record (for example, half- or three-quarters strength).

When you flush the feeding tube to maintain patency, be sure to document the time and the flushing solution (such as water or cranberry juice). If you must replace the feeding tube, document this activity as well.

Regularly assess and document the patient's gastric function and note any prescribed medications or treatments to relieve constipation or diarrhea.

When administering continuous feedings, check and document the infusion rate hourly.

Regularly record such laboratory test findings as the patient's urine and serum glucose, serum electrolyte, and blood urea nitrogen levels and serum osmolality values as well.

Be sure to document any feeding complications, such as hyperglycemia, glycosuria, and diarrhea.

If the patient will continue receiving tube feedings after discharge, document any instructions you give to the patient and appropriate caregivers and any referrals you make to suppliers or support agencies.

Withdrawal of arterial blood

When you must obtain blood for ABG analysis, keep careful records of the following: the patient's vital signs and temperature, the arterial puncture site, and the results of Allen's test. Also document any indications of circulatory impairment, such as swelling, discoloration, pain, numbness, or tingling in the bandaged arm or leg, and bleeding at the puncture site.

Document the time that the blood sample was drawn, the length of time pressure was applied to the site to control bleeding and, if appropriate, the type and amount of oxygen therapy that the patient was receiving.

1/16/95	1010	Blood drawn from Ⓡ radial
		artery p̄ + Allen's test c̄
		brisk capillary refill.
		Pressure applied to site for
		5 min. and pressure drsg.
		applied. No bleeding, hematoma,
		or swelling noted. Hand pink,
		warm c̄ 2-sec capillary refill.
		Sample for ABGs placed on
		ice and taken to lab. Pt. on
		40% CAM. T 99.2° F; Hgb 10.2.
		———— Pat Matting, RN

When filling out a laboratory request form for ABG analysis, be sure to include the following information for laboratory records: the patient's current temperature and respiratory rate, his most recent hemoglobin level, and the fraction of inspired oxygen and tidal volume if he's on mechanical ventilation.

Assistive procedures

When you assist a doctor in such procedures as bone marrow aspiration, esophageal tube insertion, insertion or removal of arterial or central venous lines, lumbar puncture, suture removal, or thoracentesis, your role also involves patient support, pa-

tient teaching, and evaluation of the patient's response.

Careful charting of these procedures is your responsibility. Document the name of the doctor performing the procedure, the patient's response to the procedure, the patient teaching provided, and any other pertinent information.

Bone marrow aspiration

When assisting the doctor with a bone marrow aspiration, document the date and time and the name of the doctor performing the procedure. Also describe the appearance of the specimen aspirated, the patient's response to the procedure, and the appearance of the aspiration site. Monitor the patient's vital signs after the procedure and observe the aspiration site for bleeding. Document any pertinent information about the specimen sent to the laboratory.

1/30/95	1000	Assisted Dr. Shelburne while
		he performed a bone marrow
		aspiration at 0915 hr. Pt.
		tolerated the procedure well
		with little discomfort. Speci-
		mens sent to lab, as ordered.
		The procedure was per-
		formed on the Ⓡ anterior iliac
		crest. No bleeding at site. VS:
		BP, 142/82; P, 88; R, 22. Afebrile.
		Bed rest being maintained.
		———— Margaret Little, RN

Esophageal tube insertion and removal

Make sure that your documentation includes the date and time that you assisted the doctor with inserting and removing the esophageal tube and the name of the doctor who performed the procedure.

As applicable, record the intragastric balloon pressure, the amount of air injected into the gastric balloon port, the amount of fluid used for gastric irrigation, and the color, consistency, and amount of gastric return both before and after lavage.

Because intraesophageal balloon pressure varies with respirations and esophageal contractions, be sure to record the baseline pressure, which is the most important pressure.

Document the patient's tolerance of both the insertion and removal procedures.

12/21/94	1210	Sengstaken-Blakemore tube
		placed w/o difficulty by Dr.
		Fasholt via ® nostril. 50 cc
		air injected into gastric bal-
		loon. Abdominal X-ray ob-
		tained to confirm placement.
		Gastric balloon inflated c̄
		500 cc air. Tube secured to
		football helmet traction. Large
		amt. BRB drainage noted. Tube
		irrigated c̄ 1800 ml of iced
		NSS till clear. NG tube placed
		in Ⓛ nostril and attached to
		8 mm of Ohio wall suction.
		Esophageal balloon inflated
		to 30 mm Hg and clamped.
		Equal BS bilat. No SOB, VSS.
		Pt. tolerated procedure.
		Emotional support given.──
		── Evelyn Sutcliffe, RN

Insertion and removal of an arterial line

When assisting the doctor who's inserting an arterial line, record the time, date, doctor's name, insertion site, and type, gauge, and length of the catheter.

12/5/94	0625	#20G arterial catheter placed
		in ® radial artery by anesthes.
		Dr. Soma on 2nd attempt
		after + Allen's test. Trans-
		ducer leveled and zeroed.
		Readings accurate to cuff
		pressures. Site w/o redness or
		swelling. 4" x 4" gauze pad c̄
		efodine ointment applied. ®
		hand and wrist taped and secured
		to armboard. Line flushes easily.
		Good waveform on monitor.
		Pt.'s hand pink and warm c̄ 2-sec
		capillary refill.-Susan Chang, RN

At removal, record the time, date, doctor's name, length of the catheter, and condition of the insertion site. If any catheter specimens were obtained for culture, be sure to document that too.

Insertion and removal of a central venous line

Typically when you assist the doctor who inserts a central venous line, you'll need to document the time and date of insertion, the length and location of the catheter, the solution infused, the doctor's name, and the patient's response to the procedure. Other measures that need to be noted include the time of the X-ray study performed to confirm the line's safe and correct placement, the X-ray results, and your notification of the doctor of the results.

12/24/94	1100	Procedure explained to pt.
		and consent obtained by Dr.
		Corona. Pt. in Trendelenburg
		position and TLC placed by
		Dr. Corona on 1st attempt in
		® SC. Cath. sutured in place
		c̄ 3-0 silk and sterile
		dressing applied per proto-
		col. All lines flushed c̄ 100
		units heparin and PC X-ray
		obtained to confirm line
		placement. VSS. Pt. tolerated
		procedure well. ———
		——— Luana Ortlip, RN

After assisting with a CV line's removal, record the time and date of removal and the type of antimicrobial ointment and dressing applied. Note the length of the catheter and the condition of the insertion site. Also document collecting any catheter specimens for culture or other analysis.

Lumbar puncture

During lumbar puncture, observe the patient closely for signs such as a change in LOC, dizziness, or changes in vital signs. Report these observations to the doctor and document them carefully.

Also record the cerebrospinal fluid (CSF) pressure initially and during the procedure. Record obtaining the test tube specimens of CSF as they are obtained. Document the patient's tolerance of the procedure and any pertinent information about the specimens in the chart.

Monitor the patient's condition, and keep him in a flat supine position for 6 to 12 hours. Encourage fluid intake, assess him for headache, and check the puncture site for leaking CSF. Document all of your observations and interventions.

Suture removal

Generally, you'll be asked to remove sutures alone (with a written medical order, of course). When documenting this procedure, note the appearance of the suture line, the date and time the sutures were removed, and whether the wound site contained purulent drainage. If you suspect infection at the site, notify the doctor, collect a specimen, and send it to the laboratory for analysis.

Thoracentesis

When assisting with a thoracentesis, assess the patient for any sudden or unusual pain, faintness, dizziness, or vital signs changes. Report these observations to the doctor immediately and record them as soon as possible. Document the date and the time, the name of the doctor performing the procedure, the amount and quality of fluid aspirated, and the patient's response to the procedure.

If later symptoms of pneumothorax, hemothorax, subcutaneous emphysema, or infection occur, notify the doctor immediately and document your observations and interventions on the chart. Also note whether you sent a fluid specimen to the laboratory for analysis.

Infection control

An important contributor to effective infection control is meticulous record keeping. Various federal agencies require documentation of infections so that the data can be assessed and used for preventing and controlling future infections. Also, the data you record help your health care facility meet national and local accreditation standards.

Typically, you must report any culture result that shows a positive infection and any surgery, drug, elevated temperature, X-ray finding, or specific treatment related to infection to your facility's infection control department. (See *Reporting diseases and infections,* pages 262 and 263.)

Document signs and symptoms of the infection and the steps you take to prevent its spread. Always follow universal precautions against direct contact with blood and body fluids, and be sure to document that you've done so.

12/28/94	1300	Wound and skin precautions maintained. Pt. temperature remains elevated at 102.3° R. Amount of purulent drainage from the incision has increased since yesterday. Dr. Levick notified. Repeat C&S ordered. Specimen obtained and sent to the lab. ————
		———— Lynne Karkoff, RN

Teach the patient and his family about these precautions, and document this also. Record the dates and times of your interventions both in the patient's chart and on the Kardex. Document any breach in an isolation technique and file an incident report should this occur. If the doctor prescribes a drug to treat the infection, record this as well.

Be sure to communicate the results of any culture and sensitivity studies to the doctor so that he may prescribe the appropriate drug to treat the infection. Record the patient's response to this drug.

Diagnostic tests

Before receiving a diagnosis, most patients undergo testing—as simple as a blood test or as complicated as magnetic resonance imaging. Enter all tests given to a patient in the chart, along with the patient's tolerance of the procedures.

Begin documenting diagnostic testing with any preliminary assessments you make of a patient's condition. For example, if your patient is pregnant or has certain allergies, record this information because it might affect the test or the test result. If the patient's age, illness, or disability requires special preparation for the test, remember to enter this information in his chart as well.

Always prepare the patient for the test and document any teaching you've done about the test itself and any follow-up care associated with it. Be sure to document the administration or withholding of drugs and preparations, special diets, food or fluid restrictions, enemas, and specimen collection.

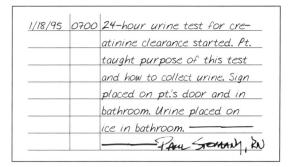

1/18/95	0700	24-hour urine test for creatinine clearance started. Pt. taught purpose of this test and how to collect urine. Sign placed on pt.'s door and in bathroom. Urine placed on ice in bathroom. ————
		———— Paul Stohany, RN

Pain control

Your primary goal is to eliminate or minimize your patient's pain. Determining its severity can be difficult, however, because pain is subjective. You can use a number of tools to assess pain; when you use

Reporting diseases and infections

The Centers for Disease Control and Prevention, the Occupational Safety and Health Administration, the Joint Committee on Accreditation of Health Care Organizations, and the American Hospital Association all require health care facilities to document and report certain diseases acquired in the community or in hospitals and other health care facilities.

Generally, the health care facility reports diseases to the appropriate local authorities. These authorities notify the state health department, which in turn reports the diseases to the appropriate federal agency or national organization.

Because regulations vary from community to community and state to state and because different agencies focus on different data, the list of reportable diseases isn't conclusive and may change periodically.

- Acquired immunodeficiency syndrome (AIDS)
- Amebiasis
- Animal bites
- Anthrax (cutaneous or pulmonary)
- Arbovirus
- Aseptic meningitis
- Botulism (food-borne, infant)
- Brucellosis
- Campylobacteriosis
- Chancroid
- Chlamydial infections
- Cholera
- Diarrhea of the newborn, epidemic
- Diphtheria (cutaneous or pharyngeal)
- Encephalitis (postinfectious or primary)
- Food poisoning
- Gastroenteritis (institutional outbreaks)
- Giardiasis
- Gonococcal infections
- Gonorrhea
- Group A beta-hemolytic streptococcal infections (including scarlet fever)
- Guillain-Barré syndrome
- Hepatitis A, infectious (include suspected source)
- Hepatitis B, serum (include suspected source)
- Hepatitis C (include suspected source)
- Hepatitis, unspecified (include suspected source)
- Histoplasmosis
- Influenza
- Kawasaki disease
- Lead poisoning
- *Legionella* infections (Legionnaires' disease)
- Leprosy
- Leptospirosis
- Listeriosis
- Lyme disease
- Lymphogranuloma venereum
- Malaria
- Measles (rubeola)
- Meningitis (specify etiology)
- Meningococcal disease
- Mumps
- Neonatal hypothyroidism
- Pertussis
- Phenylketonuria
- Plague (bubonic or pneumonic)
- Poliomyelitis (spinal paralytic)
- Psittacosis (ornithosis)
- Rabies
- Reye's syndrome

Reporting diseases and infections (continued)

- Rheumatic fever
- Rickettsial diseases (including Rocky Mountain spotted fever)
- Rubella (German measles) and congenital syndrome
- Salmonellosis (excluding typhoid fever)
- Shigellosis
- Staphylococcal infections (neonatal)
- Syphilis (congenital < 1 year)
- Syphilis (primary or secondary)

- Tetanus
- Toxic shock syndrome
- Toxoplasmosis
- Trichinosis
- Tuberculosis
- Tularemia
- Typhoid and paratyphoid fever
- Typhus (flea- and tick-borne)
- Varicella (chicken pox)
- Yellow fever

them, always document the results. (See *Assessing and documenting pain,* page 264.)

When charting pain levels and characteristics, first determine where the patient feels the pain, whether it's internal, external, localized, or diffuse. Also find out whether the pain interferes with the patient's sleep or other activities of daily living. Describe the pain in the patient's own words and enter them in the chart.

Be aware of the patient's body language and behaviors associated with pain. Does he wince or grimace? Does he move or squirm in bed? What positions seem to relieve or worsen the pain? What other measures (heat, cold, massage, drugs) relieve or heighten the pain? All of this information is important in assessing your patient's pain and should be documented.

Enter into the chart whichever interventions you take to alleviate your patient's pain and document the patient's responses to your interventions.

| 12/19/94 | 1600 | Pt. admitted to room 3042 with diagnosis of pancreatic cancer and severe pain in the LLQ. Pt. taking Percocet 2 tabs q 4 hr. at home without relief at present. Dr. Martin notified. Dilaudid 2 mg. ordered and given I.V. @ 1600 hrs. VS stable. Pt. resting at present.————— Kathy Collins, RN |

Codes

Guidelines established by the American Heart Association direct you to keep a written, chronological account of a patient's condition throughout resuscitative efforts. If you're a designated recorder for a patient's cardiopulmonary arrest record, document therapeutic interventions and the patient's responses to these as they occur. Don't rely on your memory to record

BETTER CHARTING

Assessing and documenting pain

Used appropriately, standard assessment tools, such as the McGill-Melzack Pain Questionnaire or the Initial Pain Assessment Tool (developed by McCaffery and Beebe), provide a solid foundation for your nursing diagnoses and plans of care. If your health care facility doesn't use standardized pain questionnaires, you can devise other pain measurement tools, such as the pain flow sheet or the visual and graphic rating scales that appear below. Whichever pain assessment tool you choose, remember to document its use and include the graphic record in your patient's chart.

Pain flow sheet

The flow sheet, possibly the most convenient tool for pain assessment, provides a standard for reevaluating the patient's pain at ongoing and regular intervals. It's also beneficial for patients and families who may feel too overwhelmed by the pain experience to answer a long, detailed questionnaire.

If possible, incorporate pain assessment into the flow sheet you're already using. Generally, the easier the flow sheet is to use, the more likely you and your patient will be to use it.

PAIN FLOW SHEET					
Date and time	Pain rating (0 to 10)	Patient behaviors	Vital signs	Pain rating after intervention	Comments
11/6/94 0800	7	wincing, holding head	186/88 98–22	5	Dilaudid 2 mg IM given.
11/6/94 1200	3	relaxing, reading	160/80 84–18	2	Tylox ǂ P.O. given.

Visual analog pain scale

In a visual analog pain scale, the patient marks a linear scale with words or numbers that correspond to his perceived degree of pain. Draw a scale to represent a continuum of pain intensity. Verbal anchors describe the pain's intensity; for example, "no pain" begins the scale and "pain as bad as it could be" ends it. Ask the patient to mark the point on the continuum that best describes his pain.

VISUAL ANALOG SCALE	✳	
No pain		Pain as bad as it could be

Graphic rating scales

Other rating scales have words that represent pain intensity. Use these scales as you would the visual analog scale. Have the patient mark the spot on the continuum that best describes his pain.

GRAPHIC RATING SCALE		○		
No pain	Mild	Moderate	Severe	Pain as bad as it could be

Everyday Events

the sequence of events. (See *Keeping a code record,* page 266.)

If a code is called, you'll complete a *code record,* a form that incorporates detailed information about the code (including observations, interventions, and any drugs given to the patient).

1/24/95	2100	Summoned to the pt.'s room
		@ 2020 hr. by a shout from
		roommate. Found pt. unre-
		sponsive, w/o respirations or
		pulse. Roommate stated, "He
		was talking to me; then all of
		a sudden he started gasping
		and holding his chest."
		Code called. Initiated CPR
		with Ann Gibbons, RN. Code
		team arrived @ 2023 hr.
		and continued resuscitative
		efforts. (See code record.) Pt.
		groaned and opened eyes @
		approx. 2030 hr. (see neuro-
		logic flow sheet). Notified
		Dr. Smith @ home @ 2040 hr.
		and explained situation—will
		be in immediately. Pt. trans-
		ferred to ICU @ 2035 hrs.
		Family notified of pt.'s con-
		dition and transfer.———
		———Betty Dillon, RN

Some health care facilities use a resuscitation critique form to identify actual or potential problems with the resuscitation process. This form tracks personnel responses and response times as well as the availability of appropriate drugs and functioning equipment.

Intake and output monitoring

Many patients require 24-hour intake and output monitoring. They include surgical patients, patients on I.V. therapy, patients with fluid and electrolyte imbalances, and patients with burns, hemorrhage, or edema.

You'll keep most intake and output sheets at the patient's bedside or by the bathroom door to remind you to measure and document his intake and output. If the patient is incontinent, document this as well as tube drainage and irrigation volumes.

For easy reference, list the volumes of specific containers. Infusion devices make documenting enteral and I.V. intake more accurate. But keeping track of intake that isn't premeasured—for example, food such as gelatin that is normally fluid at room temperature—requires the cooperation of the patient, family members (who may bring him snacks and soft drinks or help him to eat at the health care facility), and other caregivers.

So make sure that everyone understands how to record or report all foods and fluids that the patient consumes orally.

Don't forget to count I.V. piggyback infusions, drugs given by I.V. push, patient-controlled analgesics, and any irrigation solutions that aren't withdrawn. You'll also need to know whether the patient receives any fluids orally or intravenously while he's off of your unit.

Recording fluid output accurately requires the cooperation of the patient and staff members in any other departments your patient goes to. If he's ambulatory, remind him to use a urinal or a commode.

Loss of fluid through the GI tract is normally 100 ml or less daily. However, if the

BETTER CHARTING

Keeping a code record

Here's an example of the completed code record for inclusion in your patient's chart.

CODE RECORD

Patient Name *John Little*　　　　Weight *165 lb* Date *1/24/95*

Time	BP	Heart rate	Heart rhythm	Atropine (mg)	Calcium chloride (ampules)	Epinephrine (mg)	Lidocaine (mg)	Procainamide (mg)	Dopamine (mg/ml)	Isoproterenol (mg/ml)	Lidocaine (g/ml)	Defibrillation (joules)	CPR	Airway	PaO₂	PaCO₂	HCO₃⁻	pH
		Vital signs				Bolus meds				Infused meds			Actions		Arterial blood gas (ABG) levels			
2020	0	0											✓	mask				
2025	0	0	VF									200						
2025													✓					
2026												300						
2027												360						
2029						1	75						✓	ET tube	27	76	14	7.10
2030												360						
2031													✓					
2031												360						
2032		88	NSR															
2032		92	NSR															
2035	140/90	96					75								43	26	23	7.26

Time　**Actions**
2020　Code called. CPR initiated by Terry Cohn, RN, and Carol Gibbons, R.N.
2020　Bagged by Lynne Hart, RN.
2025　Single-channel ECG. Central line inserted via ® SC by Dr. Shaw.
2029　ABG via ® femoral artery by Dr. Nolan. Oral intubation by anesthesiologist.
2032　Converted to NSR.
2035　ABG via Ⓛ femoral artery. Pressure applied. Unresponsive.

Time code called *2020*　　☑ Informed family
☐ Arrest witnessed　　　　☑ Informed attending doctor
☑ Arrest unwitnessed
☑ Intubation *2029*
☑ Arrhythmia *VF*

Disposition
☐ SICU　　☐ OR
☑ MICU　　☐ Morgue
☐ CCU　　☐ Other

Status after resuscitation
BP 140/90
Heart rate 96. Bagged
with 100% O₂ and
transported to MICU

Clinical care nurse: *Mary Jane Belinsky, RN*　　**Code chief:** *Joel Reynolds, MD*

patient's stools become excessive or watery, they must be counted as output. Vomiting, drainage from suction devices and wound drains, and bleeding are other measurable sources of fluid loss. (See *Charting intake and output*, page 268.)

Skin and wound care

Because many patients are susceptible to pressure ulcers, always document findings related to the patient's skin condition. Clearly note in the record whether a patient had a pressure ulcer upon admission or whether the ulcer developed in the health care facility.

When a chronically ill or immobile patient enters your unit with a pressure ulcer, record its location, appearance, size, depth, and color and the appearance of exudate from that ulcer.

2/1/95	1400	Pt. admitted by stretcher
		to room 418B. Pt. lethargic.
		Skin dry. Incontinent of
		urine. 1" wide, black pressure
		ulcer noted on ® heel. Puru-
		lent, yellow drainage noted
		on ulcer's dressing. Dr. Kelly
		notified. Surgical consult or-
		dered for debridement of ulcer.
		® foot elevated on 2 pillows.
		Heel and elbow protectors
		applied. Skin lotion applied.
		Incontinent care given hour-
		ly. No other skin breakdown
		noted. Buttocks reddened but
		epidermis intact.
		————— Elaine Black, RN

If a patient's skin condition worsens during hospitalization, his stay may be ex-

tended, in which case you'll need a clear record of skin care and related factors. This is especially important because family members typically think that pressure ulcers stem from poor nursing care, although risk factors, such as obesity, decreased hemoglobin level, immobility, infection, incontinence, and fractures, are equally responsible.

If your health care facility requires you to photograph pressure ulcers found at the time of admission, always date the photographs. You can then evaluate changes in a patient's skin condition by comparing his current skin integrity with previous photographs.

Personal property

Encourage patients to send home their money, jewelry, and other valuable belongings. If a patient refuses to do so, make a list of his possessions and store them according to your hospital policy.

The list of the patient's valuables should include a description of each one. To protect yourself and your employer, ask the patient (or a responsible family member in lieu of the patient) to sign, or witness, the list that you compile so that you both understand which items you're responsible for.

Use objective language to describe each item, noting its color, approximate size, style, type, serial number, or other distinguishing feature. Don't assess the item's value or authenticity. For example, you might describe a diamond ring as a "clear, round stone set in a yellow metal band."

Besides jewelry and money, include dentures, eyeglasses or contact lenses, hearing aids, prostheses, and clothing on the list.

BETTER CHARTING

Charting intake and output

As this sample shows, you can monitor your patient's fluid balance by using an intake and output record.

Name: _Josephine Kline_
Medical record #: _49731_
Admission date: _12/13/94_

INTAKE AND OUTPUT RECORD

	INTAKE						OUTPUT				
	Oral	Tube feeding	Instilled	I.V. and IVPB	TPN	Total	Urine	Emesis	NG tubes	Other	Total
Date _12/15//94_ _0700–1500_	250	320	H₂0 50	1100		1720	1355				1355
_1500–2300_	200	320	H₂0 50	1100		1670	1200				1200
_2300–0700_	0	320	H₂0 50	1100		1470	1500				1500
24-hr total	450	960	H₂0 150	3300		4860	4055				4055
Date											
24-hr total											
Date											
24-hr total											
Date											
24-hr total											

KEY: IVPB = I.V. piggyback   NG = nasogastric   TPN = total parenteral nutrition

Standard measures

Styrofoam cup	240 ml	Water (large)	600 ml	Milk (large)	600 ml	Ice cream, sherbet, or gelatin	120 ml
Juice	120 ml	Water pitcher	750 ml	Coffee	240 ml		
Water (small)	120 ml	Milk (small)	120 ml	Soup	180 ml		

Everyday Events

12/8/94	1300	Pt. admitted to room 318 with
		one pair of brown glasses,
		upper and lower dentures,
		a yellow metal band with a
		red stone, pink bathrobe, and
		black radio. —Paul Cullen, RN

Place valuable items in an envelope and other personal belongings in approved containers; then label them with the patient's identification number. Never use garbage containers, laundry bags, or any other unauthorized receptacle for valuables; they could be discarded accidentally.

If the patient refuses to remove a ring, explain that it may have to be cut off if it compromises his circulation. If he decides to leave it on anyway, tape it in place. Be sure to document your conversation and actions.

If your patient is homeless, he may have all of his personal belongings with him. You'll need to identify and tag each item.

Shift reports

If you're the charge nurse, you'll need to complete an end-of-shift report (sometimes called a unit report). This document, which tracks both conditions and activities on the unit, provides a running record of the patient census, staff-to-patient ratio and assignments, bed utilization, patient emergencies or acute changes, patient or family problems, incidents, equipment and supply problems, number of high-risk procedures, and other important data.

The end-of-shift report sheets are typically reviewed during quality improvement investigations and referred to for other reports. They can be helpful to the nurse-manager charged with solving the day-to-day problems of a unit. (See *Documenting the events of your shift*, page 270.)

Common charting flaws

Ideally, every chart you receive from the nurses on the previous shift will be complete and accurate. Unfortunately, this is not always the case. Although you can't necessarily affect what other nurses do, you can try to make your own charting flawless so it doesn't mislead another caregiver.

Blank spaces in the chart

Don't leave any blank spaces on chart forms; fill them in completely. A blank space implies that you failed to give complete care or assess the patient fully.

If information requested on a form doesn't apply to a particular patient, write "N/A" (not applicable) or draw a line through the empty space, as shown in the example below:

1/19/95	1500	20 y/o male admitted to
		room 418B by wheelchair. #20
		angiocath inserted in ⓡ
		antecubital vein with I.V. of
		1,000 ml D5½NSS infusing at
		125 ml/hr. O₂ at 2 L/min. via
		NC. Demerol 50 mg given I.M.
		for abdominal pain. Relief
		reported.————————
		————— —David Dunn, RN

BETTER CHARTING

Documenting the events of your shift

Most health care facilities require the charge nurse to complete an end-of-shift report (or unit report sheet). Use the form below as an example of the information most hospitals need to know.

Date: _11/26/94_   **Charge nurse:** _Donna Moriarty, R.N._

Patient census: Start of shift: _38_   End of shift: _37_

Number of admissions _2_

Number of transfers _2 in, 3 out_

Deaths _2_

Codes _0_

Comments
One patient transferred to SICU postop

Staff profile: Start of shift: _9_   End of shift: _7_

RNs _4_   Orientees _0_

LPNs _3_   Students _0_

Nursing assistants _2_

Agency _0_

Other _0_

Called in sick _Unit clerk – not replaced_

Late _0_

Floated _1 aide, 1 LPN floated out halfway through shift_

Unit workload during shift

Quiet _____   Busy but steady _____   Very busy _X_   Understaffed _X_

Equipment and supply problems
IV pumps not available. No sterile drsg. kits in supply cart. Not enough linen

High-risk procedures performed
CVP line insertion, wound debridement, chest tube insertion

Assignment, personnel, or performance problems
Staff floated out 4 hr. into shift to cover sick calls on another unit – increased pt. ratio for rest of staff.

Patient or family problems
Mr. Hale in room 516-B – his condition deteriorated rapidly – developed acute abdomen and required emergency surgery. Family distraught –need time and privacy to speak with physician and clergy. Conference room is too small to accommodate more than 10 people (18 family members present). Because room doubles as staff lounge, privacy is difficult to maintain.

Number of incident reports filed: _None_   **Number of problem logs completed:** _None_

This leaves no doubt that you addressed every part of the record. It also prevents others from inserting information that could change the meaning of your original documentation.

Care given by someone else

Anyone reading your notes assumes that this record is an account of your firsthand knowledge of care provided. If it isn't, you need to say so.

When nursing assistants are working with you, for example, your role may include charting for them. In some health care settings, they aren't permitted to make formal chart entries, but they may use flow sheets to document tasks they've completed. A registered nurse (RN) or licensed practical nurse (LPN) would document any other information.

If that's the case in your facility, include the nursing assistant's name in your notes. Be sure to include the assistant's full name, not just her initials.

You may also worry about the legality of countersigning notes that were entered by LPNs or nursing assistants when you haven't actually supervised their work. Review the policy set by your employer and your state board of nursing. Does countersigning mean that the LPN or nursing assistant performed her nursing actions in your presence? If so, don't countersign unless she did.

On the other hand, if your health care facility recognizes that you don't always have the time to witness your colleagues' actions, then your countersigning indicates that the notes describe care that the LPN or nursing assistant had the authority and competence to perform. Of course, your countersigning also means that you veri-

fied that all required patient care procedures were performed.

If another nurse asks you to document her care or sign her notes, don't. Unless your employer authorizes or requires you to witness someone else's notes, your signature makes you responsible for anything you write in the notes.

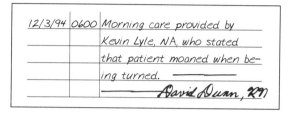

Late entries

Late entries are appropriate in several situations:
• if the chart was unavailable when you needed it (as shown below)—for example, when the patient was away from the unit (in X-ray or physical therapy)

Everyday Events

Avoid late additions

If the court uncovers alterations in a patient's chart during the course of a trial, suspicions may be aroused. The court may logically infer that additional alterations have been made. In such situations, the value of the entire medical record may be seriously discounted.

That's what happened to the nurse involved in one case. She failed to chart her observations of a postoperative patient for 7 hours during which time the patient died.

Later, the patient's family sued the hospital, charging the nurse with malpractice. The nurse insisted that she had observed the patient, but because her particular unit was understaffed and overpopulated, she wasn't able to record her observations. She explained that the assistant director of nursing instructed her at a later time about the hospital's policy on charting late additions. Then the nurse subsequently added her observations to the patient's medical record.

However, the court wasn't convinced that the nurse had indeed observed the patient during the postoperative period. Suspicious of the altered record, it ruled that the nurse's failure to chart her observations at the proper time supported the plaintiff's claim that she'd made no such observations.

• if you need to add important information after completing your notes
• if you forgot to write notes on a particular chart.

Keep in mind, however, that a late or altered chart entry can arouse suspicions and can be a significant problem in the event of a malpractice trial. (See *Avoid late additions*.)

If you must make a late entry or alter an earlier entry, find out if your health care facility has a protocol for doing so. Many do. If not, the best approach is to add the entry to the first available line, and label the entry "late entry" to indicate that it's out of sequence. Then record the time and date of the entry and, in the body of the entry, record the time and date it should have been made.

Corrections

When you make a mistake on a chart, correct it promptly. Never erase, cover, completely scratch out, or otherwise obscure an erroneous entry because this may imply a cover-up. (See *Correcting a charting error.*)

If the chart ends up in court, the plaintiff's attorney will be looking for anything that may cast doubt on the chart's accuracy. Never try to erase an error or obliterate it with correction fluid or heavy black ink. These practices are red flags.

Patient noncompliance

Suppose a patient won't comply with nursing or medical interventions. In the chart, describe any patient behavior that goes against your instructions; then report the problem to the appropriate person. Note any attempts to encourage the patient's compliance, even if unsuccessful. If the patient's care is questioned later, the record will be an important factor in your defense.

Patients may ignore common instructions, such as "Follow your diet," "Don't get out of bed without assistance," "Take your medicine as directed," or "Keep your doctor's appointment for a checkup."

Beyond explaining the importance of following these instructions or complying with restrictions and urging the patient to comply, you may be able to do little. But you must chart the noncompliance.

Dietary restrictions

If your patient is on dietary restrictions and you discover unauthorized food or beverages at his bedside, point out to him the need to follow his prescribed dietary plan. Document the noncompliance and your patient teaching, and notify the patient's doctor.

| 12/17/94 | 1400 | Pt. found with milkshake and cookies at bedside. Discussed with pt. his need to maintain 1,800-calorie ADA diet. Pt. refused to remove these foods, stating, "I'll eat what I want." Dr. Miller notified that pt. is not complying with prescribed diabetic diet. Dietitian called to see pt. and wife. ——— Claire Bowden, RN |

Out of bed against advice

Even after you've told a patient that he can't get out of bed or that he must call you for help, you may go to his room and find him climbing over the bed rails. Or

BETTER CHARTING

Correcting a charting error

When you make a mistake on the clinical record, correct it by drawing a single line through it and writing the words "mistaken entry" above or beside it. Follow these words with your initials and the date. If appropriate, briefly explain the necessity for the correction.

Be sure that the mistaken entry is still readable. This indicates that you're only trying to correct a mistake, not cover it up.

DATE	TIME	PROGRESS NOTES
12/19/94	0900	MISTAKEN ENTRY J.M. 12/19/94 Pt. walked to bathroom. States he experiences no difficulty urinating. ——— John Morris, RN

you may discover relatives helping him to the bathroom because they don't want to disturb you.

Either scenario puts the patient at risk for a fall and you at risk for a lawsuit. What can you do? You can clearly document your instructions and anything that the patient does in spite of them (see the example on page 274, top left). Be sure to include any devices that are used to ensure patient safety, such as bed alarms or leg alarms. This shows that you recognized the potential for a fall and that you tried to prevent it.

12/13/94	0300	Assisted pt. to bathroom. Weak, unsteady on feet. States she gets dizzy when she stands. Instructed pt. to call for assistance to get OOB. Side rails up. Call button within reach. ————— Robert Bellry RN
12/13/94	0430	Found pt. walking to bathroom. Stated she got OOB by herself. Reminded her to call for assistance. Said she understood. ————— Robert Bellry RN

Medication abuse or refusal

If the patient refuses or abuses prescribed medication, describe the event in his chart. Here are some examples of situations needing careful documentation:

• You discover unprescribed drugs at the patient's bedside. Document the type of medication (pills or powders), the amount of medication, and its appearance (color and shape).

• You find a supply of his prescribed drugs in his bedside table, indicating that he is hoarding his medication instead of swallowing each dose. Record the type of medication that you found and the amount.

• You try to give him prescribed medications and he refuses. Document his refusal and the reason for his refusal, assuming he tells you. Also be sure to name the medications. Taking these steps will ensure that the patient's refusal isn't misinterpreted as an omission or a medication error on your part.

• You observe that his behavior suddenly changes after he has visitors (see the example, above right), and you suspect the visitors of providing him with contraband (narcotics or other drugs, for example). Document how the patient appeared before and after you suspect his visitors gave him an unprescribed substance.

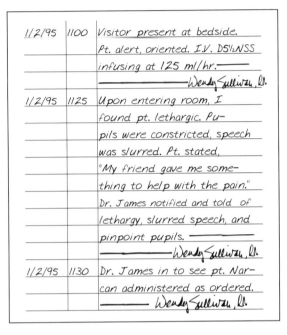

1/2/95	1100	Visitor present at bedside. Pt. alert, oriented. I.V. D5½NSS infusing at 125 ml/hr. ————— Wendy Sullivan, RN
1/2/95	1125	Upon entering room, I found pt. lethargic. Pupils were constricted, speech was slurred. Pt. stated, "My friend gave me something to help with the pain." Dr. James notified and told of lethargy, slurred speech, and pinpoint pupils. ————— Wendy Sullivan, RN
1/2/95	1130	Dr. James in to see pt. Narcan administered as ordered. ————— Wendy Sullivan, RN

Follow-up appointments

At discharge, discuss the date that the patient will see the doctor for a follow-up evaluation. Or if the patient will make the appointment himself, encourage him to do so, explaining the need for ongoing medical care.

Document the date that the patient is expected to return for a follow-up visit or the actual date of the appointment and the date you discussed the appointment with him. This protects you from claims that you neglected to inform him of the need to return for medical care.

Also document any related patient teaching that you performed and identify any written instructions that you provided, such as an appointment card (or a leaflet about when the patient should call the doctor following discharge). If feasible, mail a reminder letter with a return receipt requested.

If you should be accused of negligence related to follow-up care, you can then point to tangible evidence of your attempt to encourage the patient's compliance.

2/2/95	1300	Pt. notified to return to
		see Dr. Meade on 2/16/95 at
		0900. Discussed this with pt.
		and his wife.
		Anne Norse, RN

Refusing treatment

Infinitely more serious than minor instances of noncompliance, refusing treatment is not just an important patient care and safety issue. It's a critical documentation concern as well.

Any mentally competent adult can refuse treatment. And in most cases, the health care personnel that are responsible for the patient's care can remain free of legal jeopardy as long as they fully inform the patient about his medical condition and the likely consequences of refusing treatment.

Today's legal community recognizes a competent adult's right to refuse medical treatment, even when that refusal will clearly result in his death.

When your patient refuses treatment, inform him of the risks involved in making such a decision. If possible, inform him in writing.

If he continues to refuse, notify the doctor, who will then decide on the most appropriate plan of action.

12/8/94	2000	Pt. refusing to have I.V.
		inserted, stating that he's
		"sick and tired of being
		stuck." Explained to pt. the
		need for I.V. fluids and anti-
		biotics and likely result of
		refusing treatment. Dr.
		Bradley notified. Dr. Bradley
		spent time with pt. Pt. still
		refusing I.V. Orders written
		to force fluids, repeat
		electrolytes in morning, and
		give amoxicillin P.O.
		Barbara Timmons, RN

Make sure that you document the patient's exact words in the chart. To protect yourself legally, document that you didn't provide the prescribed treatment because the patient refused it. Then ask the patient to sign a refusal-of-treatment release form.

If the patient refuses to sign the release form, document this refusal in the progress notes. For additional protection, your facility's policy may require you to ask the patient's spouse or closest relative to sign another refusal-of-treatment release form. Document whether the spouse or another relative does this. (See Chapter 2, Legal and Ethical Implications of Documentation.)

Interdisciplinary communications

A call from the laboratory informing you of a patient's test results must be documented. You must also document a call from a patient asking you for advice and any patient information you tell a doctor over the phone. Finally, you may on occasion have to give a patient's family bad news over the telephone, and this too must be noted in the chart.

Information from other departments

When a department, such as the laboratory or X-ray department, notifies your unit of a patient's test results, document this in the patient's chart. If you need to notify the doctor of these results, be sure to document that also.

1/4/95	1400	Laboratory technician Mary
		Boyle called floor to report
		pt.'s random blood glucose level
		of 486. Dr. Denny notified.
		Stat blood glucose ordered.
		Pt. being monitored until
		results available. ⎯⎯
		⎯⎯ Anne Brwin, RN

Reports to doctors

You've just phoned the doctor to tell him about his patient's deteriorating condition. He listens as you give laboratory test results and the patient's signs and symptoms, thanks you for the information, and hangs up—without giving you an order.

Unless you properly document your conversation with him, the doctor could claim he "wasn't notified" should this patient's care subsequently come into question. (See *Ensuring clear communication.*)

Nurses often write, "Notified doctor of patient's condition." This statement is too vague. In the event of a malpractice suit, it allows the plaintiff's lawyer (and the doctor) to imply that you didn't communicate the essential data. The chart should include exactly what you told the doctor.

12/15/94	2215	Called Dr. Spencer regarding
		increased serous drainage
		from pt.'s Ⓛ chest tube. Dr.
		Spencer's order was to ob-
		serve the drainage for 1 more
		hr. and then call him.⎯⎯
		⎯⎯ Danielle Burns, RN

Telephone advice to patients

Nurses, especially those working in the emergency department (ED), frequently get requests to give advice to patients by telephone. A hospital has no legal duty to provide a telephone-advice service. And you have no legal duty to give advice to anyone who calls.

The best response to a telephone request for medical advice is to tell the caller to come to the hospital because you can't assess his condition or treat him over the phone. Like all rules, however, this too has its exceptions. One exception to this rule is a life-threatening situation when someone needs immediate care, treatment, or referral.

CHARTING GUIDELINES

Ensuring clear communication

To ensure clear communication when discussing a patient's care with a doctor on the phone, remember to keep the following points in mind:
• If you don't know the doctor, ask him to state and spell his full name.
• Include the exact time you contacted the doctor. To establish proof, you could have the hospital operator dial the number for you, or have another nurse listen in and then cosign the time of notification. If you don't note the time you called, allegations may be made later that you failed to obtain timely medical treatment for the patient.
• Always note the change, problem, or result you've reported to the doctor in the chart, along with the doctor's orders or response. Use his own words if possible.

• If you're reporting a critical laboratory test result (for example, a low serum potassium level of 3.2 mEq/liter) but don't receive an order for intervention (such as potassium replacement therapy), be sure to verify with the doctor that he doesn't want to give an order. Then document this fact on the doctor's order sheet. For example, you'd write: "Dr. Jones informed of potassium of 3.2 mEq/liter. No orders received."
• If you think that not having a doctor's order for intervention puts your patient's health at risk, follow the chain of command and notify your supervisor. Then be sure to document your action.

Accepting responsibility

If you do dispense advice over the phone, keep in mind that a legal duty arises the minute you say, "Okay, let me tell you what to do." You now have a nurse-patient relationship, and you're responsible for any advice you give. Once you start to give advice by telephone, you can't decide midway through that you're in over your head and simply hang up. That may be considered abandonment. You must give appropriate advice or a referral. You may say, "After listening to you, I strongly suggest that you come to the ED or call your doctor."

If the caller is a patient you cared for recently, you may choose to give him advice. For example, if the doctor prescribed medication and gave him an instruction sheet, you probably told him to call if he had any questions. Obviously, you won't refuse to answer his questions if he calls.

If the question is elementary, such as "Should I drink orange juice or something else when I take this diuretic?" you're probably safe answering. However, direct anything more specific to the doctor, especially if the patient's symptoms have changed.

If you do decide to give telephone advice, establish a system of documenting such calls—with a telephone log, for example. The log should include the date and time of the call, the name of the caller (if he'll give it), the address of the caller, the caller's request or chief complaint, the disposition of the call, and the name of the person who made that disposition.

The disposition will depend on the request. For example, you may give the caller a poison-control number or suggest that the person come to the ED for evaluation. Document whatever information you give.

1/6/95	1615	Jeremy Smith phoned asking how
		big a cut has to be to require
		stitches. I asked him to de-
		scribe the injury he was in-
		quiring about. He described a
		4" gash in his ⓁΤ leg from a fall.
		I recommended that he come
		into the ED to be assessed.
		————— Pat Palermo, RN

Some nurses hesitate to use a telephone log because they assume that if they don't document, they won't be responsible for the advice they give. This assumption is faulty. A patient may make only one call to the hospital, usually about something important to him. He'll remember that; you may not.

The telephone log can provide evidence and refresh your recollection of the event. It may remind you that you didn't tell the patient to take two acetaminophen tablets to lower his fever of 105° F (40.5° C). Instead you told him to come to the ED. Or maybe you told a young athlete to come to the ED for an X-ray of his injured ankle.

Once you log such information, the law presumes that it is true because you wrote it in the course of ordinary business.

Giving bad news by phone

Sometimes you may have the unpleasant task of telephoning a patient's family member with news of a patient's deteriorating condition or death. Be sure to chart the date, the time, and the name of the family member notified.

Doctors' orders

Because most of each patient's treatment requires doctor's orders, careful and accurate documentation of these orders is crucial.

Written orders

No matter who transcribes a doctor's orders—an RN, LPN, or unit secretary—a second person needs to double-check the transcription for accuracy. Your unit should also have some method of checking for transcription errors at least once every 24 hours.

Night-shift nurses usually do this by placing a line across the order sheet to indicate that all orders above the line have been checked. They also sign and date the sheet to verify that they've done the 24-hour medication check.

When checking a patient's order sheet, always make sure that the orders were written for the intended patient. Occasionally, an order sheet will be stamped with one patient's ID plate but will be inadvertently placed in another patient's chart. By double-checking, you'll avert potential mistakes.

If an order is unclear, ask the doctor who wrote it to clarify it. Don't waste time asking other people for their interpretation; they'd be guessing too. If a doctor is notorious for his poor handwriting, ask him to read his orders to you before he leaves the unit.

Preprinted orders

Many health care facilities use preprinted order forms to make doctors' orders easier to read and interpret. If this is the case in your health care facility, don't automatically assume that a preprinted order is a flawless document in the medical record; it isn't. You may still need to clarify its meaning with the doctor who made it. (See *Avoiding pitfalls of preprinted order forms,* page 280.)

Verbal orders

Errors made interpreting or documenting verbal orders can lead to mistakes in patient care and liability problems for you. Clearly, verbal orders can be a necessity—especially if you're providing home health care. But in a health care facility, try to take verbal orders only in an emergency when the doctor can't immediately attend to the patient.

In most cases, verbal orders should not include do-not-resuscitate (DNR) or no-code orders.

Carefully follow your hospital's policy for documenting a verbal order. And use a special form if one exists. Usually, you'll follow this procedure:
• If time and circumstances allow, have another nurse read the order back to the doctor.
• Record the order on the doctor's order sheet as soon as possible. Note the date; then record the order verbatim.
• On the following line, write "VO" for verbal order. Then write the doctor's name

and the name of the nurse who read the order back to the doctor.
• Sign your name and write the time.
• Draw lines through any spaces between the order and your verification of the order.
• Record in ink the type of drug, the dosage, the time you administered it, and any other information your facility's policy requires.

1/5/95	1500	Digoxin 0.125 mg P.O. now and
		daily in a.m. Furosemide 40 mg
		P.O. now and daily starting in
		a.m. V.O. Dr. Blackstein taken by
		Karen Dunn, RN §
		Danny Matthews, RN

Make sure that the doctor countersigns the order within the time limits set by your facility's policy. Without this countersignature, you may be held liable for practicing medicine without a license.

Telephone orders

Mr. Perry is having trouble breathing. Your assessment findings include bilateral crackles on auscultation and dependent edema. The doctor, who's busy in an emergency, gives you a telephone order for oxygen.

Normally, you should accept only written orders from a doctor. But in a situation like this, when the patient needs immediate treatment and the doctor isn't available to write an order, telephone orders are acceptable.

Telephone orders may also be taken to expedite care when new information is available that doesn't require a physical examination (laboratory data, for example). Keep in mind that telephone orders are

Avoiding pitfalls of preprinted order forms

When documenting the execution of a doctor's preprinted order, make sure that you've interpreted and carried out the order correctly. Even though these forms aim to prevent problems (caused by illegible handwriting, for example), they may still be misread. Here are some considerations for developing preprinted forms.

Insist on approved forms
Use only preprinted order forms that have your health care facility's approval and the seal of approval of the medical records committee. Most facilities stamp or print an identification number or code on the form. When in doubt, call the medical records department—the doctor may be using a form he developed or one provided by a drug manufacturer.

Require compliance with policies
To enhance communciation and continuity, a preprinted order form needs to comply with hospital policies and other regulations. For example, a postoperative preprinted order form shouldn't say "Renew all previous orders" if hospital policy requires specific orders. And it shouldn't allow you to select a drug dose from a range ("meperidine 50 to 100 mg I.M. q 4 h," for example) if that's prohibited in your state. Alert your nurse-manager if any order form requires you to perform duties that are outside your scope of practice.

Make sure the form is completed correctly
In most cases, a preprinted order form includes a list of orders—and more than the doctor wants you to follow. So he'll need to indicate what should be done. For example, he may check the appropriate orders, put his initials next to them, or cross out the ones he doesn't want.

Ask for clarity and precision
Make sure that the doctor orders doses in the unit of measure in which they are dispensed. For example, make sure that the form uses the metric system instead of the error-prone apothecary system. Report any errors to your nurse-manager.

Promote proper nomenclature
Ask doctors to use generic drug names, especially when more than one brand of a generic drug is available ("acetaminophen" instead of "Tylenol," for example). But if only one brand of a drug is available, its name can be included in parentheses after the generic name—for example, "dobutamine (Dobutrex)."

Bypass opportunities for misinterpretation
Unapproved, potentially dangerous abbreviations and symbols—such as q.d., U, and q.o.d.—don't belong on preprinted order forms. Improper spacing between a drug name and its dosage can also contribute to medication errors. For example, a 20-mg dose of Inderal written as "Inderal20mg" could be misinterpreted as 120 mg.

Ensure that the copy is readable
If your faciltiy uses a no-carbon-required form, make sure that the bottom copy contains an identical set of preprinted orders; this is the copy that goes to the pharmacy. All lines on it should also appear on the top copy—extra lines on the pharmacy copy can hide decimal points (making 1.5 look like 15, for example) and the tops of numbers (making 7 and 5 look like 1 and 3).

for the patient's well-being and not strictly for convenience.

They should be given directly to you, rather than through a third party. Also, carefully follow your facility's policy for documenting a telephone order. Generally, you'd follow this procedure:
• Record the order on the doctor's order sheet as soon as possible. First, note the date and time; then write the order verbatim. On the next line, write "t.o." for telephone order. (Don't use "p.o." for phone order. The abbreviation could be misinterpreted to mean "by mouth.") Then, write the doctor's name and sign your name. If another nurse listened to the order with you, have her sign the order too.

2/4/95	1100	M.S. Contin 30 mg, P.O. now and
		q 12 hr for pain. Bisacodyl
		suppos. ī R now. May repeat
		x1 if no results. ———
		T.O. Dr. Mills / Cathy Dole, R.N.
		& Ellen Waters, R.N.

• Have another nurse listen as the doctor gives the order in case he gives a no-code order or if you're having difficulty understanding him.
• Draw lines through any blank spaces in the order.
• Make sure that the doctor countersigns the order within the time limits set by your facility's policy. Without his signature, you may be held liable for practicing medicine without a license.

To save time and avoid errors, consider asking the doctor to send a copy of the order by fax machine. (See *Advantages of faxing orders,* page 282.)

Clarifying doctors' orders

Although unit secretaries may transcribe orders, the nurse is ultimately responsible for the accuracy of the transcription. Only you have the authority and the knowledge to question the validity of orders and to spot errors.

Follow your health care facility's policy for clarifying orders that are vague or possibly erroneous. If you don't have a policy to cover a particular situation, contact the prescribing doctor, and always document your actions. Then ask your nursing administrator for a step-by-step policy to follow so that if the situation ever recurs, you'll know what do.

An order may be correct when issued, but improper later because of changes in the patient's status. When this occurs, delay the treatment until you've contacted the doctor and clarified the situation. Follow your hospital's policy for clarifying an order. (See *When in doubt, question orders,* page 283.)

Clarify ambiguous orders with the doctor. Document your efforts to clarify the order and document whether the order was carried out. If you believe a doctor's order is in error, you must refuse to carry it out, until you receive clarification. Keep a record of your refusal together with the reasons and an account of all communication with the doctor. Inform your immediate supervisor. If the order is correct as written, initial and checkmark each line. Below the doctor's signature, sign your name, the date, and the time.

DNR orders

When a patient is terminally ill and his death is expected, his doctor and family (and the patient if appropriate) will agree that a DNR or a no-code order is appropri-

Advantages of faxing orders

The facsimile, or fax, network in most hospitals now includes a clinical laboratory, the pharmacy, and radiology and cardiology departments. You and other staff members can transmit exact copies of orders, laboratory test results, X-rays, and electrocardiogram (ECG) strips in as little as 15 seconds.

Speeds communication

Besides taking a doctor's order by phone, current telecommunication technology allows the doctor to back up his phone order in writing for the patient's chart.

The order can be faxed not only to you on the unit but also to the pharmacy, X-ray, or other relevant departments. The results: no more time wasted calling the department and waiting to get through and no more time spent waiting for your order to be picked up.

In return, the receiving department gets a copy of the original order (needed for filling the order and for department files).

An additional advantage comes from the fax machine itself, which prints the date and time the order was sent and the department it came from.

If an order can't be filled, the receiving department can contact the doctor for clarification or for a new order, again reducing delays in filling orders and wasting your time as a go-between.

Laboratory, X-ray, and ECG findings and other clinical information can be faxed back to you, enabling you to learn routine results almost at once.

Reduces errors

Using a fax network helps you and the other services involved to prevent errors by checking one another's work and consulting the doctor directly about unresolved problems. What's more, you have printed accounts for accurate documentation.

---

ate. The doctor writes it, and the staff carries it out when the patient goes into cardiac or respiratory arrest.

12/19/94	1900	DO NOT RESUSCITATE THIS PATIENT.————— ————Joel Reynolds, MD

This is a legal order and you'll incur no liability when you don't attempt to resuscitate such a patient and he subsequently dies. You may, however, incur liability if

you initiate resuscitation counter to the DNR order.

Although a verbal or telephoned DNR order may be taken, it must be witnessed or heard by two nurses. In all circumstances, be sure to follow your hospital's policy and procedure on DNR.

Every patient with a DNR code should have a written order on file. The order should be consistent with the hospital's policy.

Unless the doctor has written a DNR order or signed off on documentation of his telephoned verbal order, always initiate resuscitation efforts.

Increasingly, patients are deciding in advance of a crisis whether or not they want to be resuscitated. Health care facilities must provide written information to patients concerning their rights under state law to make decisions regarding their care, including the right to refuse medical treatment and the right to formulate an advance directive. (See Chapter 2, Legal and Ethical Implications of Documentation.)

This information must be provided to all patients, usually at the time of admission. You must also document that the patient has received this information and whether he has brought a written advance directive with him. (See *Documenting advance directives,* page 284.) In some instances, you can file a photocopy of the directive in the patient's record.

As a nurse, you have a responsibility to help the patient make an informed decision about continuing treatment. Sometimes his request differs from what his family or his doctor wants for him. In these situations, make sure that the discrepancies are thoroughly documented in the chart. (See *Charting the patient's final request,* page 285.)

Incidents

Chart all patient injuries caused by falls, restraints, burns, or other factors. Then, file an incident report in compliance with your health care facility's procedure.

Also file an incident report whenever a patient insists on being discharged against medical advice (AMA).

When in doubt, question orders

Always question a doctor's order if it seems strange or "not right."

In *Poor Sisters of Saint Francis Seraph of the Perpetual Adoration, et al. v. Catron* (1982), a hospital was sued for negligence because a nurse failed to question a doctor's order regarding an endotracheal tube.

The doctor ordered that the tube be left in the patient's trachea for an excessively long period: 5 days instead of the standard 2 to 3 days.

The nurse knew that 5 days was exceptionally long, but instead of clarifying the doctor's order and documenting her actions, she followed the order.

As a result, the patient's voice box was irreparably damaged, and the court ruled the hospital negligent.

An incident report serves two functions. First, it informs the administration of the incident, allowing the risk management team to consider changes that might prevent similar incidents in the future. Second, the incident report alerts the administration and the health care facility's insurance company to a potential claim and the need for further investigation.

Only a person with firsthand knowledge of an incident should file a report, and only the person making the report should sign it. Never sign a report describing circumstances or events that you didn't

Documenting advance directives

As patient self-determination bills become law, health care facilities are spurred to develop procedures to satisfy their patient's requests and to comply with the law as well. Accordingly, more and more health care facilities are requiring documentation of the patient's advance directive or lack of it.

An advance directive is a legal document by which a person tells his medical caregivers how he prefers to be treated in an illness from which he can't reasonably expect to recover. Advance directives also include living wills (which instruct the doctor to administer no life-sustaining treatment) and durable powers of attorney (which name another person to act in the patient's behalf for medical decisions in the event that the patient cannot act for himself).

Because these laws vary from state to state, be sure to find out how the law applies to your practice and to the medical record.

Previously executed directive

If a patient has previously executed an advance directive, request a copy of it for his chart. Some health care facilities routinely make this request a part of admission or preadmission procedures.

Also be sure to document the name, address, and phone number of the person entrusted with decision-making power.

Presently executed directive

If a patient wants to execute an advance directive during his stay in the health care facility, he can do so as long as he's a competent adult. In such a case, the record should include documented proof of competency (usually the responsibility of the medical, legal, social services, or risk management department) along with the signed and witnessed, newly executed advance directive.

Directives about nutrition and hydration

If you practice in an area with laws related to artificial nutrition and hydration (nourishment provided by invasive tubes and I.V. lines—not food and fluid taken by mouth), record the patient's wishes if these issues are not addressed in his advance directive.

Revocation of the directive

Legally, the patient can revoke an advance directive at any time verbally or in writing. In such a case, include a copy of the written revocation in the record or sign and date a statement in the patient's medical record that the patient made the request verbally. Consult your hospital policy and state laws pertaining to living wills and advance directives. This statement may need to be countersigned.

witness. Each person with firsthand knowledge should fill out and sign a *separate* report. Your report should:
• identify the person involved in the incident

• document accurately and objectively any unusual occurrences that you witnessed
• record details of what happened and the consequences for the persons involved; include sufficient information so that admin-

istrators can decide whether the matter requires further investigation
• avoid opinions, judgments, conclusions, or assumptions about who or what caused the incident
• avoid making suggestions about how to prevent the incident from happening again.

Such items as detailed statements from witnesses and descriptions of remedial action are normally part of an investigative follow-up: Don't include them in the incident report itself. Although the incident report isn't part of the patient's chart, it may be used later in litigation. Don't note in the chart that you filed an incident report, but do include the clinical details of the incident in the chart. Make sure that the descriptions in the incident report and the chart mirror each other. (See Chapter 2, Legal and Ethical Implications of Documentation.)

Once it's filed, the incident report may be reviewed by the nursing supervisor, the doctor called to examine the patient, appropriate department heads and administrators, the health care facility's attorney, and the insurance company. (See *What happens to an incident report,* page 286.)

Falls

Current research shows that patient falls constitute 75% to 80% of all incidents reported on clinical units. The total includes falls involving patients, visitors, and staff. Among events qualifying as falls are slips, slides, knees giving way, faints, or tripping over equipment. About 2% of all hospitalized patients fall, and of these, 2% suffer a fracture.

Charting the patient's final request

If a terminally ill patient expresses a wish not to be resuscitated, and you call a code when he goes into cardiac or respiratory arrest, you're violating his right to refuse treatment. But if you don't call a code, you're practicing medicine without a license, and you're liable for his death if he dies.

How to proceed
• If a terminally ill patient tells you he doesn't want to be resuscitated in a crisis, document his statement and chart his degree of awareness and orientation. Contact your nurse-manager immediately and request assistance from administration, legal services, or social services.
• If the doctor knows of the patient's wish and still refuses to write a do-not-resuscitate order, document this in your notes. The doctor has the same responsibility regarding the patient's right to refuse treatment that you have, and he may be liable if he doesn't comply with the patient's request.
• If your terminally ill patient has prepared an advance directive, make sure that his doctor has seen it and is aware of it.

Consequences of falls include prolonged hospitalization, increased hospital costs, and liability problems.

Risk and prevention
Because falls raise so many problems, your health care facility may require an all-out risk assessment and prevention effort. (See *Determining a patient's risk of falling,* page 287.) If so, you'll need to document

What happens to an incident report

The chart below provides a comprehensive overview of incident report routing.

Patient incident

Report significant medical and nursing facts in patient's chart.

Write incident report during the shift on which the incident took place.

Give incident report to supervisor.

Unit supervisor forwards report to appropriate administrator within 24 hours.

Administrator reviews report.

Administrator forwards pertinent information from the report to the appropriate department for follow-up action.

Incident reports are collected and summarized to detect patterns and trends and to highlight trouble spots.

Administrator reviews patterns and trends and decides whether incidents result from poor policies or staff errors.

If incidents result from policy problems, the health care facility makes appropriate policy changes.

If incidents result from staff errors, the health care facility directs appropriate personnel to investigate records to detect trends.

If the records indicate a pattern of errors or if the error being reviewed is grievous, the hospital offers appropriate remediation, such as counseling, a refresher course or, rarely, probation or suspension.

Determining a patients' risk of falling

Certain patients have a greater risk of falling than others. Using a chart such as the one below, which was developed for use with older patients, can help you determine the extent of the risk.

To use the chart, check each applicable item and total the number of points. A score of 10 or above indicates a risk of falling.

POINTS   **PATIENT CATEGORY**

Age

1	_____	80 or older
2	✓	70 to 79 years old

Mental state

0	_____	Oriented at all times or comatose
2	_____	Confused at all times
4	✓	Confused periodically

Duration of hospitalization

0	✓	Over 3 days
2	_____	0 to 3 days

Falls within the past 6 months

0	_____	None
2	✓	1 or 2
5	_____	3 or more

Elimination

0	✓	Independent and continent
1	_____	Uses catheter, ostomy, or both
3	_____	Needs help with elimination
5	_____	Independent and incontinent

1	✓	**Visual impairment**
3	_____	**Confinement to chair**
2	_____	**Blood pressure**

Drop in systolic pressure of 20 mg Hg or more between lying and standing positions

POINTS   **PATIENT CATEGORY**

Gait and balance

Assess gait by having the patient stand in one spot with both feet on the ground for 30 seconds without holding onto something. Then have him walk straight ahead and through a doorway. Next, have him turn while walking.

1	_____	Wide base of support
1	✓	Loss of balance while standing
1	_____	Balance problems when walking
1	_____	Diminished muscle coordination
1	_____	Lurching or swaying
1	_____	Holds on or changes gait when walking through a doorway
1	_____	Jerking or instability when turning
1	_____	Needs an assistive device, such as a walker

Medications

How many different drugs is the patient taking?

0	_____	None
1	_____	1
2	✓	2 or more

___	Alcohol	✓ Hypoglycemics
___	Anesthetics	___ Narcotics
___	Antihistamines	___ Psychotropics
✓	Antihyperten-	___ Sedative-hyp-
	sives	notics
___	Antiseizure	___ Other drugs
	drugs	(specify)
___	Antidiabetics	
___	Benzodiazepines	
___	Cathartics	
___	Diuretics	

1	✓	Check if the patient has changed drugs, dosage, or both in the past 5 days.

_13_ **TOTAL**

your role in this activity. For example, if your facility requires a risk assessment form for patients, complete it and keep it in the patient's chart.

Avoiding falls

There are no foolproof ways to prevent every patient from falling, but the following strategies may help. As required by your health care facility, document the following safety interventions:

• Keep the bed's side rails raised or lowered, when indicated, and include your decision to do so in the chart as part of your interventions for addressing the nursing diagnosis of "Risk for trauma."
• Monitor the patient regularly—continuously, if his condition makes this necessary—and document your findings.
• Offer a bedpan or commode regularly and chart this care measure.
• Provide an adequately lighted and clean, clutter-free environment.
• Make sure that someone helps and supports the patient whenever he gets out of bed and that he has proper footwear for walking safely.
• Make sure that adequate staff are available to transfer him, if necessary.
• Apply restraints or mechanical devices that provide a warning signal when a patient tries to climb out of bed.
• Suggest that a relative or friend stay with the patient.
• Patients taking medications that cause orthostatic hypotension, central nervous system depression, or vestibular toxicity need special nursing care when a doctor's orders require them to be up in a chair for meals. If you can't supervise such a patient while he's sitting up, make sure that another member of the health care team does.

Charting falls

If a patient falls despite precautions, be sure to chart the event and file an incident report. Check the patient for bruises, lacerations, or abrasions. Note any pain or deformity in the extremities, particularly the hip, arm, leg, or lumbar spine. Assess blood pressure while the patient is lying down and sitting up. Look for a drop of 20 to 30 mm Hg in the systolic reading, which may indicate orthostatic hypotension. Perform a neurologic assessment. Check for slurred speech, a weakness in the extremities, or a change in mental status. Notify the patient's doctor.

| 1/6/95 | 1400 | Pt. found on the floor beside her bed and chair. Pt. c/o pain in her Ⓡ hip area with difficulty moving Ⓡ leg. No abrasions or lacerations noted. BP elevated at 158/94. P, 94; R, 22. Pt. states she fell trying to get to her chair. Mental status unchanged. Dr. Burns notified. Pt. returned to bed. Hip X-ray reveals fractured Ⓡ hip. Pt. medicated for hip pain. Family notified by Dr. Burns. Pt. assessed hourly. Discussed the need for side rails with pt. Instructed in use of call button. Side rails up at present. —————Ellen Kumich, RN |

Restraints

Restraints are "prescriptive devices"—you can't use them unless you have a doctor's order. (Some states may authorize other licensed health care professionals to prescribe restraints.) You'll need to consult your hospital's policy for the correct protocol to follow in emergencies—for example, when the patient's safety is at risk and you have no time to obtain an order.

Restraints can cause numerous problems, including limited mobility, skin breakdown, impaired circulation, incontinence, and strangulation.

If you are ordered to use restraints with a patient, avoid causing pain or injury to the patient by applying them in a safe manner. (See *Using restraints safely,* page 290.)

| 12/12/94 | 0100 | Pt. getting OOB repeatedly and wandering in hallway. Confused and thinks he is at home. Even while I sat in room, he continued to climb over the side rails to get OOB. Dr. Cohen notified. Posey protective device ordered and applied. Explained the reasons for applying device with pt. Pt. checked q̄ 15 min. VS WNL. Pt. sleeping comfortably at present.————— *Mary Pomante, Rn* |
| | 0130 | Patient sleeping comfortably. ————— *Mary Pomante, Rn* |

If a competent patient makes an informed decision to refuse restraint, the hospital may require the patient to sign a release that would absolve the hospital of liability should injury result from the patient's refusal to be restrained.

Burns

Another frequent cause of injury to patients is burns. Patients are burned by spilled hot food or liquids, hot baths, and electrical equipment. Always assess the risk of burns and take appropriate precautions.

Patients who have hand tremors should be cautioned not to handle hot foods or liquids by themselves. Patients with decreased sensation in their feet or hands should be taught to test bathwater with an unaffected extremity. Explain to patients taking medication causing drowsiness that they may be more prone to burns and need to be cautious. Document these instructions in your notes and the patient's response to this information.

If a patient in your care does burn himself, always document the injury in his chart.

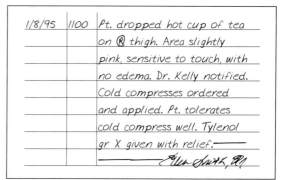

| 1/8/95 | 1100 | Pt. dropped hot cup of tea on ® thigh. Area slightly pink, sensitive to touch, with no edema. Dr. Kelly notified. Cold compresses ordered and applied. Pt. tolerates cold compress well. Tylenol gr X given with relief.——— *Ellen Smith, RN* |

Discharge AMA

Although a patient can choose to leave the hospital at any time, the law requires clear evidence that he's mentally competent to make that choice. In most hospitals, an AMA form serves as a legal document to protect you, the doctors, and the facility should any problems arise from a patient's unapproved discharge.

Using restraints safely

Improperly restraining a patient can leave you vulnerable to a host of legal charges, such as negligence, professional malpractice, false imprisonment, or battery. The case discussed below is about a nurse who failed to use restraints effectively.

The patient who slipped away
In *Robison v. Micheline Faine and Catalano's Nurse Registry, Inc.* (1987), the nurse, Micheline Faine, was required to restrain the patient, Ms. Robison, before leaving her hospital room. With the time for lunch break approaching, Faine tied the patient in a restraining device and left to find a relief nurse. Once the relief nurse entered the room, Faine left for lunch.

When Faine returned 20 minutes later, she found that Ms. Robison was gone, although the restraining device was still attached to the bed and the side rails were up. While Faine had been at lunch, Ms. Robison had slipped out of the restraint, left the hospital through an emergency stairway leading to the roof, and attempted to jump to a nearby tree. She fell to the ground and sustained serious injuries.

No exemption from liability
At the malpractice trial, the judge instructed the jury to exempt Ms. Faine from liability. But an appeals court disagreed. It ruled that Ms. Faine wasn't automatically exempt from liability because the patient would have been unable to free herself if the restraining device had been tied correctly. The appeals court ordered a new trial for Ms. Faine to determine whether she was negligent.

The AMA form should clearly document that the patient knows he's leaving against medical advice, that he's been advised of the risks of leaving and understands them, and that he knows he can come back. If a patient refuses to sign the AMA form, document this refusal on the form and enter it in his chart. Use the patient's own words to describe his refusal. Include the following information on the AMA form:
• patient's reason for leaving AMA
• names of relatives or others notified of the patient's decision and the dates and times of the notifications
• explanation of the risks and consequences of the AMA discharge, as told to the patient, including the name of the person who provided the explanation
• instructions regarding alternative sources of follow-up care given to the patient
• list of those accompanying the patient at discharge and the instructions given to them
• patient's destination after discharge.

Document any statements and actions reflecting the patient's mental state at the time he chose to leave the hospital. This will help protect you, the doctor, and the hospital against a charge of negligence. The patient may later claim that his discharge occurred while he was mentally incompetent and that he was improperly supervised while he was in that state.

1/4/95	1400	Pt. found in room, packing his
		clothes. When asked why he
		was dressed and packing, he
		stated, "I am tired of all
		these tests, and I'm not having
		any more of them. They still
		don't know what's wrong with
		me. I can't take any more of
		this. I'm going home." Dr.
		Minelli notified and came to
		speak with pt. Pt.'s wife
		notified and she came into
		the hospital. She was unable
		to persuade husband to stay.
		Pt. willing to sign AMA form.
		AMA form signed. Pt. told of
		the possible risks of his
		leaving the hospital with
		headaches and hypertension.
		Pt. agrees to see Dr. Minelli
		in his office in 2 days. Dis-
		cussed appointment with pt.
		and wife. Pt. going home
		after discharge. Accompanied
		pt. in wheelchair to main
		lobby, with wife. Pt. left
		at 1345 hr. ———
		——— *Lynn Bonell*

Also check your facility's policy regarding incident reports. If the patient leaves without anyone's knowledge or if he refuses to sign the AMA form, you'll probably be required to fill out an incident report.

Missing patient

Suppose the same patient never said anything about leaving, but on rounds you discover he's missing. First, of course, try to find him in the hospital. Attempt to contact his home. If he's gone, notify your nurse-manager, the patient's doctor, and the police, if necessary. The police are usually called if there is a possibility of the patient hurting himself or others, especially if he's left the hospital with any medical devices.

In the chart, note the time that you discovered the patient missing, your attempts to find him, and the people notified. Include any other pertinent information.

Selected references

Berryman, E.P., et al. "Point by Point: Predicting Elders' Falls," *Geriatric Nursing* 10(4):199-201, July-August 1989.

Better Documentation. Clinical Skillbuilders. Springhouse, Pa.: Springhouse Corp., 1992.

Burton, M. "Keeping Track of Intake and Output," *Nursing94* 24(4):25, April 1994.

Cohen, M.R., and Davis, N.M. "Preprinted Order Forms: Tips for Troubleshooting," *Nursing94* 24(4):49, April 1994.

Eggland, E.T. *Nursing Documentation Resource Guide.* Gaithersburg, Md.: Aspen 1993.

Everyday Events

Fischbach, F.T. *Documenting Care: Communication, the Nursing Process and Documentations Standards.* Philadelphia: F.A. Davis, 1991.

Green, E., and Katz, J.A. "A Quality-Assurance Tool That Works Overtime," *RN* 49(9):30-31, September 1989.

Iyer, P. "Documenting Telephone Orders," *Nursing92* 22(8):21, August 1992.

Iyer, P. "Thirteen Charting Rules to Keep You Legally Safe," *Nursing91* 21(6):40-45, June 1991.

Iyer, P.W., and Camp, N.H. *Nursing Documentation: A Nursing Process Approach,* 2nd ed. St. Louis: Mosby–Year Book, Inc., 1995.

Kessler, D.A. "Using Medwatch: A Better Way to Report Adverse Events," *Nursing93* 23(11):49-50, November 1993.

Leger-Krall, S. "When Restraints Become Abusive," *Nursing94* 24(3):55-56, March 1994.

Nurse's Legal Handbook, 3rd ed. Springhouse, Pa.: Springhouse Corp., 1996.

Nurse's PhotoLibrary. Springhouse Pa.: Springhouse Corp., 1994.

Nursing Procedures, 2nd ed. Springhouse, Pa.: Springhouse Corp., 1996.

Stephan, A. "Notifying the Doctor by Phone," *Nursing93* 23(11)20, November 1993.

Stephan, A. "Charting Tips: Documenting Your Patient's Valuables," *Nursing93* 23(10):31, October 1993.

Stewart, S., and Cohen, M.R. "Fast Facts About FAX," *Nursing90* 20(8):41, August 1990.

CHAPTER EIGHT

Legally Perilous Charting Practices

If you're ever named in a malpractice suit that proceeds to court, your documentation may be your best defense. It provides a running record of your patient care. How and what you documented—and even what you didn't document—will heavily influence the outcome of the trial.

Credible evidence

Typically, the outcome of every malpractice trial boils down to one question: Whom will the jury believe? The answer usually depends on the credibility of the evidence. In a malpractice suit, a plaintiff presents evidence designed to show that he was harmed or injured because care provided by the defendant (in this case, the nurse) failed to meet accepted standards of care. The nurse, of course, strives to present evidence demonstrating that she provided an acceptable standard of care. However, if she can't offer believable evidence, the jury may have no choice but to accept the plaintiff's evidence. Even worse, if the nurse's evidence—including the medical record—is discredited, the plaintiff's attorney may convince a jury of her negligence.

In a malpractice suit, jurors usually view the medical record as the best evidence of what really happened. It's often the hinge that swings the jury's verdict.

Negligent or not

If you have actually been negligent and have truthfully documented the care given, the medical record will naturally be the plaintiff's best evidence, as it should be. In such instances, the case will probably be settled out of court.

If you haven't been negligent, the medical record should be your best friend. It should provide the best evidence of quality care (even though a plaintiff's attorney can manipulate standard data and charting practices to make them *seem* negligent). If the charted record makes you *seem* negligent, however, the jurors may conclude that you *were* negligent because they base their decision on the evidence. The lesson: A "bad" medical record can be used to make a good nurse look bad. A "good" medical record should defend itself—and those who wrote it.

Because malpractice litigation is on the rise—and because more and more nurses are being specifically named in such lawsuits—you'll need to document defensively, especially in legally hazardous situations.

By knowing how to chart, what to chart, when to chart, and even who should chart, you'll avoid many legal perils. And knowing how to handle such legally sensitive situations as patient nonconformance, knowing how to protect yourself from misinterpreting written records, and knowing how computer charting affects lawsuits will offer additional safeguards.

How to chart

You may assume that every nurse knows how to chart. This isn't necessarily so. Charting is a craft that's refined with experience. A skilled nurse knows that she needs to document defensively, keeping in mind that it's not only what she charts but how she charts that's important.

Chart objectively

The medical record should contain descriptive, objective information: what you see, hear, feel, smell, measure, and count—not what you suppose, infer, conclude, or assume. The chart may also contain subjective information, but only when it's supported by documented facts.

Resist drawing conclusions

As important as reporting facts objectively is the need to resist including your opinions or drawing conclusions when you chart. If your opinions come to light in a courtroom, the plaintiff's attorney will have an opportunity to impugn your credibility and the credibility of the medical record as well. (See *Avoiding assumptions*, page 296.)

Stick with the facts

To make sure that you keep the medical record factual, follow these simple rules:
• Record only what you see and hear. For example, don't record that a patient pulled out his I.V. line if you didn't witness him doing so. Do, however, describe your findings—for example, "Found pt., arm board, and bed linens covered with blood. I.V. line and venipuncture device were untaped and hanging free...."

Similarly, don't record that a patient fell out of bed if you didn't see him fall. If you saw him lying on the floor, record that. If the patient says he fell out of bed, record that. If you heard a muffled thud, went to the patient's room, and found him lying on the floor, record that. An example of how to document a patient's fall appears above at right.

1/8/95	0600	Heard pt. scream. Found pt.
		lying beside bed. Pt. has lacer-
		ation 2 cm long on forehead.
		Side rails up. Pt. stated he
		climbed over side rails to go
		to the bathroom. BP elevated
		at 184/92, P 96, R 24. Dr.
		Phillips notified. Pt. c/o pain
		in ® hip. Pt. to X-ray for
		X-ray of ® hip.———————
		————— Mary Jo Faye, RN

• Describe—don't label—events and behavior. Expressions such as "appears spaced out," "flying high," "exhibiting bizarre behavior," or "using obscenities" mean different things to different people.

If a plaintiff's attorney asked you to define those terms, could you do it? Even if you could, would you be likely to gain or lose credibility in the process? Which will give the plaintiff's attorney more room to maneuver—objective facts or subjective conclusions?

Facts, accurately reported, give the plaintiff's attorney little room to maneuver. Subjective conclusions force you into the uncomfortable position of having to defend your own words. You will almost always lose credibility and distract the jury from your main defense in the process. Keep these considerations in mind when you chart.
• Be specific. Your goal in documenting is to describe facts clearly and concisely. To do so, use only approved abbreviations and express your observations in quantifiable terms.

For example, concluding "output adequate" isn't as helpful as giving an exact measurement of 1,200 ml. Similarly, "Pt. appears to be in pain" is vague. Ask your-

ON TRIAL

Avoiding assumptions

Strive to record the facts about a situation—not your assumptions or conclusions. In the following example, a nurse failed to document the facts—and instead charted her assumptions about a patient's fall. As a result, she has to endure this damaging cross-examination by the plaintiff's attorney.

ATTORNEY: Would you read your fifth entry for January 6th, please?
NURSE: 'Patient fell out of bed....'
ATTORNEY: Thank you. Did you actually see the patient fall out of bed?
NURSE: Actually, no.
ATTORNEY: Did the patient tell you he fell out of bed?
NURSE: No.
ATTORNEY: Did anyone actually see the patient fall out of bed?
NURSE: Not that I know of.
ATTORNEY: So these notes reflect nothing more than conjecture on your part. Is that correct?
NURSE: I guess so.
ATTORNEY: Is it fair to say then, that you charted something as fact even though you didn't know it was?
NURSE: I suppose so.
ATTORNEY: Thank you.

self why he "appears to be in pain" and document the specific findings—for example, "Pt. requested pain medication after complaining of severe lower back pain radiating to his right leg."

Similarly, avoid catchall phrases such as "Pt. comfortable." Instead, describe his comfort. Is he resting, reading, sleeping? This type of information is more helpful and informative.

Here's an example of specific, clear documentation:

2/1/95	1400	Dressing removed from ℝ mastectomy site. Incision is pink. No drainage. Measures 12.5 cm long and 2 cm wide. Slight bruising noted center of incision. Dressing dry. Drain site below mastectomy incision measures 2 cm x 2 cm. Bloody, dime-sized drainage noted on drain dressing. No edema noted. Betadine dressings applied. Pt. complaining of mild incisional pain. 2 Tylox P.O. given at 1330 hours. Pt. reports relief.——— *Joan Delaney, RN*

Use neutral language

Avoid including inappropriate comments or language in your notes. Not only are such comments unprofessional, but they can trigger difficulties in legal cases.

For example, one elderly patient's family became upset after the patient developed pressure ulcers. They complained that the patient wasn't receiving adequate care. The patient later died, probably of natural causes.

However, because the patient's family was dissatisfied with the care the patient received, they sued. In the patient's chart, under prognosis, the doctor had written "PBBB." After learning that this stood for "pine box by bedside," the insurance company was only too happy to settle for a significant sum.

Eliminate bias

Don't use words that suggest a negative attitude toward the patient. For example, don't use unflattering or unprofessional adjectives such as "obstinate," "drunk," "obnoxious," "bizarre," or "abusive" to describe the patient's behavior.

Remember, the law allows the patient to see his chart. A derogatory reference is likely to anger the patient—and an angry patient is more likely to sue.

Disparaging remarks, accusations, arguments, or name-calling could lead to a defamation of character or libel suit. Not only that, just imagine how your harsh words would sound in court. They most certainly would invite the plaintiff's attorney to attack your professionalism with an argument such as this: "Look at how this nurse felt about my client—she called him 'rude, difficult, and uncooperative.' It's right here in her own handwriting! No wonder she didn't take good care of this patient—she didn't like him."

If a patient is difficult or uncooperative, document the behavior objectively. That way, the jurors will draw their own subjective conclusions. Here's one example:

| 1/19/95 | 1400 | I attempted to give pt. medication, but he said, "I've had enough pills. Now leave me alone." Explained the importance of the medication and attempted to determine why he would not take it. Pt. became agitated and refused to talk. Dr. Ellis notified that medication was not given and that pt. is agitated. —— *Anne Curry, R.N.* |

Keep the medical record intact

Take special care to keep the patient's chart complete and intact. Discarding pages from the medical record, even for innocent reasons, is bound to raise doubt in an attorney's mind about the chart's reliability.

Suppose, for example, you spill coffee on a page, blurring several entries. You remove the original page from the chart, copy it, and place the copy in the chart. Then you discard the original. Imagine having to admit to a jury that you destroyed original evidence.

You could try to explain that you did so for an innocent reason, but the jury could be difficult to convince. Jurors are skeptical; they must be. Giving them something like that to use against you makes the plaintiff's job a lot easier and yours much more difficult.

Once something is considered part of the official record, never discard or destroy it. If you replace an original sheet with a copy, cross-reference it with lines like these: "Recopied from page..." and "Recopied on page...." Then, be sure to retain the original. (See *Consequences of missing records,* page 298.)

What to chart

When you're busy, getting your work done may seem more important than documenting every detail. But from a jury's viewpoint, an incomplete chart suggests incomplete nursing care. This is one of the most serious and frequent charting errors. It's no accident that a popular saying among malpractice attorneys is "Not charted, not done."

Consequences of missing records

The case of *Battocchi v. Washington Hospital Center,* 581 A.2d 759 (D.C. App. 1990), underscores the significance of keeping the medical record intact. In this case, the plaintiffs brought a medical malpractice suit against the hospital and a doctor for injuries sustained by their son during forceps delivery.

The nurse in attendance documented the events and her observations of the delivery immediately after the delivery and posted the record in the chart. Later, the hospital's risk management personnel obtained the chart for analysis but apparently lost the nurses' notes from the record.

The court ruled in favor of the hospital and doctor, holding that the jury couldn't presume negligence and causation against them simply because the hospital lost the attending nurse's notes.

However, on appeal, the District of Columbia Court of Appeals sent the case back to the trial court so that the lower court could rule whether the hospital's loss of the records stemmed from negligence or impropriety.

That's not literally true, of course, but it's an easy conclusion for a jury to draw. You may have performed a nursing procedure that you simply forgot to chart. If the chart doesn't back you up, though, you'll have a hard time convincing a jury to accept your version of events. Many malpractice disputes arise when a nurse is accused of not performing a necessary duty that she says she performed.

Learn to anticipate litigation whenever you give patient care. Before you document, assess the situation and decide whether your actions might become significant in light of a lawsuit. If they could, chart them. Specifically, be sure to chart anything having to do with medication administration and the patient's response to treatment, unusual events, full assessment data, and discharge teaching. For example, if you withhold a medication or omit a treatment (or perform other activities that deviate from the usual), document the reason. Also document any actions taken to address the omission, if applicable.

Failure to document everything diminishes your ability to confidently and persuasively testify about the details—any one of which could be critical to the verdict. Of course, you should never document some things, such as conflicts among the staff. (See *Keeping the record clean.*)

Record critical and extraordinary information

When you encounter a critical or an extraordinary situation, take pains to document the details. Failure to chart these situations can have serious repercussions. (See *What you don't chart can hurt you,* page 301, and *Recording critical information: A case in point,* page 302.)

For example, consider the case of Tommy York, who was left partially paralyzed and severely brain damaged after an accident. He was admitted to the hospital for an intensive rehabilitation program.

Soon after he arrived, his parents told his nurse that a support from the right side of his wheelchair was missing and that they had noticed scratches on their

Keeping the record clean

What you say and how you say it are of utmost importance in documenting defensively. Even statements you think are harmless may return to haunt you in a lawsuit. Keeping the patient's chart free of negative, inappropriate information—potential legal bombshells—can be quite a challenge when you're writing detailed narrative notes. Here are some guidelines to help you sidestep charting pitfalls—and record a more accurate account of your patient's care and status.

Avoid reporting staffing problems
Granted, staff shortages may affect patient care or contribute to an incident. But don't refer to staffing problems in a patient's chart. Instead, discuss them in a forum that can help resolve the problem. In a confidential memo or an incident report, call the situation to the attention of the appropriate personnel, such as your nurse-manager. Also review your hospital's policy and procedure manuals to determine how you're expected to handle this situation.

Keep staff conflict and rivalries out of the record
Entries about disputes with nursing colleagues (including characterization and criticism of care provided), questions about a doctor's treatment decisions, or reports of a colleague's rude or abusive behavior reflect personality clashes and don't belong in the medical record. They're not legitimate concerns about patient care. Worse, these entries may trigger further investigation by the plaintiff's attorney, who is likely to exploit any conflict among codefendants.

As you would with staffing problems, address concerns about a colleague's judgment or competence in the appropriate setting. Talk with your nurse-manager (just make sure that you have the facts). Consult with the doctor directly if an order puzzles you. Share your opinions, observations, or reservations about colleagues with your nurse-manager only; avoid mentioning them in a patient's chart.

If you discover personal accusations or charges of incompetence in a chart, speak with the writer of the criticisms and point out the implications of including such conflicts in the medical record.

Never mention an incident report in the medical record
A confidential, administrative communication, an incident report is filed separately from the patient's chart. Although you should document the facts of an incident in the patient's chart, never use the words "incident report" or indicate in the patient's chart that you have filed one.

For example, "Found pt. lying on the floor at 1250 hours. Vital signs were stable. Notified Dr. Gary Dietrich at 1253 hours, and he saw pt. at 1300 hours" is a sufficient and accurate statement of the facts.

Steer clear of words associated with errors
Terms such as "by mistake," "accidentally," "somehow," "unintentionally," "miscalculated," and "confusing" are bonus words to a plaintiff's attorney. Don't use a term that suggests an error was made or that a patient's safety was jeopardized. Instead, let the facts speak for themselves.

(continued)

Keeping the record clean *(continued)*

For example, "Pt. was given Demerol 100 mg I.M. at 1300 hours for abdominal pain. Dr. was notified but gave no orders. Pt.'s vital signs remained stable."

If the ordered drug dose was 50 mg, this entry will let other health care providers know that the patient was overmedicated without calling undue attention to it.

Avoid naming names

Naming another patient in someone else's chart violates confidentiality. Use the word "roommate," the person's initials, or a room and bed number to describe the other patient.

Never chart that you informed a colleague of a situation if you only mentioned it

Telling your nurse-manager in the elevator or a rest room about a patient's deteriorating condition doesn't qualify as informing her. She's likely to forget the details; she may not even realize you expect her to intervene. You need to clearly state why you're notifying her so she can focus on the facts and take appropriate action. Otherwise, you can't say you've informed her.

son's right arm. The nurse failed to record the parents' or her own observations.

Later, the patient's hip became red, swollen, and increasingly painful. Despite the fact that Tommy York's mother pointed out these symptoms to the nurse, she again failed to record any observations in the medical record.

Finally, the patient was diagnosed with a broken hip. The parents sued and the court ruled the hospital negligent in the keeping of files, records, and other documents. The plaintiff was awarded $250,000, the maximum allowable in the state where the lawsuit was filed.

Look at the right-hand column for an example of how to document extraordinary information correctly.

2/19/95	0900	Digoxin 0.125 mg P.O. not given because of nausea and vomiting. Dr. Kelly notified that digoxin not given. Dr. Kelly gave order for digoxin 0.125 mg I.V. Administered at 0915 hours.————Ruth Bullock, R.N.

Chart complete assessment data

Failing to perform and then document an adequate physical assessment is a key factor in many malpractice suits. Therefore, when initially assessing your patient, focus on his chief complaint. But also follow up on—and document—any other problems he might mention in passing.

After completing the initial assessment, don't underestimate the value of a well-

What you don't chart can hurt you

Only careful documentation can substantiate your version of events. Consider the situations described below.

The case of the reputed phone call

A patient was admitted to the hospital for surgery for epicondylitis (tennis elbow). After the surgery, a heavy cast was applied to the patient's arm. The patient complained to the nurse of severe pain, for which the nurse repeatedly administered pain medication.

The next morning, when the surgeon visited, he split the patient's cast. By that time, the ulnar nerve was completely paralyzed and the patient was left with a useless, clawed hand.

The patient subsequently sued the nurse for failing to notify the surgeon about his pain. At the deposition, the dialogue between the nurse and the plaintiff's attorney sounded like this:

ATTORNEY: Did you call the doctor?
NURSE: I must have called him.
ATTORNEY: Do you remember calling him?
NURSE: Not exactly, but I must have.
ATTORNEY: Do you have a record of making that call?
NURSE: No, I don't.

ATTORNEY: If you'd made such a call, shouldn't there be a record of it?
NURSE: Yes, I guess so.
ATTORNEY: 'Guess' is right; you can't really say that you made that call. You can only 'guess' that you 'must have.'

The case of the secret incident

A patient who was recuperating from a total hip replacement was being lowered into a Hubbard tank by an orderly. During the process, the metal basket holding the patient collapsed, the patient struck his hip, and his wound reopened. The orderly stopped the bleeding and took the patient back to his room.

A nurse then treated the wound, but failed to document the facts of the incident. The wound later became infected, necessitating removal of the prosthesis. As a result, the patient was left with a permanent limp.

In the subsequent lawsuit, the court ruled in the patient's favor. The court noted that a determining factor was the absence of critical information on the patient's medical record, which would have assisted the doctor and staff in providing proper care.

constructed plan of care. A well-written plan of care not only gives you a clear approach to the patient's problems, but also helps defend your care if you are sued.

Phrase each patient problem statement clearly, and don't be afraid to modify the statement as you gather new assessment data. Also state the plan of care for solving each problem, and then identify the actions you intend to implement. What's important here is that you understand and communicate what you are doing and why. (For more information, see *Using good interview techniques to improve documentation,* page 303.)

Recording critical information: A case in point

The following case illustrates why you need to do your best to practice safely—and to accurately document as proof of your care. If you do, you have a good chance of staying out of court.

Failure to chart

Patti Bailey was admitted to deliver her third child. During her pregnancy, she'd gained 63 pounds, her blood pressure had risen from 100/70 in her first trimester to 140/80 at term, and an ultrasound done at 22 weeks showed possible placenta previa.

Over the 4 hours after her admission, she received 10 units of oxytocin in 500 ml of 5% dextrose in lactated Ringer's solution. Charting during this period was scant—her blood pressure was never recorded, and there were only single notations of the fetal heart rate and how labor was progressing. The nurses failed to record either the baby's reaction to the drug or the nature of Mrs. Bailey's contractions.

Suddenly, after complaining of nausea and epigastric pain, Mrs. Bailey suffered a generalized tonic-clonic seizure. Because her condition was so unstable, she couldn't undergo a cesarean section. So her baby girl was delivered by low forceps. Mrs. Bailey developed disseminated intravascular coagulation and required 20 units of whole blood, platelets, and packed red blood cells within 8 hours of delivery.

Incredibly, Mrs. Bailey's nurse had essentially documented nothing on the labor or delivery records or the progress notes.

Deficient policy and procedure manuals

When the unit's policy and procedure manuals were reviewed, no protocol for administering oxytocin and assessing the patient was included. At the very least, the manuals should have recommended using an oxytocin flow sheet to record vital signs, labor progress, fetal status, and changes in the drug administration rate.

The payoff

Although Mrs. Bailey recovered, her daughter has seizures and is developmentally disabled. Now age 15, the daughter can't walk or talk and she has a gastrostomy tube for nutrition. The case was settled out of court for $450,000, with the nurse and hospital responsible for one-third of the amount; the doctor paid the rest.

Document discharge instructions

Because of insurance constraints, the hospital commonly discharges patients earlier than in years past. As a result, the patient and his family must change dressings, assess wounds, and perform other functions that a nurse traditionally performed.

To perform these functions properly, the patient and his home caregiver must receive adequate instruction. The responsibility for these instructions is usually the nurse's. If a patient receives improper instructions and an injury results, you could be held liable.

Using good interview techniques to improve documentation

Assessing a patient's condition adequately is part of your professional and legal responsibility. That means following up and documenting each of the patient's complaints. Documenting your data can be easier when you know how to ask questions that evoke the most information from your patient. What follows is an example of an open-ended interview with a patient being assessed for abdominal pain.

NURSE: How would you describe the pain in your abdomen?
PATIENT: Well, it's dull but constant. Actually, it doesn't bother me as much as my blurry eyesight.
NURSE: Tell me about your blurry eyesight.
PATIENT: When I work long hours at my computer, all the words and lines seem to blend together. Sometimes it happens when I watch television too. I probably should see my eye doctor, but I haven't had the time.

NURSE: We'll be sure to follow up on your blurred vision. Now let's get back to that abdominal pain. How does it affect your daily routine and your ability to sleep?

A lot of things went right in this interview.
• First, the nurse didn't dismiss the patient's vision problem. If she had and it turned out to be serious, she may have been judged negligent.
• Second, she asked open-ended questions so that the patient could explain his answers rather than simply saying yes or no.
• Third, she didn't put words in the patient's mouth. For example, she avoided saying, "The abdominal pain bothers you when you try to sleep, doesn't it?" That would have been a leading question. And the patient, assuming the nurse knows the right answer because she's a nurse, might have answered yes— even if the correct answer was no.

Many hospitals distribute printed instruction sheets describing treatments and home care procedures that provide adequate instruction.

Courts typically consider these teaching materials as evidence that instruction took place. However, to support testimony that instructions were given, the materials should be tailored to each patient's specific needs and contain any verbal or written instructions you provide.

When to chart

Finding the time to chart can be a problem during a busy shift. But timely entries are of crucial concern in malpractice suits.

Ideally, you'll document your nursing care and other relevant activity when you perform it, or not long after—but never before performing it. (See *Understanding the importance of timely documentation,* pages 304 and 305.) Documenting ahead of time makes your notes inaccurate and also leaves out information about the pa-

Understanding the importance of timely documentation

Although you would never document care before providing it, you may wait until the end of your shift or until your dinner break to complete your nurses' notes. That's what one nurse did. Some time later she was summoned to court as a witness in a malpractice suit. She took the witness stand, answered the attorney's questions, and regularly referred to and read from the chart while doing so. She relied heavily on it for her defense and, in the process, implicitly asked the jury to do the same.

The plaintiff's attorney began his cross-examination by asking the nurse to read from her entries. After a few minutes, listen to what happened:

ATTORNEY: Excuse me, may I interrupt? As I listened to you read these entries, a question occurred to me. Maybe it occurred to the jury, too. Would you tell us whether you make the entries you are reading at the time of the events they describe?
NURSE: Well, no, I would have made them sometime later.
ATTORNEY: You're sure?
NURSE: Yes.
ATTORNEY: Thank you. Now, I'd like you to look at the chart and tell the jury whether you noted the time that you actually gave the patient his medication.
NURSE: No, I didn't.
ATTORNEY: Now, I'd like you to look at the chart again and tell the jury whether you indicated the time that you made the entry.
NURSE: No.
ATTORNEY: Given the absence of those two pieces of information, how could you so promptly and confidently respond to my origi-

nal question? How can you remember so clearly now that you made the entry sometime after the event it describes? Is it because your regular practice is to wait until the end of your shift to chart each and every detail of every event that transpired over your entire shift, and that you rely solely on your memory when making all these entries?
NURSE: Well, yes, that's true.
ATTORNEY: Would you tell the jury how long a shift you worked that day?
NURSE: A 10-hour shift.
ATTORNEY: And how many patients did you see over that 10-hour period?
NURSE: About 15.
ATTORNEY: Now, each of these 15 patients was different, correct? Each had his own individualized plan of care that corresponded to his particular health problems, isn't that right?
NURSE: That's right.
ATTORNEY: And how many different times did you see each of these different patients over the 10-hour period?
NURSE: I probably saw each one, on average, about once an hour.
ATTORNEY: In other words, you probably had 150 patient contacts on that shift alone, is that correct?
NURSE: I suppose so.
ATTORNEY: Now, during the course of your shift, do unexpected events sometimes develop? Unanticipated developments that must be attended to?
NURSE: Sometimes, yes.
ATTORNEY: And when these situations occur, do they distract you from things you had planned to do?
NURSE: Sometimes.

(continued)

Understanding the importance of timely documentation (continued)

ATTORNEY: After working such a long shift, do you sometimes feel tired?

NURSE: Yes.

ATTORNEY: And at the end of a shift, are you sometimes in a hurry? With things to do, places to go, people to see?

NURSE: Yes.

ATTORNEY: Now, would you tell the jury the purpose of the chart you keep for each patient?

NURSE: Well, we want to communicate information about the patient to others on the health care team, and we want to develop a historic account of the patient's problems, what's been done for him, and his progress.

ATTORNEY: So, other people rely on the information in this chart when they make their own decisions about the patient's care?

NURSE: Yes, that's true.

ATTORNEY: So you'd agree that the chart must be reliable?

NURSE: Yes.

ATTORNEY: And you'd agree that it must be factual and accurate in all respects?

NURSE: Yes.

ATTORNEY: And you'd agree that it needs to be comprehensive and complete, wouldn't you?

NURSE: Yes, I would.

ATTORNEY: So you're trying to develop a record that is factual, accurate, and complete at a time when you are sometimes tired, sometimes in a hurry, after working 10 consecutive hours and seeing 15 different patients 10 different times, and after having dealt with unexpected and distracting events. Is that the essence of your testimony?

NURSE: Well...yes.

ATTORNEY: Thank you. You may continue to read your entries to the jury.

By attacking the timeliness of charted entries, the attorney undermined their reliability, accuracy, and completeness. The jurors will now probably be skeptical of the chart.

How to prevent untimely entries

So, how do you prevent an attorney from exploiting this rather common charting practice resulting from limited time and a heavy workload? By routinely carrying a notepad and keeping personal, working notes. If you normally write notes while events are fresh in your mind, you won't have to deal with even the suggestion that your recollections at the end of the shift were uncertain, confused, mistaken, or otherwise unreliable. You've denied the opposition the opportunity.

When you make your official entries, use your working notes. Be sure, however, that your chart entries are consistent with them. During a lawsuit, a plaintiff's attorney could subpoena your notes, hoping to find discrepancies between them and the chart. If he succeeds, he'll use those discrepancies to discredit the chart.

Legally Perilous Practices

tient's response to intervention. Even though you may subsequently do what you charted, the practice leads to an attorney's question such as: "Is it your regular or even occasional practice to chart something in anticipation of doing it?" If you answer yes, the jury won't perceive the chart as a reliable indicator of what you actually did. From that point on, your credibility and that of the medical record will be compromised.

Who should chart

You, and only you, should chart your nursing care and observations. At times, because of understaffing or other circumstances, you may be tempted to ask another nurse to complete your portion of the medical record. However, doing so is a dangerous practice that's prohibited by your state's nurse practice act.

Do your own charting

Having someone else chart for you can result in disciplinary actions that range from reprimand to suspension of your nursing license. It may also cause harm to your patient if your coworker makes an error or misinterprets information.

If the patient sued you for negligence, you would be held accountable, along with your employer, because delegated documentation does not meet the standards of *average, reasonable, and prudent* nurses in a similar circumstance.

Delegating documentation duties has another consequence. It destroys the credibility and value of the medical record, leading reasonable nurses and doctors to doubt the accuracy of the chart, and it diminishes the record's value as legal evidence. A judge will give little, if any, weight to a medical record that contains secondhand observations or hearsay evidence. To avoid this unsafe practice, do your own charting and refuse to do anyone else's.

Countersign cautiously

Countersigning, or signing off on someone else's entry, is also a sticky practice, especially in court. Although countersigning doesn't imply that you performed the procedure, it does represent that you reviewed the entry and approved the care given, assuming that the entry is accurate.

To act correctly and to protect yourself, review your employer's policy on countersigning and proceed accordingly. Does the health care facility interpret countersigning to mean that the licensed practical nurse (LPN), graduate nurse, or nurse's aide performed the nursing actions in the countersigning registered nurse's presence? If so, don't countersign unless you were there when the actions occurred.

On the other hand, if your hospital acknowledges that you don't necessarily have time to witness your coworkers' actions, then your countersignature implies that the documentation describes care that the LPN or nurse's aide had the authority and competence to perform. In countersigning, you verify that all required patient care procedures were carried out.

If hospital policy does require you to countersign a subordinate's entries, be careful. Review each entry, and make sure it clearly identifies who did the procedure. If you sign off without reviewing an entry, or if you overlook a problem the entry raises, you could share liability for any patient injury that results.

What should you do if another nurse asks you to document her care or sign her notes? In a word, don't. Unless your hospital policy authorizes or requires you to witness someone else's notes, your signature will make you responsible for anything written in the notes above it.

Charting legally sensitive situations

Among the most legally charged situations are those involving dissatisfied and litigious patients and those related to nonconforming behavior. Especially difficult patients may refuse treatment or leave the health care facility against medical advice.

Handle difficult patients with care

No doubt you've cared for dissatisfied patients and heard remarks like these: "I've been ringing and ringing for a nurse. I could have died before you got here!" or "This food is terrible—take it away!" or "I've never seen such filth in my life. What kind of a hospital is this, anyway?" These are the sounds of unhappy, complaining patients. If you tend to dismiss them, you may be increasing your risk of a lawsuit.

Try to put out the fire

Not every dissatisfied patient sues for malpractice, but a few do. Recognizing these patients and taking positive action may be what's needed to avert a lawsuit.

The first step in defusing a potentially troublesome situation is to recognize that it exists. A postoperative recovery period riddled with complications, for example, is likely to create a dissatisfied patient—and his dissatisfaction spills onto everyone who cares for him.

Most nurses know the signs: constant grumpiness, endless complaints, no response to friendly remarks, not a trace of a smile when you try a little humor. You don't have to accept the situation; instead,

try to improve it. Here are three simple strategies:

• Continue reaching out to the patient, even if he doesn't respond.
• Ask your colleagues to support and reinforce your efforts.
• Record the details of all patient contacts. (See *Documenting precisely,* page 308.)

Attorneys will tell you that many prospective litigants are determined to sue the hospital and doctor but not the nurse, whom the litigant views as sympathetic, attentive, friendly, and communicative. What better protection against a lawsuit than a bond of trust and mutual respect?

Record threats

If a patient suggests he's going to sue you and other caregivers, document this on the progress notes and report it to your nurse-manager or your employer's legal department or attorney. If a patient states that he sued a health care facility in the past, document this information too and inform the appropriate personnel. For example, you might chart this:

1/26/95	1000	Pt. stated that he sued Lincoln Hospital and the nurses and Drs. who cared for him 2 years ago, when he had surgery there.——Dave Bevins, R.N.

Chart nonconforming behavior

Occasionally, a patient may do something—or fail to do something—that may contribute to his injury or explain why he hasn't responded to nursing and medical care. Documenting these behaviors will support your defense in a malpractice suit. Jurors usually have little sympathy for pa-

Documenting precisely

Careful documentation of every contact with a problem patient can help you defend yourself and the patient's care in court—or better yet, keep you out of court altogether. Here's an example of how precise documentation saved the day for one nurse.

A prospective client wanted to sue a hospital and nurse for an incident involving his elderly father, who had been hospitalized for a cholecystectomy. Several days after surgery, his father became disoriented and disorderly, fell out of bed, and broke both hips. He never walked again.

In talking with his attorney the client claimed, "That nurse either didn't know or didn't care that Dad was confused and agitated. She did nothing to protect him from harm. I want to sue."

The son's description of the father's care sounded like nursing negligence for sure—until the attorney reviewed the patient's record and the nurse's notes.

The nurse provided a detailed account of the events preceding the fall. Clearly, she not only knew about the patient's problem but also did everything she could to protect him. Specifically, she:
• confined him to bed with a Posey restraint
• assigned a volunteer to stay with him when he became agitated
• made sure the side rails were always up
• applied a chest restraint when the patient continued trying to climb out of bed
• notified coworkers at the nurses' station about the problem and asked them to watch the patient (his bed was visible from the nurses' station).

The record established that the nurse not only acted properly but also showed concern for the patient. The patient's son was convinced that this unfortunate accident was just that—an accident.

But even if the case had gone to court, that nurse would have been well prepared to meet any challenge to her memory—the details were all there, in black and white.

tients who don't follow instructions from a nurse or doctor.

Although patients have the right to refuse medical and nursing care—unless the refusal places them at risk for harming themselves or others—be sure to document on the progress notes the behavior that contradicts medical instructions.

Note failure to provide information

You may occasionally encounter a patient who refuses to provide accurate or complete information about his health history, current medications, or treatments. He may be uncooperative for various reasons: He thinks too many caregivers have asked him the same questions too many times, he doesn't understand the significance of the information, he's fearful or disoriented, or he's suspicious of why you want him to divulge personal information. Or he may have severe pain, a psychiatric problem, or a language barrier.

In such situations, try to obtain the information from other sources or forms.

Clearly document any trouble you've had in communicating with the patient.

Here's an example of what to chart when a patient refuses to answer questions:

2/5/95	0830	When asked for a list of his current medications, the pt. said, "Why do you want to know? What business is it of yours? I don't know why I have to answer that question." ———— Nora Martin, RN

Document bedside contraband

Document any unauthorized personal belongings discovered in the patient's possession (including alcoholic beverages, tobacco, heating pads, medications, vitamins, and other items that should be checked by the biomedical department before use). Describe the object and how you disposed of it. Here's an example:

2/9/95	1100	Found 3 cans of beer in pt.'s bedside table when checking his soap supply. Explained to pt. that beer was not allowed in the hospital. Took beer to nurses' station to be sent home with family. Dr. Kennedy notified at 1140 hours. He stated he would discuss this with pt. on rounds later today.——— Elaine Bannister, RN

Record misuse of equipment

At times, a patient may manipulate equipment or misuse supplies without understanding the consequences (pressing keys on a pump or monitor, detaching tubing,

or playing with switches, for example). When misuse occurs, document in the progress notes what you saw the patient do. Include a description of what you did about the problem. Here's an example:

2/6/95	0930	I.V. rate set at 60 ml/hour, 1,000 ml in bag. Doris Kohnsler, R.N.
2/6/95	1000	Checked I.V. 840 ml left in bag. Pt. stated, "I flicked the switch because I didn't see anything happening. Then I pressed the green button and the arrow." No change in BP, no signs of fluid overload. Breath sounds clear bilaterally. Instructed pt. not to touch the pump or I.V. Dr. Hentgen notified at 1030 hours. ——— Doris Kohnsler, R.N.

Chart unauthorized discharge and elopements

If a patient decides to leave the hospital against medical advice, try to elicit the reason for leaving. Then notify your nurse-manager, the patient's doctor, and possibly a member of his family, who may be able to persuade the patient to stay.

Expect the patient's doctor to inform the patient of the risks posed by refusing further treatment. Then, if the patient still intends to leave, have him sign a release form indicating that he understands the risks. (For more information on documenting against-medical-advice discharges, see Chapter 7, Documentation of Everyday Events.)

Suppose the patient never says anything about leaving, but elopes from the health care facility. On rounds you discover that he's missing. First, look for the patient within the unit and beyond. If you can't find him, notify security, your nurse-manager, the patient's doctor, and the patient's family. If the patient is at risk for harming himself or others, notify the police. Document the time you discovered the patient missing, your attempts to find him, and the people notified.

The legal consequences of a patient leaving the health care facility without medical permission can be particularly severe if he is confused or mentally incompetent, especially if he's injured or dies of exposure as a result of his absence.

Interpreting medical record entries

Of course keeping your own documentation neat and legible should be a primary goal. But what about other caregivers who aren't careful about their handwriting?

Misinterpreting medical record entries can lead to mistakes in care. Medication errors are a typical example. A doctor's sloppy handwriting, along with the ever-increasing number of drugs on the market, can complicate your job and put you in legal jeopardy.

To avoid making an error, always be certain you clearly understand a written order before carrying it out. If you have questions, clarify the order with the doctor who wrote it. Don't ask other nurses or doctors on the unit—they would be guessing, too. And if you're transferred or assigned to another unit where you're unfamiliar with the drugs being administered, ask an experienced nurse on the unit to give them for you.

An assistant director of nursing at a well-known general hospital learned this lesson when she decided to help out on an understaffed pediatric unit. A doctor ordered 3 ml of a digitalis glycoside for an infant. Not realizing that he meant the pediatric elixir, she administered 3 ml of an injectable, adult-strength digitalis glycoside. This was equivalent to about five times what the doctor intended. When the infant died, her parents successfully sued the nurse and the hospital. (See Chapter 7, Documentation of Everyday Events, for more on clarifying orders.)

Minimizing legal risks with computer charting

The legal implications of computerized medical records are still evolving. In most cases, computer records serve as legitimate substitutes for handwritten ones. But some state laws require health care facilities with electronic records to maintain handwritten records as well.

The most pressing legal questions concern the threat to patient privacy and confidentiality (see *Maintaining confidentiality with computer charting*). With traditional record keeping, access to information is restricted simply by keeping the record on the unit. With a computerized system of record keeping, such information can be retrieved by anyone who has the proper entry code.

Health care professionals and computer programmers have devised some safeguards to protect a patient's privacy. The primary safeguard is the signature code. By developing a series of access codes,

Maintaining confidentiality with computer charting

The American Nurses' Association, the American Medical Records Association, and the Canadian Nurses Association offer these guidelines and strategies for maintaining the confidentiality of computerized medical records.

Never share your password or computer signature
Never give your personal password or computer signature to anyone—including another nurse in the unit, a nurse serving temporarily in the unit, or a doctor. Your health care facility can issue a short-term password authorizing access to certain records for infrequent users.

Log off if not using your terminal
Don't leave a computer terminal unattended after you've logged on. (Some computers have a timing device that shuts down a terminal after a certain period of disuse.)

Follow protocol for correcting errors
Follow your health care facility's protocol for correcting errors. Computer entries are part of the patient's permanent record and, as such, can't be deleted. In most cases, however, you can correct an entry error before storing the entry. To correct an error after storage, mark the entry "error" or "mistaken entry," add the correct information, and date and initial the entry. If you record information in the wrong chart, write "error," and "wrong

chart," and sign off. Here's an example: 2/14/95, 1400 hours. Pt. out of bed to sit in chair for first time. Pt. followed directions well, but needed help of 2 nurses. Pulse 74 before transfer, 86 after transfer. Stayed in chair 1 hr. Required less help on return. Error, wrong chart. _____ Beth Marshall, RN

Make backup files
Make sure that stored records have backup files—an important safety feature. If you inadvertently delete part of the permanent record (which is hard to do because the program always asks if you're sure), type an explanation into the file with the date, time, and your initials. Submit an explanation in writing to your nurse-manager.

Never display patient information
Don't leave information about a patient displayed on a monitor where others can see it. Also, don't leave print versions or excerpts of the patient's medical record unattended. Keep a log that accounts for every copy of a computer file that you've printed.

Remember, a diagnosis of acquired immunodeficiency syndrome or human immunodeficiency virus infection is part of the patient's confidential record. Disclosing this information to unauthorized people may have significant legal implications. If the diagnosis is entered as any other diagnosis, follow your health care facility's confidentiality procedures.

programmers can limit access to the records. For example, a nurse's code would allow her to view a patient's entire record, but a lab technician's code would produce only the doctor's orders for laboratory studies.

Despite signature codes, more people have access to computerized records than have access to handwritten records. This expanded access provides greater opportunity for a patient's private medical information to be available to others.

Various laws protect the privacy of a patient's medical records. The Federal Privacy Act of 1974 protects the confidential medical information of patients in VA hospitals and, in some states, nurse practice acts impose an ethical duty to safeguard patients' privacy. However, no one can fully guarantee that unauthorized persons will not gain access to computerized records.

Selected references

Calfee, B. E. "Seven Things You Should Never Chart," *Nursing94* 24(3):43, March 1994.

Calfee, B. E. "Protecting Yourself from Allegations of Nursing Negligence," *Nursing91* 21(12):34-39, December 1991.

Iyer, P. "Charting Tips: Computer Charting: Minimizing Legal Risks." *Nursing93* 23(5):86, May 1993.

Iyer, P. "Six More Charting Rules to Keep You Legally Safe," *Nursing91* 21(7):34-39, July 1991.

Iyer P., and Camp, N. *Nursing Documentation: A Nursing Process Approach,* 2nd ed. St Louis: Mosby–Year Book, Inc., 1995.

Malpractice Lawsuits

Every practicing nurse is at risk for a malpractice suit. To protect yourself legally, you must do more than provide quality care—you must also document it clearly and accurately. Faulty documentation represents one of the leading causes of malpractice suits against nurses. (See *Why nurses are sued.*)

If you fail to document, chart haphazardly, or tamper with a patient's record, the court is likely to conclude that you also failed to provide care or that you have something to hide. What kind of documentation can withstand legal scrutiny? Documentation that shows you provided care meeting standards set forth by federal regulations, state laws, hospital policies, and your profession.

Each state has laws that define malpractice. Although these laws are worded differently, they all stipulate that malpractice occurs when a patient suffers because of a health care professional's wrongful conduct, improper discharge of duties, or failure to meet standards of care. These standards are the minimum criteria for job proficiency. They guide others in judging the quality of care you and your colleagues provide.

In a malpractice claim, the suing party's (plaintiff's) attorney tries to prove that a standard of care wasn't met. Documentation that fails to provide evidence that the standard was met makes the attorney's job that much easier. (See *Spotlight on documentation in court,* pages 316 and 317.)

If you're ever involved in a malpractice suit, you'll feel more secure if you know that your documentation stands on its own merit. You'll also feel more secure if you know what happens before a trial.

Pretrial preparations include what to do and what not to do if your patient's medical record is subpoenaed, what steps you and your attorney should take if you're sued, and how to conduct yourself during a deposition and, later, during a trial.

Your pretrial role

Your involvement in the pretrial process starts when you're served a subpoena and ends when you testify at the deposition. The patient's medical record—and your documentation—will be scrutinized at every turn.

Understanding subpoenas

You may first learn that you're involved in a lawsuit when you're served legal notification—a subpoena, or summons—that a plaintiff has made charges against you (the defendant) and that you must appear at a certain time and place to testify and respond to these charges.

The court can subpoena not only your presence but also the medical record (which includes your nursing documentation). A *subpoena duces tecum* is a command to produce certain documents (such as medical records) that may be used as evidence at trial. This type of subpoena is usually served on a hospital, a clinic, or an office, but it may be served on a nurse if she possesses the documents, as in the case of a nurse practitioner who maintains her own files.

Medical records are considered critical legal evidence. They describe (or fail to describe) acts, events, conditions, diagnoses, and opinions at or near the time of

Why nurses are sued

Malpractice charges against a nurse can result from various situations. In many of these situations, the lawsuit-triggering mishap may have been out of your control. What remains in your control, however, is your timely and accurate documentation of the patient's condition, your nursing interventions, and other relevant data.

If you accurately document that you provided appropriate care, the record should protect you and your employer and may go a long way toward averting a malpractice suit. Such a suit most commonly results in the areas described below.

Medication administration
• Incorrect medications and dosages
• Incorrect injection site (I.V., I.M., S.C.)
• Administration to the wrong patient
• Injury from injections

Obstetric and related care
• Nursing error or negligence causing injury during delivery
• Delay in notifying doctor, causing injury
• Failure to monitor mother's progress in labor
• Failure to monitor neonate's condition
• Failure to provide proper neonatal care

Patient falls
• Side rails left down
• Medicated patients left unattended
• Injury caused when moving or turning patient
• Patient left unattended on stretcher or examination table

Surgery and related care
• Foreign object left in patient
• Failure to monitor patient after surgery
• Negligent postoperative care

Care involving I.V. lines, catheters, and tubes
• Infiltration
• Negligence causing emboli
• Improper insertion causing injury
• Injection of improper solution
• Improper inflation of catheter bulbs

Record keeping
• Inaccuracy, or failure to record information
• Failure to use standard abbreviations
• Failure to communicate with doctor
• Breach of confidentiality

Personal liability
• Damage to insured's property
• Malicious acts
• Intentional tortious conduct

the alleged mishap and are kept by a person with firsthand knowledge or a duty to record. They're considered trustworthy because entries are made during the normal course of business, because employees have developed habits of precision in gathering and reporting information, and be-

cause they're maintained and filed in a specific location. The courts assume that the information in medical records is true. Although this presumption can be challenged in court, it's hard to rebut.

Spotlight on documentation in court

In a malpractice suit, a patient's medical record testifies to the quality of care you provided. Its importance in the courtroom can't be exaggerated—as you'll see from the following cases.

Inadequate care

In *Collins v. Westlake Community Hospital,* 312 N.E.2d 614 (1974), a minor patient successfully sued a nurse and hospital for negligence. The boy was hospitalized with a fractured left leg, which was set in a cast and placed in traction. The evening nurse documented the condition of the boy's toes several times during her shift. The night nurse, however, didn't record the condition of his toes until morning, even though the medical record contained a doctor's order to "Watch condition of toes." At 0600 hours, the nurse documented that the boy's toes were dusky and cold and that the doctor had been contacted.

Ultimately, the boy's leg had to be amputated at the knee because of ischemic necrosis resulting from a blood clot in the femoral artery. The plaintiff claimed the amputation was necessary because the night nurse failed to observe the condition of the boy's toes during the night.

A nurse expert for the defense testified that only abnormal findings needed to be documented, although the progress notes for the same time period the previous night contained circulation checks that didn't reflect abnormal findings. To the jury, the blank chart spoke louder than the expert's words: The jury inferred that no documentation meant no observation and found the nurse liable for malpractice.

Lax assessment

In *Arant et al. v. St. Francis Medical Center, Inc., et al., v. Cage,* 605 So.2d 622 (1992), a malpractice suit was filed against nurses, a doctor, and the hospital after a patient died from a kidney infarction. The plaintiff, Mrs. Arant, contended that nurses failed to monitor and assess her husband adequately, resulting in his death, and that inadequate monitoring and assessment made it harder for the doctor to treat the patient.

Although the plaintiff raised concerns about the nurses' record keeping, expert witness testimony failed to prove that deficient monitoring or record keeping caused or contributed to the patient's death.

Too late

In *Stevens v. Humana of Delaware, Inc.,* 832 P.2d 1076 (1992), a family sued a Delaware hospital for malpractice because their newborn sustained oxygen deprivation at birth.

Documentation was a key factor in the outcome. The medical record contained an entry made by the transport nurse, stating that the nurse-anesthetist didn't arrive in the labor and delivery room until 5 minutes after the baby was born. The transport nurse testified that she routinely recorded the events surrounding the birth of every child she transported. And she routinely took the history from the nurse who was present at the birth and had firsthand knowledge of the events.

The court ruled that the baby suffered from severe oxygen deprivation from the moment of birth and that the presence of a professional (such as a nurse-anesthetist) trained in infant resuscitation was essential to prevent serious neurologic damage.

Spotlight on documentation in court *(continued)*

Insufficient information
In *St. Paul Marine Insurance Co. v. Prothro,* 266 Ark. 1020, 590 S.W.2d 35 (Ark. Ct. App. 1979), a patient was injured in physical therapy after hip replacement. Through a series of mishaps in the hospital, the patient sustained a serious wound infection. Ultimately, he was left with a limp and a shortened leg. At the trial, the patient's doctor had to rely on the medical record to aid his memory of events.

In a ruling that favored the patient, the court found that those in the hospital with a duty to record (the nurses) failed to document reliable, complete, or critical information that would have helped the doctor and staff provide proper care for the patient.

Preserving the medical record

If you're being sued by a patient, you'll naturally want to scrutinize his medical record. If you notice gaps or missing information, don't panic and try to fill in the blanks. (See *Types of tampering,* page 318.) This would be unethical and grounds for revocation of your nursing license.

What's more, today's experts have sophisticated techniques for detecting altered records. Using sophisticated equipment, they can look beneath changes made over correction fluid to reveal the original writing, and they can date ink samples the size of a pinprick.

In addition, by the time a lawsuit has been filed, the patient's attorney already has a copy of the medical record and knows the contents so well that he'll notice any alterations immediately.

Tampering with a patient's medical record to protect yourself can only create problems and suspicion. Even if you consider correcting an error that may have nothing to do with the focus of the lawsuit, you'll damage your credibility and that of the record—and you could end up losing a case you should have won.

For example, suppose you hung the wrong I.V. solution. That fact might have no bearing on a malpractice suit brought by a patient with a postoperative wound infection unrelated to the I.V. infusion. However, if you tamper with the record to conceal your error, the entire case becomes suspect. As a result, your insurance company might have to make an expensive out-of-court settlement, which wouldn't have been necessary if you hadn't tampered with the medical record.

The case of *Pyle v. Morrison,* 716 S.W. 2d 930 (1986), illustrates the point. A malpractice suit was brought against doctors for their treatment of a child's fractured arm. The jury decided in favor of the plaintiffs—$400,000 for the child and $15,000 for the father. The deciding factor was the testimony of a nurse who said that she thought a portion of the medical record had been altered after the child's surgery. Her testimony cast doubt on the

Types of tampering

Tampering with the medical record is both unethical and illegal. But exactly what constitutes tampering?

Filing an incident report after the fact

If your employer asks you to fill out an incident report long after the fact (or in response to a lawsuit), consult your attorney. Incident reports should be filed at the time of the incident and should contain factual information.

Adding to an existing record

Because the medical records department is responsible for trying to obtain a complete patient record within a short period, you may be asked to fill in the blanks on your charts. Signing an entry that you know is yours is probably safe. However, trying to remember and document assessment data, times, or other details is risky.

This added information may be inaccurate. And, in court, your actions may be viewed not as a simple completion of the record but as an instance of tampering with the record.

Omitting significant information

Don't let anyone pressure you into omitting or concealing information. A hospital administrator and the hospital's attorney can assist you if you can't get help from your nurse-manager or through the usual channels. If your employer doesn't have nurse-managers, consult your state nursing board.

The consequences of bowing to pressure could be devastating because you might face civil charges for concealing information.

Most malpractice insurance policies don't cover acts involving willful violation of the law, so your insurance company won't help you.

Rewriting the record

Never rewrite your notes and discard the original, even for an innocent reason like spilling coffee on a page. In a lawsuit, you'd have trouble convincing the plaintiff's lawyer that your actions were so innocent. Both the attorney and the jury would assume the evidence in the missing document was so damaging that you had to destroy it.

If you must copy an unreadable page, follow this procedure:
• At the top of the page, identify that the page was rewritten: "Notes copied from original of 1/17/95."
• Give a reason for the rewrite, such as "Original illegible due to coffee spill." Sign and date the entry.
• Retain the original page, and place it in the record with the copied page.

Adding to someone else's notes

Never alter another person's documentation. In court, the other person may deny making the erroneous entry that you changed—so the jurors may be suspicious of the full record.

Nor should anyone else try to fix a charting error you've made. Again, this jeopardizes the record's credibility and accuracy. If you discover someone has altered your notes, talk with your nurse-manager and follow through until the problem is corrected. The person who made the change may be unaware of the legal implications of tampering with records.

As a precaution, write every entry in ink, date it, record the time, sign it, and write on consecutive lines. Don't leave any space between the last word of your entry and your signature—and draw a line to fill up the space so that no one can insert words at the end of your entry.

credibility of the medical record in the minds of the jurors.

Tampering with the medical record also can extend the statute of limitations — the time period each state gives an injured party to file a lawsuit. Because tampering can be interpreted as a form of fraud, and fraud has a longer statute of limitations than malpractice, the plaintiff's attorney would have more time to build his case against you — perhaps as long as 10 years.

You could even face charges of "aggravated and outrageous conduct" if the plaintiff's attorney successfully argues that the record was intentionally altered because of conspiracy or fraud. The judge could then allow the jury to award punitive damages to the plaintiff — a penalty that's intended to punish you. Punitive damages exceed the actual damages and may not be covered by your insurance policies, so you'd end up paying out of your own pocket.

In addition, if medical records were destroyed, you and your employer could be fined for failing to comply with a court order to produce documents.

Dealing with your insurer

If you're covered by your employer's insurance, immediately contact the legal services administrators for instructions on how to proceed. Be sure to find out how much insurance your employer carries on you and whether your employer's attorney will represent you or whether you'll need to retain your own.

Be forewarned: If the hospital's attorney represents you, he may decide to settle the case out of court. (See *Settling out of court.*) This may be in the hospital's best interest, but not in yours, especially if you

Settling out of court

Malpractice attorneys estimate that only 10% of all malpractice lawsuits actually go to trial — the rest are settled out of court. Of the 10% that go to trial, only about 10% actually end with a final judgment. So if you're ever involved in a malpractice suit, your chances for settling out of court are good. When you discuss out-of-court settlement with your attorney, remember these points:
• If you're covered by professional liability insurance, the terms of your policy determine whether you, your attorney, or your insurer controls the settlement. Most policies don't permit the nurse to settle a case without the consent of the insurer. In fact, many policies permit the insurer to settle without the consent of the nurse being sued.
• Always review your policy to determine your settlement rights. Provide your insurer's representative and your attorney with all the information you can about the case. Then they can evaluate the plaintiff's and your liabilities and determine the best settlement with the plaintiff.
• Remember, settling out of court doesn't mean that you admit any wrongdoing. The law regards settlement as a compromise between two parties to end a lawsuit and avoid further expense. In other words, you may choose to reach a settlement rather than incur greater financial and emotional expenses by defending your innocence at a trial.
• Ask your attorney about the settlement's terms. For example, you'll usually be expected to keep the settlement agreement confidential.

Choosing liability insurance

To find the professional liability coverage that fits your needs, compare the features of a number of policies. Understanding insurance policy basics will enable you to shop more aggressively and intelligently for the coverage you need. You should work with an insurance agent who's experienced in this type of insurance. If you already have professional liability insurance, the information below may help you better evaluate your coverage.

Type of coverage

Ask your insurance agent if the policy only covers claims made before the policy expires (claims-made coverage), or if it covers any negligent act committed during the policy period (occurrence coverage). Keep in mind that an occurrence policy provides more coverage than a claims-made policy.

Coverage limits

All malpractice insurance policies cover professional liability. Some also cover personal liability, medical payments, assault-related bodily injury, and all property damage.

The amount of coverage varies, as does your premium. For example, depending on your nursing speciality, a policy costing about $100 a year may provide up to $1 million for each incident (single-occurrence limit) and up to $3 million per year (the maximum annual protection).

Remember that professional liability coverage is limited to acts and practice settings specified in the policy. Be sure your policy covers your nursing role, whether you're a student, a graduate nurse, or a working nurse with advanced education and specialized skills.

Options

Check whether the policy would provide coverage for the following incidents:
• negligence on the part of nurses under your supervision
• misuse of equipment
• errors in reporting or recording care
• failure to properly teach patients
• errors in administering medication
• mistakes made while providing care in an emergency outside your employment setting.

Also ask if the policy provides protection if your employer (the hospital) sues you.

Definition of terms

Definition of terms can vary from policy to policy. If your policy includes restrictive definitions, you won't be covered for actions outside those guidelines. For the best protection, seek broad definitions and ask for examples of actions the company hasn't covered.

Duration of coverage

Insurance is an annual contract that can be renewed or canceled each year. The policy usually specifies how it can be canceled—in writing by either you or the insurance company. Some contracts require 30 days' notice for cancellation. If the company is canceling the policy, you'll probably be given at least 10 days' notice.

Exclusions

Ask your agent about exclusions—areas not covered by the insurance policy. For example, "This policy does not apply to injury arising out of performance of the insured of a criminal act" or "This policy does not apply to nurse-anesthetists."

Choosing liability insurance   *(continued)*

Other insurance clauses

All professional liability insurance policies contain "other insurance" clauses that address payment obligations when a nurse is covered by more than one insurance policy, such as the institution's policy and the nurse's personal liability:

• The *pro rata* clause states that two or more policies in effect at the same time will pay any claims in accordance with a proportion established in the individual policies.

• The *in excess* clause states that the primary policy will pay all fees and damages up to its limits, at which point the second policy will pay any additional fees or damages up to its limits.

• The *escape clause* relieves an insurance company of all liability for fees or damages if another insurance policy is in effect at the same time; in effect, the clause states that the other company is responsible for all liability.

If you are covered by more than one policy, be alert for "other insurance" clauses and avoid purchasing a policy with an escape clause for liability.

Additional tips

Here is some additional information that will guide you in the purchase of professional liability insurance:

• The insurance application is a legal document. If you provide any false information, it may void the policy.

• If you are involved in nursing administration, education, research, or advanced or nontraditional nursing practice, be especially careful in selecting a policy because routine policies may not cover these activities.

• After selecting a policy that ensures adequate coverage, stay with the same policy and insurer, if possible, to avoid potential lapses in coverage that could occur when changing insurers.

• No insurance policy will cover you for acts outside your scope of practice or licensure. Nor will insurance cover you for intentional torts if intent to do harm is proved.

• Be prepared to uphold all obligations specified in the policy; failure to do so may void the policy and cause personal liability for any damages. Remember that any act of willful wrongdoing on your part renders the policy null and void and may lead to a breach of contract lawsuit.

weren't negligent. In this situation, consider consulting your own attorney to advise you.

If you have your own professional liability insurance, find your representative's name on your policy and notify him right away. If you don't do this within the time specified on your policy, your insurance company (insurer) may refuse to cover you. (See *Choosing liability insurance.*)

Document the time, the date, the representative's name, and his instructions. Then hand-deliver the lawsuit papers to him and get a signed and dated receipt, or send the papers by certified mail with a return receipt requested.

Usually, the policy requires the health care facility or your private insurer to provide legal counsel, to pay all the expenses related to the lawsuit, and to pay damages in a settlement or as awarded in a judgment. The contract also spells out your and the insurer's rights and obligations and contains exclusionary clauses (acts that exclude you from coverage).

When you notify your insurer that you've been sued, the company will first consider whether it must cover you at all. This is done by checking for any policy violations—for example, giving late notice of the lawsuit, giving false information on your insurance application, or failing to pay a premium on time. If your insurer is certain you've committed such a violation, it can refuse to cover you. The reasons the insurer gives—concerning how well you've maintained your policy—are called a policy defense.

Suppose your insurer thinks you've committed a violation but isn't sure it has the evidence to support a policy defense? Then it will probably send you a certified letter saying that it may not have to defend you but will do so while reserving the right to deny coverage later, withdraw from the case, or take other actions. Meanwhile, the company will seek a declaration of its rights from the court.

If the court decides your insurer doesn't have to defend you, the company will withdraw from the case. Usually, an insurer takes this action only after careful consideration, because refusing to defend you may give you grounds for suing the insurance company. In the rare event that your insurer does refuse to cover you, find your own attorney to defend you in the malpractice suit and advise you in your dealings with your insurer. If your case is sound, the attorney may suggest suing your insurer.

Finding an attorney

In the absence of a policy defense, your insurer will select and retain an attorney or a law firm specializing in medical malpractice cases to defend you. The attorney selected—called your "attorney of record"—is legally bound to do everything necessary to defend you. Your health care facility will almost certainly be named as a codefendant in the lawsuit. If this isn't the case, you'll still need to immediately alert your employer that you're being sued because your private insurer may try to involve your employer as a defendant.

If you don't have insurance, don't even consider trying to defend yourself. Quickly find yourself an experienced malpractice attorney. (See *Selecting an attorney.*)

Of course, you have the right to change attorneys at any time. You may feel that the attorney selected by your insurer seems more interested in protecting the insurer than you. If so, discuss this problem with a company representative. If you can't reach an agreement, hire your own attorney. You may have grounds for suing your insurer and the attorney it appointed.

Examining the records

Once you have an attorney, get a copy of the plaintiff's medical record. Examine the complete record, including nurses' and consultation notes, X-ray and laboratory reports, flow sheets, and doctors' orders. On a separate sheet of paper, make notes on key entries or omissions. Don't make any marks or changes on the records themselves—you'll destroy your own case by undermining your credibility.

Create your own legal file by asking your attorney to send you copies of all documents and correspondence pertaining to the case. Try to maintain a file that's as complete as your attorney's. If you don't understand a document, ask your attorney to explain it. File documents in chronological order in your own file system (such as folders or a looseleaf notebook).

Protecting your property

Ask your attorney about the legal devices you can use to protect your property. Many states have homestead laws that permit you to protect a substantial part of the equity in your house, as well as other property, from any judgment against you. Such protection is essential if you don't have malpractice insurance or if you lose your case and the damages awarded exceed your insurance coverage.

Your attorney's pretrial role

Your attorney will explain the legal process to you from complaint to appeal. (See *Understanding the legal process,* pages 324 and 325.) He'll file the appropriate legal documents in response to the subpoena you were served. He'll ask for your help in preparing the response to the allegations made against you and in preparing your defense, and will ask you to present your position in detail and question you to

Selecting an attorney

If you're sued for malpractice, you may be faced with the added worry of hiring your own attorney. This can happen if you don't have malpractice insurance, if you're dissatisfied with the attorney your insurer provides, or if your insurer uses a policy defense and doesn't cover you.

Here are several suggestions for finding and selecting an attorney to meet your needs.
• If you work in a health care facility with a legal services department, find out if your employer will provide you with an attorney or refer you to one.
• If you have a relative or friend who is an attorney or judge, ask him for a referral to a competent malpractice attorney.
• If you belong to a professional association, seek a referral to an attorney from the association.
• If none of these solutions applies to you, ask for a referral from your local bar association, lawyer referral service, or area law school (listed in the telephone book). Try to find an attorney who's experienced in medical malpractice cases.
• Before you hire anyone to defend you, ask other health care professionals if they've heard of the attorney you're thinking of using, and go by his reputation.
• Interview more than one attorney. Ask how long he thinks the lawsuit will take and how much money he'll charge.
• Finally, try to choose an attorney who you feel understands your case and will work in your best interest.

Understanding the legal process

Being named as a defendant in a malpractice lawsuit can be confusing as well as stressful. One of the best antidotes is knowing what to expect.

This chart summarizes the basic legal process from complaint to appeal. If you're ever involved in a lawsuit, your attorney will explain the specific procedures that your case requires.

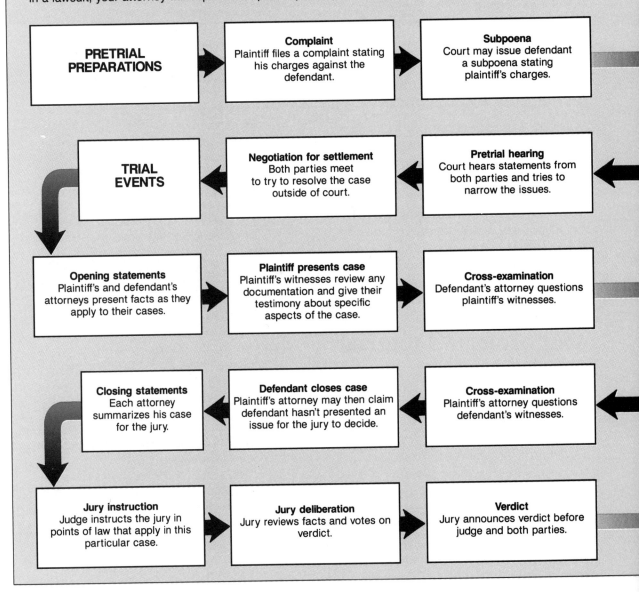

PRETRIAL PREPARATIONS	**Complaint** Plaintiff files a complaint stating his charges against the defendant.	**Subpoena** Court may issue defendant a subpoena stating plaintiff's charges.

TRIAL EVENTS	**Negotiation for settlement** Both parties meet to try to resolve the case outside of court.	**Pretrial hearing** Court hears statements from both parties and tries to narrow the issues.

Opening statements Plaintiff's and defendant's attorneys present facts as they apply to their cases.	**Plaintiff presents case** Plaintiff's witnesses review any documentation and give their testimony about specific aspects of the case.	**Cross-examination** Defendant's attorney questions plaintiff's witnesses.

Closing statements Each attorney summarizes his case for the jury.	**Defendant closes case** Plaintiff's attorney may then claim defendant hasn't presented an issue for the jury to decide.	**Cross-examination** Plaintiff's attorney questions defendant's witnesses.

Jury instruction Judge instructs the jury in points of law that apply in this particular case.	**Jury deliberation** Jury reviews facts and votes on verdict.	**Verdict** Jury announces verdict before judge and both parties.

Answer or counterclaim
Defendant files an answer or counterclaim to plaintiff's charges.

Discovery
Plaintiff's and defendant's attorneys develop their cases by gathering information during depositions and interrogatories and by reviewing other documents.

Plaintiff closes case
Defendant's attorney may then make a motion to dismiss the case, claiming plaintiff's evidence is insufficient.

Defendant presents case
Defendant's witnesses testify, explaining what they saw, heard, and know. Expert witnesses review any documentation and give their opinions about specific aspects of the case.

Appeal (optional)
Attorneys review transcripts. The party against whom the court ruled may appeal if he feels the judge didn't interpret the law properly, instruct the jury properly, or conduct the trial properly.

clarify specific points. Remember—all discussions between you and your attorney are privileged (confidential) communications that are protected by law. He can't disclose any information that you give him without your permission.

Because discussions with other people might result in information leaks that could compromise your case, your attorney will tell you not to discuss the lawsuit with anyone but him. He'll advise you not to mention the lawsuit to colleagues and, above all, not to contact the person suing you. Your chances of convincing the plaintiff to drop the case are very slim, and every word you say to him can be used against you in court. All communication between you and the plaintiff should be through the attorneys who represent you.

Your attorney will also obtain complete copies of pertinent medical records and any other documents that you and he determine are important to your defense. He'll uncover every relevant detail about the case against you by using discovery devices—legal procedures for obtaining information.

Discovery devices include an interrogatory (questions written to the plaintiff that require answers under oath), a deposition (oral cross-examination of the plaintiff, under oath and before a court reporter), and a defense medical examination (an examination of the injured party by a doctor selected by your attorney or your insurer).

The plaintiff's attorney will also use discovery devices, so you may have to answer interrogatories, with your attorney's help, and appear for a deposition as well. Your attorney will carefully prepare you to participate in these procedures and to testify at the trial.

Malpractice Lawsuits

He'll stress the importance of credibility by appearance—dressing appropriately and presenting a professional demeanor—and will rehearse with you the questions he'll ask at trial or the questions that he believes the plaintiff's attorney will ask you. He'll probably discuss the best way to phrase your answers, emphasizing that you should answer only the question asked and not volunteer other information.

Remember, your attorney is your advocate, and he wants to win your case. But he needs your cooperation to put forth a good defense. If you fail to cooperate with the attorney provided by your insurer, the company can use this as a policy defense. However, this doesn't mean that you must follow all your attorney's requests. If you think that he's asking you to do or say things that aren't in your best interest or that might damage your professional reputation, tell him so. Just get your differences ironed out *before* you go to court.

Surviving the deposition

During a deposition, the plaintiff's attorney questions you in the presence of your attorney and a court reporter. This enables both parties to review each other's cases to see if one is stronger than the other. The attorneys also observe the plaintiff and defendant during their separate depositions and gauge their credibility. If one party is a much stronger witness, the opposing party may decide to settle the case out of court.

Your attorney will explain the deposition procedure to you beforehand. He'll advise you to review all medical records in the case, which may help you recall important facts. During the actual deposition, the plaintiff's attorney has the right to inspect and copy any material you bring with you to aid your memory. Be sure that your attorney gets to inspect and approve this material first.

At the start of the deposition, you'll be sworn in by the court reporter. As you answer questions under oath, the court reporter records everything so that a written transcript can be prepared later. This transcript may be used at trial to challenge your credibility on the stand, or the facts revealed in the deposition may cause the case to be settled before it goes to trial.

Your attorney will probably advise you to respond to all questions with simple answers and not to volunteer any information. If you have any doubts when responding to the other attorney's questions, avoid absolute answers. If you don't understand a question, ask the plaintiff's attorney for clarification. If you don't know the answer to a question, state honestly that you don't know.

Memory fades with time, and even with the aid of medical records you won't be expected to recall the details of conversations that took place months or years ago. If the case goes to court, however, you'll be held accountable for the answers you gave at the deposition.

Your attorney may object to some of the questions you're asked at the deposition. So before answering anything, hesitate for a moment to give him time to state his objection. If his objection is sustained (accepted), you won't have to answer the question. If he raises an objection but you still answer the question, the judge will rule on the objection at a later time. If that objection is sustained, your answer will be stricken from the record. Unless your attorney instructs you not to answer a question, you must give a response.

Defending yourself on the witness stand

While you're on the witness stand, the plaintiff's attorney will use several tactics to throw you off guard. Your attorney should discuss the following strategies with you.

Creating false security

The plaintiff's attorney knows that most jurors like and sympathize with nurses. So he won't want to antagonize the jury by being too hard on you. Instead, he'll try to make you "self-destruct" by creating a false sense of security, lulling you with politeness, respect, and even compliments. Before long, you'll let down your defenses and start thinking: "This guy's really nice. He's only trying to be fair with me, so why was I so worried?" Then, in the same friendly way, he'll ask a question like: "Isn't it possible that you didn't document giving Mr. Smith his heart medication *because you didn't give it*, not because you forgot? Isn't it just possible?"

If you concede, you'll set the stage for one of two things. Either the attorney will carry his argument further, gently giving you enough rope to hang yourself, or he'll end his cross-examination abruptly, then pick up the point later, with a vengeance, in his summation to the jury. Always remember: The plaintiff's attorney is no

friend of yours. Don't be lulled by his friendly demeanor or his winning personality. Stay on guard. If you just answer the questions directly and briefly, you'll be off the stand soon and never have to see him again.

Asking leading questions

A leading question is one that suggests an answer—for example, "Isn't it true that the medication was green?" In direct questioning (when your attorney questions you), leading questions aren't allowed. However, in cross-examination (when the plaintiff's attorney questions you), just about every question is a leading question. The attorney will never ask you something like, "What happened when you examined the patient?" That offers you too much leeway to give an answer he doesn't want the jury to hear. Instead, he'll say something like, "Isn't it true that the patient was sweating?" or "Isn't it a fact that Mrs. Smith complained about her arm?" Your answer should be a simple yes or no. Of course, the attorney is hoping that you'll say more and give him the chance to charge ahead and upset you and disrupt your testimony.

Most nurses want to be helpful. Attorneys recognize this and try to use it to their advantage. You may want the jury to hear more than a simple yes or no. But wait until redirect questioning—when your own attorney questions you again after cross-examination. If he thinks you should expand on an answer, he'll ask the appropriate questions.

Before you answer a question from either attorney, take time to formulate your answer. Keep your answers to the absolute minimum—yes or no whenever possible.

Malpractice
Lawsuits

Don't stray from the main point; answer only the question that was asked.

Questioning your recollection

Because most cases don't come to trial until several years after the incident, one of the plaintiff's attorney's most effective techniques is to attack your recollection in a deceptively polite way. The questioning might go like this:

ATTORNEY: Mrs. Brown, how many years ago did this happen?

NURSE: 5.

ATTORNEY: How many patients do you see a week?

NURSE: About 80.

ATTORNEY: Then that would be about 4,000 patients a year, would it not?

NURSE: Yes.

ATTORNEY: Which would come to 20,000 patients in 5 years, wouldn't it?

NURSE: Yes.

If you never charted the incident, the attorney might not attack your memory of it directly. Instead, he might just end the questioning abruptly and pick up the point again during his closing statement. If you *did* chart the incident, he might question you further, hoping that you'll contradict yourself.

Obviously, the wise approach is to chart everything that might be important. But suppose you didn't record a particular incident that you remember well? Inform your attorney of this before the trial, and tell him why the incident is so vivid in your mind. Do you remember it because of certain people involved or because of where it occurred? This information will give him the chance, either before or after cross-examination, to let you explain to the jury why you remember the incident even though you didn't document it.

The importance of charting everything is illustrated in this case: A patient died a few days after leaving the hospital against medical advice (AMA). Yet, his family filed suit against the hospital alleging that the medical staff had failed to adequately warn him about the risks of leaving. A nurse testified that the patient had told her he was leaving no matter what the doctors said, but she hadn't noted this on the chart.

Instead of accusing the nurse of giving false testimony, the plaintiff's attorney questioned her about the importance of nurses' notes. He got her to concede that she wasn't likely to remember every patient she treated years ago. But under redirect questioning by the hospital's attorney, the nurse explained that even though she cared for hundreds of patients each year, she remembered those who were especially belligerent, such as the patient who'd left AMA.

Catching you in a contradiction

You can be sure that any competent attorney will carefully read the patient's chart and your signed pretrial deposition before the case comes to court. Naturally, you should also read this information before the trial. If you haven't read it, or you're not sure how to answer a question, always ask to see the chart to refresh your memory. And if you don't know something, simply say that you don't. In either case, the jury won't hold it against you.

If you read your deposition before the trial and disagree with something you said, tell your attorney. This allows him to defuse a potentially damaging situation.

During his questioning, he'll let you explain why you've changed your mind. For example, you might say, "I've had a lot of time to recollect since the deposition. Then, I was a little confused and didn't understand the question." This perfectly logical explanation would look like a mighty poor excuse if it came out for the first time under cross-examination.

Uncovering your bias

Another common technique is to weaken the nurse's testimony by trying to show that she's biased toward the hospital or someone she works with who also is involved in the lawsuit.

Besides having a professional relationship with her nurse-manager, she may also have social or business relationships with members of a doctor's family or with a hospital administrator. This tactic usually works very effectively on witnesses who haven't been adequately prepared by their attorneys. It usually unnerves and embarrasses them.

For example, in one case, a nurse testified that a patient arrived in the emergency department intoxicated and on diazepam but refused to be admitted to the hospital. The nurse said that she gave the patient the hospital's number to call if she needed help, but that she never documented this. When the patient died 4 days later, the family alleged that she'd never been told she could be admitted and had never been given the hospital's number.

While the plaintiff's attorney didn't directly accuse the nurse of lying, here's how the questioning went:
ATTORNEY: You know the hospital administrator pretty well, don't you? The fact is, you bought a house from him, didn't you?

NURSE: Yes.
ATTORNEY: And isn't it a fact that your children play with his children?
NURSE: Yes.
ATTORNEY: You wouldn't want to do anything to hurt his or the hospital's reputation, would you?
NURSE: No.

The nurse's answers were absolutely correct. But she hesitated, blushed, and was obviously ill at ease—a mistake. Although the jury believed her and returned a verdict for the hospital, the nurse's credibility could have been seriously damaged.

Having social or business relationships with people you work with is normal, and jurors expect it. So don't be afraid to admit such relationships—just don't act evasive about it. If the plaintiff's attorney tries to give the impression that you're afraid of losing your job, simply state, "I took the oath, and I'm here to tell the truth as I know it."

Uncovering bias against the patient

The plaintiff's attorney may also try to undermine your testimony by showing that you disliked the patient. Don't deny the truth—if the patient was hard to like, admit it. Just be sure to explain why you felt this way and that your feelings didn't interfere with your giving him the best possible care. Jurors don't expect you to like everyone. They'll empathize with you for providing good nursing care under difficult conditions and may even respect you for it. If you have a difficult patient, document it in objective terms. These patients are almost always the ones who sue.

Malpractice Lawsuits

Baiting you

If you give the plaintiff's attorney the opportunity, he'll get tough with you—very sweetly. For example, in one case, an attorney asked a nurse why she hadn't immediately recorded a patient's vital signs when he was admitted to the emergency department. The nurse explained that the patient had needed immediate care, so she'd jotted his vital signs on the bed sheet, where everyone could see them. Under cross-examination, the nurse said that she resented being accused of "incompetence." The attorney gave her a surprised look and replied, "Did you ever hear me use the word 'incompetence'? You're saying it, but I'm not thinking that." Although the facts won this case for the hospital, the nurse could have lost her credibility with the jurors by planting the word "incompetence" in their minds.

If a plaintiff's attorney is ever rude to you, don't be rude in return, and don't lose your temper. This will only make the jurors think, "If she's like this here, what's she like in the hospital?" Don't disagree with an attorney just to disagree. This will only create more problems for you and cause you to be on the stand longer.

A final thought

As you expand your nursing expertise and take on more patient care responsibilities, you'll also be accepting greater legal risks. But you don't have to accept the inevitability of being sued. If you give high-quality care and chart meticulously, you'll be doing everything in your power to avoid a lawsuit.

Selected references

Aiken, T.D., and Catalano, J.T. *Legal, Ethical, and Political Issues in Nursing.* Philadelphia: F.A. Davis Co., 1994.

Calfee, B.E. "Steering Clear of Trouble: Litigation Lesson," *Nursing94* 24(1):47, January 1994.

Iyer, P.W. "Six More Charting Rules to Keep You Legally Safe," *Nursing91* 21(7): 34-39, July 1991.

Nurse's Handbook of Law and Ethics. Springhouse, Pa.: Springhouse Corp., 1992.

Appendices

NANDA Taxonomy I, Revised

The North American Nursing Diagnosis Association (NANDA) endorsed its first nursing diagnosis taxonomic structure, NANDA Taxonomy I, in 1986. In 1989 and 1994, this taxonomy was revised. The revised taxonomy represents the currently accepted classification system for nursing diagnoses. The nine human response patterns and their definitions are: Exchanging: Mutual giving and receiving; Communicating: Sending messages; Relating: Establishing bonds; Valuing: Assigning worth; Choosing: Selection of alterations; Moving: Activity; Perceiving: Reception of information; Knowing: Meaning associated with information; and Feeling: Subjective awareness of information.

Pattern 1: Exchanging

1.1.2.1	Altered nutrition: More than body requirements
1.1.2.2	Altered nutrition: Less than body requirements
1.1.2.3	Altered nutrition: Potential for more than body requirements
1.2.1.1	Risk for infection
1.2.2.1	Risk for altered body temperature
1.2.2.2	Hypothermia
1.2.2.3	Hyperthermia
1.2.2.4	Ineffective thermoregulation
1.2.3.1	Dysreflexia
1.3.1.1	Constipation
1.3.1.1.1	Perceived constipation
1.3.1.1.2	Colonic constipation
1.3.1.2	Diarrhea
1.3.1.3	Bowel incontinence
1.3.2	Altered urinary elimination
1.3.2.1.1	Stress incontinence
1.3.2.1.2	Reflex incontinence
1.3.2.1.3	Urge incontinence
1.3.2.1.4	Functional incontinence
1.3.2.1.5	Total incontinence
1.3.2.2	Urinary retention
1.4.1.1	Altered (specify type) tissue perfusion (renal, cerebral, cardiopulmonary, gastrointestinal, peripheral)
1.4.1.2.1	Fluid volume excess
1.4.1.2.2.1	Fluid volume deficit
1.4.1.2.2.2	Risk for fluid volume deficit
1.4.2.1	Decreased cardiac output
1.5.1.1	Impaired gas exchange
1.5.1.2	Ineffective airway clearance
1.5.1.3	Ineffective breathing pattern
1.5.1.3.1	Inability to sustain spontaneous ventilation

1.5.1.3.2	Dysfunctional ventilatory weaning response
1.6.1	Risk for injury
1.6.1.1	Risk for suffocation
1.6.1.2	Risk for poisoning
1.6.1.3	Risk for trauma
1.6.1.4	Risk for aspiration
1.6.1.5	Risk for disuse syndrome
1.6.2	Altered protection
1.6.2.1	Impaired tissue integrity
1.6.2.1.1	Altered oral mucous membrane
1.6.2.1.2.1	Impaired skin integrity
1.6.2.1.2.2	Risk for impaired skin integrity
1.7.1	Decreased adaptive capacity: Intracranial
1.8	Energy field disturbance

Pattern 2: Communicating

2.1.1.1	Impaired verbal communication

Pattern 3: Relating

3.1.1	Impaired social interaction
3.1.2	Social isolation
3.1.3	Risk for loneliness
3.2.1	Altered role performance
3.2.1.1.1	Altered parenting
3.2.1.1.2	Risk for altered parenting
3.2.1.1.2.1	Risk for altered parent/infant/child attachment
3.2.1.2.1	Sexual dysfunction
3.2.2	Altered family processes
3.2.2.1	Caregiver role strain
3.2.2.2	Risk for caregiver role strain

3.2.2.3.1	Altered family process: Alcoholism
3.2.3.1	Parental role conflict
3.3	Altered sexuality patterns

Pattern 4: Valuing

4.1.1	Spiritual distress (distress of the human spirit)
4.2	Potential for enhanced spiritual well being

Pattern 5: Choosing

5.1.1.1	Ineffective individual coping
5.1.1.1.1	Impaired adjustment
5.1.1.1.2	Defensive coping
5.1.1.1.3	Ineffective denial
5.1.2.1.1	Ineffective family coping: Disabling
5.1.2.1.2	Ineffective family coping: Compromised
5.1.2.2	Family coping: Potential for growth
5.1.3.1	Potential for enhanced community coping
5.1.3.2	Ineffective community coping
5.2.1	Ineffective management of therapeutic regimen (individual)
5.2.1.1	Noncompliance (specify)
5.2.2	Ineffective management of therapeutic regimen: Families
5.2.3	Ineffective management of therapeutic regimen: Community
5.2.4	Ineffective management of therapeutic regimen: Individual
5.3.1.1	Decisional conflict (specify)
5.4	Health-seeking behaviors (specify)

Pattern 6: Moving

6.1.1.1	Impaired physical mobility

6.1.1.1.1	Risk for peripheral neurovascular dysfunction
6.1.1.1.2	Risk for perioperative positioning injury
6.1.1.2	Activity intolerance
6.1.1.2.1	Fatigue
6.1.1.3	Risk for activity intolerance
6.2.1	Sleep pattern disturbance
6.3.1.1	Diversional activity deficit
6.4.1.1	Impaired home maintenance management
6.4.2	Altered health maintenance
6.5.1	Feeding self-care deficit
6.5.1.1	Impaired swallowing
6.5.1.2	Ineffective breast-feeding
6.5.1.2.1	Interrupted breast-feeding
6.5.1.3	Effective breast-feeding
6.5.1.4	Ineffective infant feeding pattern
6.5.2	Bathing or hygiene self-care deficit
6.5.3	Dressing or grooming self-care deficit
6.5.4	Toileting self-care deficit
6.6	Altered growth and development
6.7	Relocation stress syndrome
6.8.1	Risk for disorganized infant behavior
6.8.2	Disorganized infant behavior
6.8.3	Potential for enhanced organized infant behavior

Pattern 7: Perceiving

7.1.1	Body image disturbance
7.1.2	Self-esteem disturbance
7.1.2.1	Chronic low self-esteem
7.1.2.2	Situational low self-esteem
7.1.3	Personal identity disturbance
7.2	Sensory-perceptual alterations (specify as visual, auditory, kinesthetic, gustatory, tactile, olfactory)
7.2.1.1	Unilateral neglect
7.3.1	Hopelessness
7.3.2	Powerlessness

Pattern 8: Knowing

8.1.1	Knowledge deficit (specify)
8.2.1	Impaired environmental interpretation syndrome
8.2.2	Acute confusion
8.2.3	Chronic confusion
8.3	Altered thought processes
8.3.1	Impaired memory

Pattern 9: Feeling

9.1.1	Pain
9.1.1.1	Chronic pain
9.2.1.1	Dysfunctional grieving
9.2.1.2	Anticipatory grieving
9.2.2	Risk for violence: Self-directed or directed at others
9.2.2.1	Risk for self-mutilation
9.2.3	Posttrauma response
9.2.3.1	Rape-trauma syndrome
9.2.3.1.1	Rape-trauma syndrome: Compound reaction
9.2.3.1.2	Rape-trauma syndrome: Silent reaction
9.3.1	Anxiety
9.3.2	Fear

ANA Standards of Nursing Practice

In 1991, the American Nurses' Association (ANA) developed standards of clinical nursing practice that provide guidelines for determining quality nursing care. In updating previous standards, the ANA addressed not only care but also performance standards and established measurement criteria for evaluating whether a nurse's activities meet those standards.

Standards of care

Nursing care standards are based on the steps of the nursing process—assessment, nursing diagnosis, planning, implementation, and evaluation.

Standard I: Assessment
The nurse collects health data about the client. Measurement criteria are as follows:
• The nurse bases data collection priorities on the client's immediate health condition and needs.
• The nurse uses appropriate assessment techniques in collecting data.
• Data collection involves the client, significant others, and health care providers when appropriate.
• The data collection process is systematic and ongoing.
• Relevant data are documented in a retrievable form.

Standard II: Diagnosis
The nurse analyzes the assessment data in determining diagnoses. Measurement criteria are as follows:
• Diagnoses derive from the assessment data.
• Diagnoses are validated with the client, significant others, and health care providers when possible.
• Diagnoses are documented in a manner that facilitates the determination of expected outcomes and plan of care.

Standard III: Outcome identification
The nurse identifies expected outcomes individualized to the client. Measurement criteria are as follows:
• Outcomes derive from the diagnoses.
• Outcomes are documented as measurable goals.
• Outcomes are mutually formulated with the client and health care providers when possible.
• Outcomes are realistic and related to the client's present and potential capabilities.
• Outcomes are attainable in relation to resources available to the client.
• Outcomes include a time estimate for attainment.
• Outcomes provide direction for continuity of care.

Standard IV: Planning
The nurse develops a plan of care that pre-scribes interventions to attain expected out-comes. Measurement criteria are as follows:
• The plan of care is individualized to the client's condition or needs.
• The plan of care is developed with the client, significant others, and health care providers when appropriate.
• The plan of care reflects current nursing practice.
• The plan of care is documented.
• The plan of care provides for continuity of care.

Standard V: Implementation
The nurse implements the interventions identi-fied in the plan of care. Measurement criteria are as follows:
• Interventions are consistent with the estab-lished plan of care.
• Interventions are implemented in a safe and appropriate manner.
• Interventions are documented.

Standard VI: Evaluation
The nurse evaluates the client's progress to-ward attainment of outcomes. Measurement criteria are as follows:
• Evaluation is systematic and ongoing.
• The client's responses to interventions are documented.
• The effectiveness of interventions is evaluated in relation to outcomes.
• Ongoing assessment data are used to revise diagnoses, outcomes, and the plan of care as needed.
• Revisions in diagnoses, outcomes, and the plan of care are documented.
• The client, significant others, and health care providers are involved in the evaluation pro-cess when appropriate.

Standards of professional performance

Nursing performance standards include guide-lines for quality of care, performance appraisal, education, collegiality, ethics, collaboration, re-search, and resource utilization.

Standard I: Quality of care
The nurse systematically evaluates the quality and effectiveness of nursing practice. Measure-ment criteria are as follows:
• The nurse participates in quality-of-care activ-ities as appropriate to the individual's position, education, and practice environment. Such ac-tivities may include:
—identification of aspects of care important for quality monitoring
—identification of indicators used to monitor quality and effectiveness of nursing care
—collection of data to monitor quality and ef-fectiveness of nursing care
—analysis of quality data to identify opportu-nities for improving care
—formulation of recommendations to improve nursing practice or client outcomes
—implementation of activities to enhance the quality of nursing practice
—participation on interdisciplinary teams that evaluate clinical practice or health services
—development of policies and procedures to improve quality of care.
• The nurse uses the results of quality-of-care activities to initiate changes in practice.
• The nurse uses the results of quality-of-care activities to initiate changes throughout the health care delivery system as appropriate.

Standard II: Performance appraisal
The nurse evaluates nursing practice in relation to professional practice standards and relevant

statutes and regulations. Measurement criteria are as follows:

• The nurse engages in performance appraisal on a regular basis, identifying areas of strength as well as areas for professional and practice development.

• The nurse seeks constructive feedback regarding practice.

• The nurse takes action to achieve goals identified during performance appraisal.

• The nurse participates in peer review as appropriate.

Standard III: Education

The nurse acquires and maintains current knowledge in nursing practice. Measurement criteria are as follows:

• The nurse participates in ongoing educational activities related to clinical knowledge and professional issues.

• The nurse seeks experiences to maintain clinical skills.

• The nurse seeks knowledge and skills appropriate to the practice setting.

Standard IV: Collegiality

The nurse contributes to the professional development of peers, colleagues, and others. Measurement criteria are as follows:

• The nurse shares knowledge and skills with colleagues and others.

• The nurse provides peers with constructive feedback regarding their practice.

• The nurse contributes to an environment that is conducive to clinical education of nursing students as appropriate.

Standard V: Ethics

The nurse's decisions and actions on behalf of clients are determined in an ethical manner. Measurement criteria are as follows:

• The nurse's practice is guided by the standard nurses' code.

• The nurse maintains client confidentiality.

• The nurse acts as a client advocate.

• The nurse delivers care in a nonjudgmental and nondiscriminatory manner that is sensitive to client diversity and that preserves and protects the client's autonomy, dignity, and rights.

• The nurse seeks available resources to help formulate ethical decisions.

Standard VI: Collaboration

The nurse collaborates with the client, significant others, and health care providers in providing client care. Measurement criteria are as follows:

• The nurse communicates with the client, significant others, and health care providers regarding client care and nursing's role in the provision of care.

• The nurse consults with health care providers for client care as needed.

• The nurse makes referrals, including provisions for continuity of care as needed.

Standard VII: Research

The nurse uses research findings in practice. Measurement criteria are as follows:

• The nurse uses interventions substantiated by research as appropriate to the individual's position, education, and practice environment.

• The nurse participates in research activities as appropriate to the individual's position, education, and practice environment. Such activities may include:

— identification of clinical problems suitable for nursing research

— participation in data collection

— participation in a unit, organization, or community research committee or program

— sharing of research activities with others

— conducting research

— critiquing research for application to practice

— using research findings in the development of policies, procedures, and guidelines for client care.

Standard VIII: Resource utilization

The nurse considers factors related to safety, effectiveness, and cost in planning and delivering client care. Measurement criteria are as follows:
• The nurse evaluates factors related to safety, effectiveness, and cost when two or more practice options would result in the same expected client outcome.
• The nurse assigns tasks or delegates care based on the needs of the client and the knowledge and skill of the provider selected.
• The nurse assists the client and significant others in identifying and securing appropriate services available to address health-related needs.

Commonly Accepted Abbreviations

ABBREVIATION	MEANING
AAA	abdominal aortic aneurysm
Ab	antibody
ABC	airway, breathing, circulation
ABG	arterial blood gas
a.c.	before meals
AC	assist control
ACE	angiotensin-converting enzyme
ACh	acetylcholine
ACLS	advanced cardiac life support
AD	Alzheimer's disease auris dextra (right ear)
ADA	American Diabetes Association
ADH	antidiuretic hormone
ADL	activities of daily living
AFIB	atrial fibrillation
AFL	atrial flutter
AFP	alpha-fetoprotein
Ag	antigen
A-G	albumin-globulin (ratio)
AGA	appropriate for gestational age
AHD	arteriosclerotic heart disease autoimmune hemolytic disease
AHF	antihemophilic factor (factor VIII)
AICD	automatic implantable cardioverter-defibrillator
AIDS	acquired immunodeficiency syndrome

ABBREVIATION	MEANING
ALL	acute lymphocytic leukemia
ALS	amyotrophic lateral sclerosis
ALT	alanine aminotransferase (formerly called serum glutamic pyruvic transaminase [SGPT])
a.m.	morning
AMA	against medical advice American Medical Association
AMI	acute myocardial infarction
AML	acute myelocytic leukemia
amt.	amount
ANA	American Nurses' Association antinuclear antibody
AP	anteroposterior apical pulse
APTT	activated partial thromboplastin time
ara-A	adenine arabinoside (vidarabine)
ara-C	cytosine arabinoside (cytarabine)
ARDS	acute respiratory distress syndrome
ARF	acute renal failure acute respiratory failure acute rheumatic fever
AS	aortic sounds aqueous solution astigmatism auris sinistra (left ear)
ASA	acetylsalicylic acid (aspirin)
ASD	atrial septal defect
ASO	antistreptolysin-O

ABBREVIATION	MEANING
AST	aspartate aminotransferase (formerly called serum glutamic oxaloacetic transaminase [SGOT])
ATP	adenosine triphosphate
A.U.	each ear
AV	arteriovenous atrioventricular
AVM	arteriovenous malformation
BBB	bundle-branch block
BCG	bacille Calmette-Guérin
BCNU	carmustine
BE	barium enema base excess
b.i.d.	twice daily
BJ	Bence Jones
BLS	basic life support
BM	bowel movement
BMR	basal metabolic rate
BP	blood pressure
BPH	benign prostatic hyperplasia (or hypertrophy)
BPM	beats per minute
BRB	bright red blood
BRP	bathroom privileges
BSA	body surface area
BUN	blood urea nitrogen
C	Celsius centigrade certified cervical
CA	cardiac arrest
CABG	coronary artery bypass grafting
CAD	coronary artery disease
CAM	cool aerosol mask
cAMP	cyclic adenosine monophosphate

ABBREVIATION	MEANING
CAPD	continuous ambulatory peritoneal dialysis
caps	capsules
CBC	complete blood count
cc	cubic centimeter
CC	Caucasian child chief complaint common cold creatinine clearance critical care critical condition
CCNU	lomustine
CCU	cardiac care unit critical care unit
CDC	Centers for Disease Control and Prevention
CEA	carcinoembryonic antigen
CF	cardiac failure cystic fibrosis
CFS	chronic fatigue syndrome
CGL	chronic granulocytic leukemia
CHB	complete heart block
CHD	childhood disease congenital heart disease congenital hip disease
CHF	congestive heart failure
CK	creatine kinase
CK-BB	creatine kinase, brain
CK-MB	creatine kinase, heart
CK-MM	creatine kinase, skeletal muscle
cm	centimeter
CML	chronic myelogenous leukemia
CMV	continuous mandatory ventilation cytomegalovirus
CNS	central nervous system
CO	cardiac output

ABBREVIATION	MEANING
c/o	complains of
COLD	chronic obstructive lung disease
comp	compound
COPD	chronic obstructive pulmonary disease
CP	capillary pressure cerebral palsy cor pulmonale creatine phosphate
CPAP	continuous positive airway pressure
cpm	counts per minute cycles per minute
CPR	cardiopulmonary resuscitation
CRIS	controlled-release infusion system
C & S	culture and sensitivity
CSF	cerebrospinal fluid
CT	chest tube clotting time coated tablet compressed tablet computed tomography corneal transplant
CV	cardiovascular central venous
CVA	cerebrovascular accident costovertebral angle
CVP	central venous pressure
CXR	chest X-ray
d	day
/d	per day
D	dextrose
dB	decibel
D/C	discharge discontinue
D & C	dilatation and curettage
DD	differential diagnosis discharge diagnosis dry dressing
D & E	dilatation and evacuation

ABBREVIATION	MEANING
DES	diethylstilbestrol
D & I	dry and intact
DIC	disseminated intravascular coagulation
dil	dilute
disp	dispense
DJD	degenerative joint disease
DKA	diabetic ketoacidosis
dl	deciliter
DM	diabetes mellitus
DNA	deoxyribonucleic acid
DNR	do not resuscitate
$D_5\frac{1}{2}NSS$	dextrose 5% in 0.45% normal saline solution
DOA	date of admission dead on arrival
DS	double-strength
DSA	digital subtraction angiography
DSM-IV	*Diagnostic and Statistical Manual of Mental Disorders*, 4th ed.
DTP	diphtheria and tetanus toxoids and pertussis vaccine
DTR	deep tendon reflexes
DVT	deep vein thrombosis
D_5W	dextrose 5% in water
EBV	Epstein-Barr virus
EC	enteric-coated
ECF	extended care facility extracellular fluid
ECG	electrocardiogram
ECHO	echocardiography
ECMO	extracorporeal membrane oxygenator
ECT	electroconvulsive therapy
ED	emergency department
EDTA	ethylenediamine tetra-acetic acid
EEG	electroencephalogram

ABBREVIATION	MEANING
EENT	eyes, ears, nose, throat
EF	ejection fraction
ELISA	enzyme-linked immunosorbent assay
elix.	elixir
EMG	electromyography
EMIT	enzyme-multiplied immunoassay technique
ENG	electronystagmography
EOM	extraocular movement
ER	emergency room expiratory reserve
ERCP	endoscopic retrograde cholangio-pancreatography
ERV	expiratory reserve volume
ESR	erythrocyte sedimentation rate
ESWL	extracorporeal shock-wave lithotripsy
et	and
ETT	endotracheal tube
ext.	extract
F	Fahrenheit
FDA	Food and Drug Administration
FEF	forced expiratory flow
FEV	forced expiratory volume
FFP	fresh frozen plasma
FHR	fetal heart rate
fl., fld.	fluid
Fr.	French
FRC	functional residual capacity
FSH	follicle-stimulating hormone
FSP	fibrinogen-split products
FT_3	free triiodothyronine
FT_4	free thyroxine

ABBREVIATION	MEANING
FTA	fluorescent treponemal antibody (test)
FTA-ABS	fluorescent treponemal antibody absorption (test)
FUO	fever of undetermined origin
FVC	forced vital capacity
G	gauge
g, gm, GM	gram
GFR	glomerular filtration rate
GI	gastrointestinal
G6PD	glucose-6-phosphate dehydrogenase
gr	grain (about 60 mg)
gt.	gutta (drop)
GU	genitourinary
GVHD	graft-versus-host disease
GYN	gynecologic
h., hr.	hour
H	hypodermic injection
Hb	hemoglobin
HBD	alpha-hydroxybutyrate dehydrogenase
HBIG	hepatitis B immunoglobulin
HBsAg	hepatitis B surface antigen
hCG	human chorionic gonadotropin
Hct	hematocrit
HDL	high-density lipoprotein
HDN	hemolytic disease of the newborn
heme +	Hematest positive
heme −	Hematest negative
Hgb	hemoglobin
hGH	human growth hormone
HIV	human immunodeficiency virus
HLA	human leukocyte antigen
HMO	health maintenance organization
HNKS	hyperosmolar nonketotic syndrome
HOB	head of bed

ABBREVIATION	MEANING
hPL	human placental lactogen
h.s.	at bedtime
HS	half-strength hour of sleep house surgeon
HSV	herpes simplex virus
HVA	homovanillic acid
Hz	hertz
HZV	herpes zoster virus
IA	internal auditory intra-arterial intra-articular
IABP	intra-aortic balloon pump
IC	inspiratory capacity
ICF	intracellular fluid
ICHD	Inter-Society Commission for Heart Disease
ICP	intracranial pressure
ICU	intensive care unit
ID	identification initial dose inside diameter intradermal
I & D	incision and drainage
IDDM	insulin-dependent diabetes mellitus
IgM	immunoglobulin
IM	infectious mononucleosis
I.M.	intramuscular
IMV	intermittent mandatory ventilation
in.	inch
IND	investigational new drug
IPPB	intermittent positive-pressure breathing
IRV	inspiratory reserve volume
IU	International Unit
IUD	intrauterine device

ABBREVIATION	MEANING
I.V.	intravenous
IVGTT	intravenous glucose tolerance test
IVH	intravenous hyperalimentation (now called total parenteral nutrition [TPN])
IVP	intravenous pyelography
IVPB	intravenous piggyback
J	joule
JCAHO	Joint Commission on Accreditation of Healthcare Organizations
JP	Jackson-Pratt (drain)
JVD	jugular venous distention
JVP	jugular venous pressure
kg	kilogram
17-KGS	17-ketogenic steroids
17-KS	17-ketosteroids
KUB	kidney-ureter-bladder
KVO	keep vein open
L	liter, lumbar
LA	left atrium long-acting
LAP	left atrial pressure leucine aminopeptidase
lb.	pound
LBBB	left bundle-branch block
LD	lactate dehydrogenase
LDL	low-density lipoprotein
LE	lupus erythematosus
LES	lower esophageal sphincter
LGL	Lown-Ganong-Levine variant syndrome
LH	luteinizing hormone
LLL	left lower leg left lower lobe
LLQ	left lower quadrant
L/min	liters per minute

ABBREVIATION	MEANING
LOC	level of consciousness
LR	lactated Ringer's solution
LSB	left scapular border left sternal border
LSC	left subclavian
LTC	long-term care
LUQ	left upper quadrant
LV	left ventricle
LVEDP	left ventricular end-diastolic pressure
LVET	left ventricular ejection time
LVF	left ventricular failure
m	meter
M	molar (solution)
m²	square meter
MAO	maximal acid output monoamine oxidase inhibitor
MAR	medication administration record
MAST	medical antishock trousers (pneumatic antishock garment)
mcg	microgram
MCH	mean corpuscular hemoglobin
MCHC	mean corpuscular hemoglobin concentration
MCV	mean corpuscular volume
MD	manic depressive medical doctor muscular dystrophy
mEq	milliequivalent
mg	milligram
mgtt	microdrip or minidrop
MI	mental illness mitral insufficiency myocardial infarction myocardial ischemia
ml	milliliter
μl	microliter
MLC	mixed lymphocyte culture

ABBREVIATION	MEANING
mm	millimeter
mm³	cubic millimeter
MMEF	maximal midexpiratory flow
mmol	millimole
MRI	magnetic resonance imaging
M.R. × 1	may repeat once
MS	mitral sounds mitral stenosis morphine sulfate multiple sclerosis musculoskeletal
MUGA	multiple-gated acquisition (scanning)
MVI	multivitamin infusion
MVP	mitral valve prolapse
MVV	maximal voluntary ventilation
NC	nasal cannula
ng	nanogram
NG	nasogastric
NICU	neonatal intensive care unit
NIDDM	non-insulin-dependent diabetes mellitus (Type II diabetes)
NKA	no known allergies
NMR	nuclear magnetic resonance
Noct.	night
NP	nasopharynx nerve palsy new patient not palpable
NPN	nonprotein nitrogen
N.P.O.	nothing by mouth
NR	nerve root nonreactive no refills no report no respirations
N/R	not remarkable
NS, NSS	normal saline solution (0.9% sodium chloride solution)

ABBREVIATION	MEANING
¼ NS	¼ normal saline solution (0.225% sodium chloride solution)
½ NS	½ normal saline solution (0.45% sodium chloride solution)
NSAID	nonsteroidal anti-inflammatory drug
NSR	normal sinus rhythm
N/V	nausea and vomiting
OB	obstetric
OD	occupational disease oculus dexter (right eye) overdose
OGTT	oral glucose tolerance test
OOB	out of bed
OR	operating room
OS	oculus sinister (left eye)
OTC	over-the-counter
OU	oculus uterque (each eye)
oz.	ounce
P	pulse
PA	pernicious anemia posteroanterior pulmonary artery
PABA	para-aminobenzoic acid
PAC	premature atrial contraction
$PaCO_2$	partial pressure of arterial carbon dioxide
PACU	perioperative acute care unit postanesthesia care unit
PaO_2	partial pressure of arterial oxygen
PAP	Papanicolaou smear passive-aggressive personality primary atypical pneumonia pulmonary artery pressure
PAT	paroxysmal atrial tachycardia
PAWP	pulmonary artery wedge pressure
p.c.	after meals
PCA	patient-controlled analgesia
PC X-ray	portable chest X-ray

ABBREVIATION	MEANING
PDA	patent ductus arteriosus
PE	pelvic examination physical examination pulmonary edema pulmonary embolism
PEARL	pupils equal and reactive to light
PEEP	positive end-expiratory pressure
PEFR	peak expiratory flow rate
PEP	preejection period
per	by or through
PET	positron-emission tomography
pg	picogram
PICC	peripherally inserted central catheter
PID	pelvic inflammatory disease
PKU	phenylketonuria
p.m.	afternoon
PMI	point of maximum impulse
PML	progressive multifocal leukoencepha-lopathy
PMS	premenstrual syndrome
PND	paroxysmal nocturnal dyspnea postnasal drip
P.O.	by mouth postoperative
PP	partial pressure peripheral pulses postpartum postprandial presenting problem
PR	by rectum
PRBC	packed red blood cells
p.r.n.	as needed
PROM	passive range of motion premature rupture of the membranes
pt., Pt.	patient pint

ABBREVIATION	MEANING
PT	prothrombin time
PTCA	percutaneous transluminal coronary angioplasty
PTH	parathyroid hormone
PTT	partial thromboplastin time
PUD	peptic ulcer disease pulmonary disease
PVC	polyvinylchloride premature ventricular contraction
q	every
q a.m.	every morning
q.d.	every day
q.h.	every hour
q.i.d.	four times daily
q.n.	every night
QNS	quantity not sufficient
q.o.d.	every other day
QS	quantity sufficient
qt.	quart
R	by rectum respiration
RA	renal artery rheumatoid arthritis right atrium
RAF	rheumatoid arthritis factor
RAP	right atrial pressure
RAST	radioallergosorbent test
RBBB	right bundle-branch block
RBC	red blood cell
RDA	recommended daily allowance
RE	rectal examination right ear
REM	rapid eye movement
RES	reticuloendothelial system
Rh	rhesus blood factor

ABBREVIATION	MEANING
RHD	relative hepatic dullness rheumatic heart disease
RIA	radioimmunoassay
RL	right lateral Ringer's lactate (lactated Ringer's solution)
RLQ	right lower quadrant
RNA	ribonucleic acid
R/O	rule out
ROM	range of motion right otitis media rupture of membranes
RR	respiratory rate
RRR	regular rate and rhythm
RSC	right subclavian
RSV	respiratory syncytial virus right subclavian vein Rous sarcoma virus
R/T	related to
RUQ	right upper quadrant
RV	residual volume right ventricle
RVEDP	right ventricular end-diastolic pressure
RVEDV	right ventricular end-diastolic volume
RVP	right ventricular pressure
Rx	prescription
SA	sinoatrial
SaO_2	arterial oxygen saturation
sat.	saturated
SC	subclavian
S.C., SQ	subcutaneous
SCID	severe combined immunodeficiency syndrome
sec.	second

ABBREVIATION	MEANING
SGOT	serum glutamic oxaloacetic transaminase (now called aspartate aminotransferase [AST])
SGPT	serum glutamic pyruvic transaminase (now called alanine aminotransferase [ALT])
SHBG	sex hormone-binding globulin
SI	Système International d'Unités (International System of Units)
SIADH	syndrome of inappropriate antidiuretic hormone
SIDS	sudden infant death syndrome
Sig	write on label
SIMV	synchronized intermittent mandatory ventilation
Sl., SL	slight sublingual
SLE	systemic lupus erythematosus
SOB	shortness of breath
sol., soln.	solution
sp.	spirits
SR	sustained release
SRS-A	slow-reacting substance of anaphylaxis
stat.	immediately
STD	sexually transmitted disease
supp.	suppository
susp.	suspension
SV	stroke volume
$S\bar{v}O_2$	mixed venous oxygen saturation
syr.	syrup
T	temperature
T, Tbs., tbsp.	tablespoon
t, tsp.	teaspoon
tab.	tablet
TBG	thyroxine-binding globulin

ABBREVIATION	MEANING
TCA	tricyclic antidepressant
TENS	transcutaneous electrical nerve stimulation
TIA	transient ischemic attack
t.i.d.	three times daily
TIL	tumor-infiltrating lymphocyte
tinct., tr.	tincture
TLC	total lung capacity triple lumen catheter
TM	temporomandibular tympanic membrane
TMJ	temporomandibular joint
TNF	tumor necrosis factor
TO	telephone order
tol.	tolerate tolerates tolerated
t-PA	tissue plasminogen activator
TPN	total parenteral nutrition
TRH	thyrotropin-releasing hormone
TSH	thyroid-stimulating hormone
UA	urinalysis
UCE	urea cycle enzymopathy
USP	United States Pharmacopeia
UTI	urinary tract infection
UV	ultraviolet
V, vag.	vaginal
VAD	vascular access device ventricular assist device
VAP	vascular access port
VDRL	Venereal Disease Research Laboratory (test)
VLDL	very-low-density lipoprotein
VMA	vanillylmandelic acid
VO	verbal order

ABBREVIATION	MEANING
V/Q	ventilation-perfusion ratio
VS	vital signs
VSD	ventricular septal defect
VSS	vital signs stable
V_T, Vt	tidal volume
WBC	white blood cell
WNL	within normal limits
w/o	without
WPW	Wolff-Parkinson-White syndrome
Z/G, ZIG	zoster immune globulin

A P P E N D I X   D

Commonly Accepted Symbols

SYMBOL	MEANING
Pulses	
0	absent; not palpable
+1	weak or thready; hard to feel; easily obliterated by slight finger pressure
+2	normal; easily palpable; obliterated only by strong finger pressure
+3	bounding; readily palpable; forceful; not easily obliterated
Reflexes	
++++	very brisk; hyperactive
+++	increased, but not necessarily abnormal
++	average; normal
+	present, but diminished
0	absent
Heart murmurs	
1/6 or I/VI	faint; barely audible even to the trained ear; may not be heard in all positions
2/6 or II/VI	soft and low; easily audible to the trained ear
3/6 or III/VI	moderately loud; approximately equal to the intensity of normal heart sounds
4/6 or IV/VI	very loud, with a palpable thrill at the murmur site
5/6 or IV/VI	very loud, with a palpable thrill; audible with stethoscope in partial contact with chest
6/6 or VI/VI	extremely loud, with a palpable thrill; audible with stethoscope over but not in contact with chest

SYMBOL	MEANING
Apothecary symbols	
mx	minim (about 0.06 ml)
Rx	prescription
ℨ	dram
z or ℨ	ounce
Other symbols	
ā	before
āā	of each
@	at
c̄	with
Ca	calcium
Cl	chloride
CO	carbon monoxide
CO_2	carbon dioxide
Hg	mercury
K	potassium
Ⓛ	left
⒧	left arm
⒧	left leg
Na	sodium
NaCl	sodium chloride
O_2	oxygen
Ⓡ	right
⒭	right arm
⒭	right leg
♀	female
♂	male
"	inches
#	number, pound

SYMBOL	MEANING
Other symbols *(continued)*	
$\wedge$	diastolic blood pressure (commonly used on graphic forms)
$\vee$	systolic blood pressure
$\cong$	approximately equal to
$\approx$	approximately
$\uparrow$	increase
$\downarrow$	decrease
?	questionable
$\emptyset$, $\bar{\text{o}}$	none, no
1°	primary, first degree
2°	secondary, second degree
3°	tertiary, third degree
1:1	one-to-one
$\bar{\text{p}}$	after
$\bar{\text{s}}$	without
ss, $\bar{\text{s}}\bar{\text{s}}$, $\acute{\text{s}}\acute{\text{s}}$	one-half
$\times$	times
$\dot{\bar{\text{i}}}$	one
$\overset{..}{\text{ii}}$	two, etc.

JCAHO Nursing Care and Documentation Standards

In 1993, the Joint Commission on Accreditation of Healthcare Organizations (JCAHO) revamped certain nursing standards. The *selected* standards listed below apply to documented nursing assessment and care, programs, staffing requirements, and management in the hospital setting.

Assessment and care standards

Patients receive nursing care based on a documented assessment of their needs.

• Each patient's need for nursing care related to hospital admission is assessed by a registered nurse.

— The assessment is conducted either at the time of admission or within a time frame specified by hospital policy.

— Aspects of data collection may be delegated by the registered nurse.

— Needs are reassessed when warranted by the patient's condition.

• Each patient's assessment includes consideration of biophysical, psychosocial, environmental, self-care, educational, and discharge planning factors.

— When appropriate, data from the patient's significant other(s) are included in the assessment.

• Each patient's nursing care is based on identified nursing diagnoses or patient care needs and patient care standards and is consistent with the therapies of other disciplines.

— The patient and significant other(s) are involved in the patient's care as appropriate.

• Nursing staff members collaborate, as appropriate, with physicians and other clinical disciplines in making decisions regarding each patient's need for nursing care.

• In preparation for discharge, continuing care needs are assessed and referrals for such care are documented in the patient's medical record.

• The patient's medical record includes documentation of:

— initial assessments and reassessments

— nursing diagnoses, patient care needs, or both

— interventions identified to meet the patient's nursing care needs

— nursing care provided

— the patient's response to, and the outcomes of, the care provided

— the abilities of the patient and, as appropriate, significant other(s) to manage continuing care needs after discharge.

• Nursing care data related to patient assessments, nursing diagnoses or patient needs (or both), nursing interventions, and patient outcomes are permanently integrated into the clinical information system (for example, the medical record).

— Nursing care data can be identified and retrieved from the clinical information system.

Nursing program standards

The nurse executive and other appropriate registered nurses develop hospital-wide patient care programs, policies, and procedures that describe how the nursing care needs of patients or patient populations are assessed, evaluated, and met.

• Policies and procedures, based on nursing standards of patient care and standards of nursing practice, describe and guide the nursing care provided.

—The nurse executive has the authority and responsibility for establishing standards of nursing practice.

• The policies, procedures, nursing standards of patient care, and standards of nursing practice are:

—developed by the nurse executive, registered nurses, and other designated nursing staff members

—defined in writing

—approved by the nurse executive or designee(s)

—used, as indicated, in the assessment of the quality of patient care.

• Review of policies and procedures includes information about the relevance of policies; procedures, nursing standards of patient care, and standards of nursing practice in actual use; ethical and legal concerns; current scientific knowledge; and findings from quality assessment and improvement activities and other evaluation mechanisms as appropriate.

—Nursing staff members have a defined mechanism designed to address ethical issues in patient care.

—When the hospital has an ethics committee or other defined structures designed to address ethical issues in patient care, nursing staff members participate.

• Policies and procedures are developed in collaboration with other clinical and administrative groups when appropriate.

—The nurse executive or designee(s) participates in the hospital admissions system to coordinate patient requirements for nursing care with available nursing resources.

—In making the decision when or where to admit or transfer a patient, consideration is given to the ability of the nursing staff to assess and meet the patient's nursing care needs.

Nursing staffing standards

Nursing policies and procedures describe the mechanism used to assign nursing staff members to meet patient care needs.

• There are sufficient qualified nursing staff members to meet the nursing care needs of patients throughout the hospital.

• The criteria for employment, deployment, and assignment of nursing staff members are approved by the nurse executive.

• Nurse staffing plans for each unit define the number and mix of nursing personnel in accordance with current patient care needs.

—In designing and assessing nurse staffing plans, the hospital gives appropriate consideration to the utilization of registered nurses, licensed practical or vocational nurses, nursing assistants, and other nursing personnel and to the potential contribution these personnel can make to the delivery of efficient and effective patient care.

—The staffing schedules are reviewed and adjusted as necessary to meet defined patient needs and unusual occurrences.

—Appropriate and sufficient support services are available to allow nursing staff members to meet the nursing care needs of patients and their significant other(s).

—Staffing levels are adequate to support participation of nursing staff members, as assigned, in committees and meetings and in educational and quality assessment and improvement activities.

• The hospital's plan for providing nursing care is designed to support improvement and innovation in nursing practice and is based on both the needs of the patients to be served and the hospital's mission.

—The plan for nurse staffing and the provision of nursing care is reviewed in detail on an annual basis and receives periodic attention as warranted by changing patient care needs and outcomes.
• Registered nurses prescribe, delegate, and coordinate the nursing care provided throughout the hospital.
• Consistent standards for the provision of nursing care within the hospital are used to monitor and evaluate the quality of nursing care provided throughout the hospital.
• The appropriateness of the hospital's plan for providing nursing care to meet patient needs is reviewed as part of the established budget review process.
• The review includes:
—an analysis of actual staffing patterns
—findings from quality assessment and improvement activities.
• The allocation of financial and other resources is assessed to determine whether nursing care is provided appropriately, efficiently, and effectively.
• The allocation of financial and other resources is designed to support improvement and innovation in nursing practice.

Nursing management standards
The nurse executive and other nursing leaders participate with leaders from the governing body, management, medical staff, and clinical areas in the hospital's decision-making structures and processes.
• Nursing services are directed by a nurse executive who is a registered nurse qualified by advanced education and management experience.
• If the hospital utilizes a decentralized organizational structure, there is an identified nurse leader at the executive level to provide authority and accountability for, and coordination of, the nurse executive functions.
• The nurse executive and other nursing leaders participate in developing and implementing mechanisms for collaboration between nursing staff members, doctors, and other clinical practitioners.
• The nurse executive or designee(s) participates in evaluating, selecting, and integrating health care technology and information management systems that support patient care needs and the efficient utilization of nursing resources.
• The use of efficient interactive information management systems for nursing, other clinical (for example, dietary, pharmacy, and physical therapy), and nonclinical information is facilitated wherever appropriate.

Nursing Organizations

Academy of Medical-Surgical Nurses
East Holly Avenue, Box 56
Pitman, NJ 08071-0056
(609) 256-2323

Alabama State Nurses' Association
360 N. Hull Street
Montgomery, AL 36104-3658
(205) 262-8321

Alaska Nurses' Association
237 E. 3rd Avenue
Anchorage, AK 99501
(907) 274-0827

American Association of Critical-Care Nurses*
101 Columbia
Aliso Viejo, CA 92656-1491
(800) 899-2226

American Association of Neuroscience Nurses*
224 N. Des Plaines, Suite 601
Chicago, IL 60661
(312) 993-0043

American Association of Nurse Anesthetists*
222 S. Prospect Avenue
Park Ridge, IL 60068-4001
(708) 692-7050

*Certification program available

American College of Nurse-Midwives*
1522 K Street, NW
Suite 1000
Washington, DC 20005
(202) 289-0171

American Nurses' Association
600 Maryland Avenue, SW
Suite 100 West
Washington, DC 20024-2571
(202) 554-4444

American Radiological Nurses Association
2021 Spring Road
Suite 600
Oak Brook, IL 60521
(708) 571-9072

American Society of Postanesthesia Nurses*
11512 Allecingie Parkway
Richmond, VA 23235
(804) 379-5516

Arizona Nurses' Association
1850 E. Southern Avenue
Suite 1
Tempe, AZ 85282
(602) 831-0404

Arkansas Nurses' Association
117 S. Cedar Street
Little Rock, AR 72205
(501) 664-5853

Association of Operating Room Nurses*
2170 S. Parker Road
Suite 300
Denver, CO 80231-5711
(303) 755-6300

Association for Practitioners in Infection Control
505 E. Hawley Street
Mundelein, IL 60060
(708) 949-6052

Association of Rehabilitation Nurses*
5700 Old Orchard Road
First Floor
Skokie, Il 60077-1057
(708) 966-3433

Association of Women's Health, Obstetric, and Neonatal Nurses
700 14th Street, NW
Washington, DC 20005
(202) 662-1600

California Nurses' Association
1145 Market Street
Suite 110
San Francisco, CA 94103
(414) 864-4141

Colorado Nurses' Association
5453 E. Evans Place
Denver, CO 80222
(303) 757-7483

Connecticut Nurses' Association
377 Research Parkway
Suite 2D
Meriden, CT 06450
(203) 238-1207

Delaware Nurses' Association
2634 Capitol Trail
Suite A
Newark, DE 19711
(302) 368-2333

District of Columbia Nurses' Association
5100 Wisconsin Avenue, NW
Suite 306
Washington, DC 20016
(202) 244-2705

Emergency Nurses Association
216 Higgins Road
Park Ridge, IL 60068
(708) 698-9400

Florida Nurses' Association
P.O. Box 536985
Orlando, FL 32853-6985
(407) 896-3261

Georgia Nurses' Association
1362 W. Peachtree Street, NW
Atlanta, GA 30309
(404) 876-4624

Guam Nurses' Association
35 Rota Street
Agana, GU 96910
(671) 734-7103

Hawaii Nurses' Association
677 Ala Moana Boulevard
Suite 301
Honolulu, HI 96813
(808) 531-1628

Idaho Nurses' Association
200 N. 4th Street
Suite 20
Boise, ID 83702-6001
(208) 345-0500

*Certification program available

Illinois Nurses' Association
300 S. Wacker Drive
Suite 2200
Chicago, IL 60606
(312) 236-9708

Indiana State Nurses' Association
2915 N. High School Road
Indianapolis, IN 46224
(317) 299-4575

Intravenous Nurses Society, Inc.*
2 Brighton Street
Belmont, MA 02178
(617) 489-5205

Iowa Nurses' Association
1501 42nd Street
Suite 471
Des Moines, IA 50266
(515) 225-0495

Kansas State Nurses' Association
700 S.W. Jackson
Suite 601
Topeka, KS 66603
(913) 233-8638

Kentucky Nurses' Association
1400 S. 1st Street
P.O. Box 2616
Louisville, KY 40201
(502) 637-2546

Louisiana State Nurses' Association
712 Transcontinental Drive
Metairie, LA 70001
(504) 889-1030

Maine State Nurses' Association
P.O. Box 2240
Augusta, ME 04338-2240
(207) 622-1057

Maryland Nurses' Association
849 International Drive
Airport Square 21, Suite 255
Linthicum Heights, MD 21090
(410) 859-3000

Massachusetts Nurses' Association
340 Turnpike Street
Canton, MA 02021
(617) 821-4625

Michigan Nurses' Association
2310 Jolly Oak Road
Okemos, Ml 48864
(517) 349-5640

Minnesota Nurses' Association
1295 Bandana Boulevard, North
Suite 140
St. Paul, MN 55108-0927
(612) 646-0927

Mississippi Nurses' Association
135 Bounds Street
Suite 100
Jackson, MS 39206
(601) 982-9182

Missouri Nurses' Association
206 E. Dunklin Street
P.O. Box 325
Jefferson City, MO 65102-0325
(314) 636-4623

Montana Nurses' Association
104 Broadway
Suite G-2
P.O. Box 5718
Helena, MT 59601
(406) 442-6710

*Certification program available

National Association of Nephrology Technologists
60 Revere Drive
Suite 500
Northbrook, IL 60062
(708) 480-7675

National Association of Orthopaedic Nurses, Inc.
East Holly Avenue, Box 56
Pitman, NJ 08071-0056
(609) 256-2310

National Association of Pediatric Nurse Associates and Practitioners*
1101 Kings Highway, North
Number 206
Cherry Hill, NJ 08034
(609) 667-1773

National Association of School Nurses, Inc.*
P.O. Box 1300
Scarborough, ME 04070-1300
(207) 883-2117

Nebraska Nurses' Association
941 O Street
Suites 707-711
Lincoln, NE 68508
(402) 475-3859

Nevada Nurses' Association
3660 Baker Lane
Suite 104
Reno, NV 89509
(702) 825-3555

New Hampshire Nurses' Association
48 West Street
Concord, NH 03301
(603) 255-3783

*Certification program available

New Jersey State Nurses' Association
320 W. State Street
Trenton, NJ 08618
(609) 392-4884

New Mexico Nurses' Association
909 Virginia, NE
Suite 101
Albuquerque, NM 87108

New York State Nurses' Association
2113 Western Avenue
Guilderland, NY 12084
(518) 450-5371

North Carolina Nurses' Association
103 Enterprise Street
Box 12025
Raleigh, NC 27605-2025
(919) 821-4250

North Dakota Nurses' Association
212 N. 4th Street
Bismarck, ND 58501
(701) 223-1385

Ohio Nurses' Association
4000 E. Main Street
Columbus, OH 43213-2950
(614) 237-5414

Oklahoma Nurses' Association
6414 N. Santa Fe
Suite A
Oklahoma City, OK 73116
(405) 840-3476

Oncology Nursing Society*
501 Holiday Drive
Pittsburgh, PA 15220
(412) 921-7373

Oregon Nurses' Association
9600 S.W. Oak Street
Suite 550
Portland, OR 97223
(503) 293-0011

Appendices

Pennsylvania Nurses' Association
2578 Interstate Drive
P.O. Box 68525
Harrisburg, PA 17105-8525
(717) 657-1222

Rhode Island State Nurses' Association
300 Ray Drive
Suite 5
Providence, RI 02906-4861
(401) 421-9703

South Carolina Nurses' Association
1821 Gadsden Street
Columbia, SC 29201
(803) 252-4781

South Dakota Nurses' Association
1505 S. Minnesota
Suite 6
Sioux Falls, SD 57105
(605) 338-1401

Tennessee Nurses' Association
545 Mainstream Drive
Suite 405
Nashville, TN 37228-1201
(615) 254-0350

Texas Nurses' Association
7600 Burnet Road
Suite 440
Austin, TX 78757-1292
(512) 452-0645

Utah Nurses' Association
455 East 400, South
Salt Lake City, UT 84111
(801) 322-3439

Vermont State Nurses' Association
Champlain Mill, Box 26
1 Main Street
Winooski, VT 05404-2230
(802) 655-7123

*Certification program available

Virginia Nurses' Association
1311 High Point Avenue
Richmond, VA 23230
(804) 353-7311

Virgin Islands Nurses' Association
583 Christiansted
St Croix, VI 00821-0583

Washington State Nurses' Association
2505 2nd Avenue
Suite 500
Seattle, WA 98121
(206) 443-9762

West Virginia Nurses' Association
101 Dee Drive
P.O. Box 1946
Charleston, WV 25327
(304) 342-1169

Wisconsin Nurses' Association
6117 Monona Drive
Madison, WI 53716
(608) 221-0383

**Wound, Ostomy and Continence Nurses:
An Association of ET Nurses**
2755 Bristol Street,
Suite 110
Costa Mesa, CA 92626
(714) 476-0268

Wyoming Nurses' Association
Majestic Bldg.
1603 Capitol Avenue, Room 305
Cheyenne, WY 82001
(307) 635-3955

Documentation Guidelines for Common Nursing Diagnoses

Once you've explored your patient's chief complaints, performed an assessment, and analyzed the findings, you can formulate your nursing diagnoses (or problem list) and develop a plan of care. This plan will specify patient outcomes and the interventions to achieve them. Completing the process requires documenting your findings and activities. For your reference, this appendix provides documentation guidelines for the most commonly used nursing diagnoses.

Activity intolerance, high risk for

related to immobility

Definition
Accentuated risk of extreme fatigue or other physiologic effects following simple activity

Documenting assessment findings
Chart assessment findings related to the following:
• History of present illness
• Age
• Past experience with immobility or prescribed bed rest
• Cardiovascular status, including blood pressure, heart rate and rhythm at rest and with activity, complete blood count, skin temperature and color, edema, chest pain or discomfort

• Respiratory status, including arterial blood gases, auscultation of breath sounds, pain or discomfort associated with respiration, and rate, rhythm, depth, and pattern of respirations at rest and with activity
• Neurologic status, including level of consciousness, orientation, mental status, sensory status, motor status
• Musculoskeletal status, including range of motion (ROM), muscle size, strength, tone, and functional mobility as follows:
    0 = completely independent
    1 = requires use of equipment or device
    2 = requires help, supervision, or teaching from another person
    3 = requires help from another person and equipment or device
    4 = dependent; doesn't take part in activity.

Documenting patient outcomes
Record appropriate patient outcomes on the plan of care. Possible outcomes include:
• Patient maintains muscle strength and ROM.
• Patient carries out isometric exercise regimen.
• Patient communicates understanding of rationale for maintaining activity level.
• Patient avoids risk factors that may lead to activity intolerance.
• Patient performs self-care activities to tolerance level.
• Vital signs remain within prescribed range during periods of activity (specify).

Documenting interventions

Chart interventions related to:
• patient's expressed motivation to maintain maximum activity level within restrictions imposed by illness
• patient's physiologic response to increased activity (times and dates of vital signs: blood pressure, respirations, heart rate and rhythm)
• patient repositioning and turning (include times and assistive devices used)
• patient's functional level (use a functional mobility scale)
• prescribed ROM and other exercises (include times and assistive devices used, such as trapezes)
• patient teaching (reason for treatment regimen, signs and symptoms of overexertion, such as dizziness, chest pain, and dyspnea) and patient's response
• evaluation of expected outcomes.

Airway clearance, ineffective

related to decreased energy or fatigue

Definition

Anatomic or physiologic obstruction of the airway that interferes with normal ventilation

Documenting assessment findings

Chart the patient's complaints and your physical assessment findings, for example:
• **Chief complaints:** breathing problems and congestion, anxiety, apprehension, chest pain, choking or gasping, shortness of breath, fever, inability to cough, fatigue, decreased activity tolerance
• History of present illness
• Patient's perception of ability to clear airway
• Knowledge of physical condition
• Neurologic status, including level of consciousness, orientation, sensory status, and motor status
• Respiratory status, including symmetry of chest expansion; use of accessory muscles; cough (productive or nonproductive); respiratory rate, depth, and pattern; sputum characteristics (color, consistency, amount, odor, and changes from patient's norm); palpation for fremitus; percussion of lung fields; auscultation for breath sounds; arterial blood gas (ABG) levels; hemoglobin and hematocrit
• Pulmonary function studies
• Psychosocial status, including interest, motivation, and knowledge.

Documenting patient outcomes

Record appropriate patient outcomes on the plan of care. Possible outcomes include:
• Airway remains patent.
• Adventitious breath sounds are absent.
• Chest X-ray shows no abnormality.
• Oxygen level in normal range.
• Patient breathes deeply and coughs to remove secretions.
• Patient expectorates sputum.
• Patient demonstrates controlled coughing techniques.
• Ventilation is adequate.
• Patient shows no signs of pulmonary compromise.
• Patient demonstrates skill in conserving energy while attempting to clear airway.
• Patient states understanding of changes needed to diminish oxygen demands.

Documenting interventions

Chart interventions related to:
• patient's perceptions of ability to cough
• observed respiratory status and other physical findings
• patient positioning and repositioning (including times)
• airway and pulmonary clearance maneuvers such as coughing and deep-breathing, suctioning to stimulate cough and clear airways, aerosol treatments, postural drainage, percussion, and vibration
• sputum characteristics (including amount, odor, consistency)

• prescribed medication administration (including expectorants, bronchodilators, and other drugs)
• amount of fluid intake to help liquefy secretions
• oxygen administration (including times, dates, equipment, and supplies)
• test results, including ABG levels and hemoglobin values, and reportable deviations from baseline levels
• endotracheal intubation
• patient teaching
• evaluation of expected outcomes.

Anxiety

related to situational crisis

Definition
Feeling of threat or danger to self arising from an unidentifiable source

Documenting assessment findings
Chart the patient's complaints and your physical assessment findings, for example:
• **Chief complaints:** shortness of breath or smothering sensation; palpitations; sweating; cold, clammy hands; dry mouth; dizziness; lightheadedness; nausea, diarrhea, other abdominal distress; flushes (hot flashes) or chills; frequent urination; difficulty swallowing; tenseness, including trembling, twitching, shakiness, muscle tension, aches, soreness, restlessness; easy fatigue; keyed-up feeling; difficulty concentrating; insomnia; irritability
• Reason for hospitalization, including patient's perception of problem, onset of problem, recent stressors, life changes, other precipitants
• Mental status, including orientation to time, place, or person; insight regarding current situation; judgment; abstract thinking; general information; mood; affect; recent and remote memory; thought processes; thought content
• Coping, problem-solving ability
• Ability to perform activities of daily living
• Sleep habits
• Dietary and nutritional status
• Available support systems, including family or significant other, friends, clergy, health care agencies.

Documenting patient outcomes
Record appropriate expected outcomes on the plan of care. Possible outcomes include:
• Patient identifies factors that elicit anxious behaviors.
• Patient discusses activities that tend to decrease anxious behaviors.
• Patient practices progressive relaxation techniques _____ times a day.
• Patient copes with current medical situation (specify) without demonstrating severe signs of anxiety (specify for individual).

Documenting interventions
Chart interventions related to:
• patient's statement of anxiety and feelings of relief
• observed signs of patient's anxiety
• time spent with patient and duration of anxious episodes
• comfort measures
• patient teaching (including clear, concise explanations of anything about to occur, relaxation techniques such as guided imagery, progressive muscle relaxation, and meditation)
• referrals to counselor or support groups
• evaluation of expected outcomes.

Body image disturbance
Definition
Negative perception of self that makes healthful functioning more difficult

Documenting assessment findings

Chart the patient's complaints and your physical assessment findings, for example:
• **Chief complaints:** actual change in structure or function, missing body part, inability to look at or touch body part
• Physiologic changes
• Behavioral changes
• Patient's and family's perception of the patient's present health problem
• Patient's usual pattern of coping with stress
• Patient's role in the family
• Patient's past experiences with health problems
• Sleep pattern
• Appetite
• Hobbies and interests
• Occupational history
• Ethnic background and cultural perceptions.

Documenting patient outcomes

Record appropriate expected outcomes on the plan of care. Possible outcomes include:
• Patient acknowledges change in body image.
• Patient participates in decision making about his care (specify).
• Patient communicates feelings about change in body image.
• Patient expresses positive feelings about self.
• Patient talks with someone who has experienced the same problem.
• Patient demonstrates ability to practice two new coping behaviors.

Documenting interventions

Chart interventions related to:
• patient's observed coping patterns and responses to change in structure or function of body part (such as touching or not touching)
• patient's participation in self-care
• patient's description of self, prostheses, adaptive equipment, or limitations
• patient's focus on or denial of specific body parts

• patient's response to nursing interventions
• patient teaching (including information on how bodily functions are improving or stabilizing and specific coping strategies)
• referrals to a counselor, a support group, or another person who had a similar problem
• evaluation of expected outcomes.

Breathing pattern, ineffective

related to decreased energy or fatigue

Definition

Change in rate, depth, or pattern of breathing that alters normal gas exchange

Documenting assessment findings

Chart the patient's complaints and your physical assessment findings, for example:
• **Chief complaints:** increased breathing effort; cough; shortness of breath, especially on exertion; decreased energy; and fatigue
• History of respiratory disorder
• Respiratory status, including rate and depth of respiration, symmetry of chest expansion, use of accessory muscles, presence of cough, anterior-posterior chest diameter, palpation for fremitus, percussion of lung fields, auscultation of breath sounds, pulmonary function studies
• Neurologic and mental status, including level of consciousness and emotional status
• Knowledge, including current understanding of physical condition and physical, mental, and emotional readiness to learn.

Documenting patient outcomes

Record appropriate expected outcomes on the plan of care. Possible outcomes include:
• Patient's respiratory rate stays within ±5 of baseline.
• Arterial blood gas (ABG) levels return to baseline.
• Patient reports feeling comfortable when breathing.

• Patient reports feeling rested each day.
• Patient demonstrates diaphragmatic pursed-lip breathing.
• Patient achieves maximum lung expansion with adequate ventilation.
• Patient demonstrates skill in conserving energy while carrying out activities of daily living.

Documenting interventions
Chart interventions related to:
• patient's expressions of comfort in breathing, emotional state, understanding of medical diagnosis, and readiness to learn
• physical condition related to pulmonary assessment (including respiratory rate and depth, auscultated breath sounds, reportable changes)
• test results such as ABG levels
• prescribed medication and oxygen administration (including dates, times, dosages, routes, adverse effects, equipment, and supplies)
• comfort measures (including supporting upper extremities with pillows, providing an over-bed table with a pillow to lean on, or elevating the head of the bed)
• airway suctioning to remove secretions
• patient teaching (including pursed-lip breathing, abdominal breathing, relaxation techniques, medications, reportable adverse effects of medication, activity and rest, and diet)
• evaluation of expected outcomes.

Cardiac output, decreased

related to reduced stroke volume as a result of mechanical or structural problems

Definition
Cardiovascular or respiratory symptoms resulting from insufficient blood being pumped by the heart

Documenting assessment findings
Chart the patient's complaints and your physical assessment findings, for example:

• **Chief complaints:** problems with urination, abdominal swelling, cold and clammy skin, cough and congestion, breathlessness, fatigue, frothy sputum, abdominal tenderness, difficulty in breathing unless head is elevated
• Mental status, including orientation and level of consciousness (LOC)
• Cardiovascular status, including history of valvular disorder, heart failure, or myopathy; skin color, temperature, turgor, and capillary refill time; jugular vein distention; hepatojugular reflux; heart rate and rhythm; heart sounds; blood pressure; peripheral pulses; electrocardiogram (ECG); exercise ECG; echocardiogram; and phonocardiogram
• Respiratory status, including respiratory rate and depth, breath sounds, chest X-ray, and arterial blood gas levels
• Renal status, including weight, intake and output, and urine specific gravity.

Documenting patient outcomes
Record appropriate expected outcomes on the plan of care. Possible outcomes include:
• Patient maintains hemodynamic stability: pulse not less than _____ and not greater than _____; blood pressure not less than _____ and not greater than _____.
• Patient exhibits no arrhythmias.
• Skin remains warm and dry.
• Patient exhibits no pedal edema.
• Patient achieves activity within limits of prescribed heart rate.
• Patient expresses sense of physical comfort after activity.
• Heart's workload diminishes.
• Patient maintains adequate cardiac output.
• Patient performs stress-reduction techniques every 4 hours while awake.
• Patient states understanding of signs and symptoms, prescribed activity level, diet, and medications.

Documenting interventions

Chart interventions related to:
• patient's needs and perception of problem
• observed physical findings (include LOC, heart rate and rhythm, blood pressure, auscultated heart and breath sounds)
• reports of abnormal findings (include times, dates, and names)
• intake and output measurements, daily weight (include observation of pedal or sacral edema)
• interventions for life-threatening arrhythmias as ordered
• skin care measures to enhance skin perfusion and venous flow
• increasing patient's activity level within limits of prescribed heart rate
• patient's response to activity
• dietary restrictions as ordered
• patient teaching, including desired skills related to diet, prescribed activity, and stress management; procedures and tests; chest pain and other reportable symptoms; medications (name, dosage, frequency, therapeutic and adverse effects); simple methods for lifting and bending
• evaluation of expected outcomes.

Constipation

related to personal habits

Definition

Interruption of normal bowel movements resulting in infrequent or absent stools

Documenting assessment findings

Chart the patient's complaints and your physical assessment findings, for example:
• **Chief complaints:** decreased appetite; fever; decreased bowel movement frequency; hard, formed stools; straining during defecation; reported decreased intake of fluid, food, or fiber
• History of bowel disorder or surgery
• GI status, including nausea and vomiting, usual bowel habits, change in bowel habits, stool characteristics (color, amount, size, consistency), pain, inspection of abdomen, auscultation of bowel sounds, palpation for masses and tenderness, percussion for tympany and dullness, laxative or enema use, medications (iron, narcotics)
• Nutritional status, including dietary intake, appetite, current weight, and change from normal weight
• Activity status, type and duration of exercise, and occupation (sedentary, having restricted access to bathroom)
• Knowledge, including understanding of need for regular bowel habits, ability and motivation to change current patterns, and understanding of relationship between laxative and enema use, activity, and constipation.

Documenting patient outcomes

Record appropriate expected outcomes on the plan of care. Possible outcomes include:
• Elimination pattern returns to normal.
• Patient moves bowels every _____ day(s) without laxative or enema.
• Patient states understanding of causative factors of constipation.
• Patient gets regular exercise.
• Patient describes changes in personal habits to maintain normal elimination pattern.
• Patient states plans to seek help resolving emotional or psychological problems.

Documenting interventions

Chart interventions related to:
• frequency of bowel movements and characteristics of stools
• administration of laxatives or enemas
• patient's weight
• referrals or consultations with nutritional staff
• patient's expressions of concern about change in diet, activity level, use of laxatives or enemas, and bowel pattern

• observed characteristics of stools, diet, and activity tolerance
• patient teaching (diet, dietary fiber, exercise, long-term effects of laxatives or enemas)
• evaluation of expected outcomes.

Coping, ineffective individual

related to situational crisis

Definition
Inability to use adaptive behaviors in response to such difficult life situations as loss of health, a loved one, or job

Documenting assessment findings
Chart the patient's complaints and your physical assessment findings, for example:
• **Chief complaints:** reported or observed change in usual communication patterns, chronic fatigue, chronic worry, evidence of situational crisis, excessive drinking, inappropriate use of defense mechanisms, insomnia, irritability, irritable bowel, muscular tension, overeating or loss of appetite, verbal expression of inability to cope or seek help, verbal manipulation, inability to fulfill role expectations, meet basic needs, or solve problems
• Coping behaviors
• Degree of physical and emotional impairment
• Diversional activities
• Financial resources
• Occupation
• Patient's perception of present health problem or crisis
• Problem-solving techniques usually employed to cope with life problems
• Support systems, including family, companion, friends, and clergy.

Documenting patient outcomes
Record appropriate expected outcomes on the plan of care. Possible outcomes include:
• Patient communicates feelings about the present situation.

• Patient becomes involved in planning own care.
• Patient expresses feeling of having greater control over present situation.
• Patient uses available support systems, such as family and friends, to aid in coping.
• Patient identifies at least two coping behaviors.
• Patient demonstrates ability to use two healthful coping behaviors.

Documenting interventions
Chart interventions related to:
• patient's efforts at self-care
• patient's coping behaviors and patient's evaluation of their effectiveness
• patient's perception of current situation and what it means
• patient's verbal expression of feelings indicating comfort or discomfort
• observed patient behaviors
• nursing interventions to help patient cope and patient's responses
• patient teaching (about treatments and procedures)
• referrals to counselors and support groups
• evaluation of expected outcomes.

Denial

related to fear or anxiety

Definition
Conscious or unconscious attempt to disavow the knowledge or meaning of an event to reduce anxiety or fear to the detriment of health

Documenting assessment findings
Chart the patient's complaints and your physical assessment findings, for example:
• **Chief complaints:** doesn't admit impact of disease on life pattern, doesn't admit fear of death or invalidism, doesn't perceive personal relevance or danger of symptoms, minimizes

symptoms, reports self-treatment to relieve symptoms
• Perception of present health, including awareness of diagnosis, perception of personal relevance or impact on life pattern, and description of symptoms
• Degree of physical and emotional functional impairment
• Mental status, including general appearance, affect, mood, memory, orientation, communication, thinking process, perception, abstract thinking, judgment, and insight
• Coping behaviors
• Problem-solving strategies
• Support systems, including family or significant other, friends, and clergy; financial resources
• Belief system, including values, norms, and religion
• Self-concept, including self-esteem and body image.

Documenting patient outcomes

Record appropriate expected outcomes on the plan of care. Possible outcomes include:
• Patient describes knowledge and perception of present health problem.
• Patient describes life pattern and reports any recent changes.
• Patient expresses knowledge of stages of grief.
• Patient demonstrates behavior associated with grief process.
• Patient discusses present health problem with doctor, nurses, and family or significant other.
• Patient indicates by conversation or behavior an increased awareness of reality.

Documenting interventions

Chart interventions related to:
• patient's perception of health problem
• mental status (baseline and ongoing)
• communications with doctor (to assess what patient has been told about illness)

• patient's knowledge of grief process
• patient's behavioral responses
• interventions implemented to assist patient
• patient's response to nursing interventions
• patient teaching and patient's response
• evaluation of expected outcomes.

Diarrhea

related to malabsorption, inflammation, or irritation of bowel

Definition
Interruption of normal elimination pattern characterized by frequent, loose stools

Documenting assessment findings
Chart the patient's complaints and your physical assessment findings, for example:
• **Chief complaints:** abdominal pain and cramping, loud bowel sounds, increased frequency of defecation, loose liquid stools, urgency
• History of bowel disorder or surgery
• GI status, including nausea and vomiting, usual bowel habits, change in bowel habits, stool characteristics (color, amount, size, consistency), pain, inspection of abdomen, auscultation of bowel sounds, palpation for masses and tenderness, percussion for tympany and dullness, laxative and enema use, medications (especially antibiotics), stool culture, upper GI series, barium enema
• Nutritional status, including dietary intake, change from normal diet, appetite, current weight, change from normal weight, and food irritants and contaminants
• Fluid and electrolyte status, including intake and output, urine specific gravity, skin turgor, mucous membranes, serum potassium and sodium, and blood urea nitrogen
• Psychosocial status, including personality, stressors (finances, job, marital discord, disease process), coping mechanisms, support systems, lifestyle, and recent travel.

Documenting patient outcomes

Record appropriate expected outcomes on the plan of care. Possible outcomes include:
• Patient controls diarrhea with medication.
• Elimination pattern returns to normal.
• Patient regains and maintains fluid and electrolyte balance.
• Skin remains intact.
• Patient discusses causative factors and preventive measures.
• Patient practices stress-reduction techniques daily.
• Patient seeks out persons with similar condition or joins a support group.

Documenting interventions

Chart interventions related to:
• patient's expressions of concern about diarrhea, causative factors, and adaptation to changes in body image if diarrhea results from colorectal surgery.
• administration and observed effects of antidiarrheal medications
• intake and output measurements and daily weight
• observed stool characteristics and frequency and skin condition
• skin condition (especially decreased skin turgor or excoriation)
• bowel sounds (auscultation findings)
• patient teaching (including causes, prevention, cleanliness and comfort, dietary restrictions, stress reduction, preoperative instruction about ileostomy or colostomy, postoperative instructions about ostomy equipment)
• referrals to support groups (such as ostomy clubs)
• evaluation of expected outcomes.

Fluid volume deficit

related to active loss

Definition

Excessive loss of body fluid and electrolytes

Documenting assessment findings

Chart the patient's complaints and your physical assessment findings, for example:
• **Chief complaints:** dry mucous membranes; dry or cold, clammy skin; fever; rapid breathing; thirst; weakness; weight loss
• History of fluid loss, such as vomiting, nasogastric (NG) tube drainage, diarrhea, hemorrhage
• Vital signs
• Fluid and electrolyte status, including weight, intake and output, urine specific gravity, skin turgor, mucous membranes
• Laboratory studies, including serum electrolytes, blood urea nitrogen, hemoglobin, hematocrit, stool cultures.

Documenting patient outcomes

Record appropriate expected outcomes on the plan of care. Possible outcomes include:
• Vital signs remain stable.
• Skin color and temperature are normal.
• Electrolyte levels stay within normal range.
• Fluid volume remains adequate.
• Patient produces adequate urine volume.
• Patient has normal skin turgor and moist mucous membranes.
• Urine specific gravity remains between 1.005 and 1.010.
• Fluid and blood volume return to normal.
• Patient expresses understanding of factors that caused fluid volume deficit.

Documenting interventions

Chart interventions related to:
• vital signs
• patient's complaints of thirst, weakness, dizziness, and palpitations; interventions to control fluid loss
• observed skin and mucous membrane condition and other physical findings (including signs of fluid and electrolyte imbalances, such as tachycardia, dyspnea, or hypotension)

• intake and output and significant changes (include amount and type—urine, stools, vomitus, wound drainage, NG drainage, chest tube drainage, and any other)
• urine specific gravity values (include times and date)
• administration of any fluids, blood or blood products, or plasma expanders and patient's response
• patient's daily weight and abdominal girth
• patient's response to interventions
• patient teaching (about fluid loss, ways to monitor fluid volume at home by measuring intake and output and body weight daily)
• evaluation of expected outcomes.

Gas exchange impairment

related to altered oxygen supply

Definition
Interference in cellular respiration resulting from inadequate exchange or transport of oxygen and carbon dioxide

Documenting assessment findings
Chart the patient's complaints and your physical assessment findings, for example:
• **Chief complaints:** anxiety, confusion, breathlessness, inability to move secretions, irritability, decreased mental acuity, restlessness, sleepiness
• Neurologic status, including level of consciousness, orientation, mental status
• Respiratory status, including respiratory rate and depth, symmetry of chest expansion, use of accessory muscles, cough, sputum, palpation for fremitus, percussion of lung fields, auscultation of breath sounds, arterial blood gas (ABG) levels, pulmonary function studies
• Cardiovascular status, including skin color and temperature, heart rate and rhythm, blood pressure, complete blood count

• Activity status, including such functional capabilities as range of motion and muscle strength, activities of daily living (ADLs), occupation.

Documenting patient outcomes
Record appropriate expected outcomes on the plan of care. Possible outcomes include:
• Patient maintains respiratory rate within ±5 of baseline.
• Patient expresses a feeling of comfort in maintaining air exchange.
• Patient coughs effectively.
• Patient expectorates sputum.
• Patient sustains sufficient fluid intake to prevent dehydration: _____ml/24 hours.
• Patient performs ADLs to level of tolerance.
• Patient has normal breath sounds.
• Patient's ABG levels return to baselines: _____ pH; _____ PaO_2; _____ $PaCO_2$.
• Patient performs relaxation techniques every 4 hours.
• Patient correctly uses breathing devices to improve gas exchange and increase oxygenation.

Documenting interventions
Chart interventions related to:
• patient's complaints of dyspnea, headache, or restlessness or expression of well-being
• observed physical findings (including vital signs, auscultation results, pulmonary status, cardiac rhythm)
• medication and oxygen administration (including times, dates, dosages, route, adverse effects, equipment and supplies) and patient's response
• patient positioning and repositioning and times; bronchial hygiene measures, such as coughing, percussion, postural drainage, suctioning
• intake and output measurements
• reportable signs of dehydration or fluid overload
• test results, including ABG levels

- endotracheal intubation and mechanical ventilation measures (including equipment and supplies used)
- patient teaching (including relaxation techniques and other measures to lower demand for oxygen)
- evaluation of expected outcomes.

Hopelessness

related to failing or deteriorating physiologic condition

Definition

Subjective state in which an individual sees few or no available alternatives or personal choices and cannot mobilize energy on own behalf

Documenting assessment findings

Chart the patient's complaints and your physical assessment findings, for example:
- **Chief complaints:** decreased appetite, initiative, and daily involvement (nonverbal cues include minimal eye contact, shrugging in response to questions, turning away from speaker; verbal cues include frequent sighing and negativity); increased sleep
- Nature of current medical diagnosis
- Patient's and responsible caregiver's knowledge of diagnosis and prognosis
- Actual or perceived self-care deficits (specify)
- Mental status, including cognitive functioning, affect, mood
- Communication, including verbal (speech content, quality, quantity) and nonverbal (body positioning, eye contact, facial expression)
- Available support systems, including clergy, family, friends
- Past experience with loss, including body part or function, death, residence, employment
- History of depression, bipolar disease, other psychiatric illness
- Coping mechanisms and decision-making ability
- Nutritional status, including alteration in appetite or body weight
- Sleep pattern
- Motivation level, including personal hygiene, therapies (physical and occupational therapy), and use of diversional activities
- Developmental stage (Erikson's model), including age and role in family.

Documenting patient outcomes

Record appropriate expected outcomes on the plan of care. Possible outcomes include:
- Patient identifies feelings of hopelessness regarding current situation.
- Patient demonstrates more effective communication skills, including direct verbal responses to questions and increased eye contact.
- Patient resumes appropriate rest and activity pattern.
- Patient participates in self-care activities and in decisions regarding care planning.
- Patient uses diversional activities (specify).
- Patient identifies social and community resources for continued assistance.

Documenting interventions

Chart interventions related to:
- patient's mental status
- patient's verbal and nonverbal behaviors
- patient's medical regimen
- increasing patient's feelings of hope, self-worth, and initiative in self-care and patient's response (including time spent communicating—talking or sitting—with patient)
- medication administration and comfort measures
- referrals to ancillary services, such as dietitian, social worker, clergy, mental health clinical nurse specialist, or support groups
- patient teaching (including diversional activities, self-care instruction, and discharge planning)
- evaluation of expected outcomes.

Incontinence, functional

related to sensory or mobility deficits

Definition

Involuntary and unpredictable passage of urine in socially unacceptable situations, in which patient usually does not recognize warning signs of bladder fullness

Documenting assessment findings

Chart the patient's complaints and your physical assessment findings, for example:
• **Chief complaints:** nocturia, voiding that occurs before reaching an appropriate site or receptacle, sensation of bladder fullness usually not recognized
• History of mental retardation, trauma, alcohol abuse, medication use
• Age
• Sex
• Vital signs
• Genitourinary status, including volume of urine output, extent of clothing wetness from urine, frequency, palpation of bladder, urine leakage when standing or sitting, voiding pattern
• Fluid and electrolyte status, including blood urea nitrogen, creatinine, intake and output, mucous membranes, serum electrolytes, skin turgor, urine specific gravity
• Neuromuscular status, including manual dexterity, mental status, mobility, motor ability to start and stop urine stream, rectal exam (muscle tone, prostate size, fecal impaction), sensory ability to perceive bladder fullness
• Psychosocial status, including behavior before and after voiding, coping skills, support from family or significant other, perception of health problem, self-concept, stressors (finances, job, change in environment).

Documenting patient outcomes

Record appropriate expected outcomes on the plan of care. Possible outcomes include:
• Patient voids at specific times.

• Patient voids in appropriate situation using suitable receptacle.
• Patient has no wet episodes.
• Patient maintains fluid balance; intake equals output.
• Complications are avoided or minimized.
• Patient and responsible caregivers demonstrate skill in managing incontinence.
• Patient discusses impact of incontinence on self and others.
• Patient and responsible caregivers identify resources to assist with care following discharge.

Documenting interventions

Chart interventions related to:
• patient's expression of concern about incontinence problem and motivation to participate in self-care
• patient's voiding pattern
• intake and output
• hydration status
• bladder elimination procedures (including bladder training, commode use times, toileting schedule, episodic wetness or dryness, use of external catheter)
• skin condition and care (including use of protective pads and garments)
• patient teaching (including toileting environment, time, and place; alcohol and fluid intake; techniques for stimulating voiding reflexes; techniques for reducing anxiety)
• patient's response to treatment regimen and patient teaching
• referrals to appropriate counselors and support groups
• evaluation of expected outcomes.

Infection, high risk for

related to external factors

Definition

Presence of internal or external hazards that threaten physical well-being

Documenting assessment findings

Chart assessment findings related to the following:
• Health history, including accidents, allergies, falls, hyperthermia, hypothermia, poisoning, seizures, trauma, exposure to pollutants
• Sensory or perceptual changes (auditory, gustatory, kinesthetic, olfactory, tactile, visual)
• Circumstances of present situation that could lead to infection
• Neurologic status, including level of consciousness, mental status, orientation
• Laboratory studies, including clotting factors, hemoglobin and hematocrit, platelet count, serum albumin, white blood cell (WBC) count, and cultures of blood, body fluid, sputum, urine, wounds.

Documenting patient outcomes

Record appropriate expected outcomes on the plan of care. Possible outcomes include:
• Temperature stays within normal range.
• WBC count and differential stay within normal range.
• No pathogens appear in cultures.
• Patient maintains good personal and oral hygiene.
• Respiratory secretions are clear and odorless.
• Urine remains clear yellow, odorless, with no sediment.
• Patient shows no evidence of diarrhea.
• Wounds and incisions appear clean, pink, and free of purulent drainage.
• I.V. sites show no signs of inflammation.
• Patient shows no evidence of skin breakdown.
• Patient takes _____ ml of fluid and _____ g of protein daily.
• Patient states infection risk factors.
• Patient identifies signs and symptoms of infection.
• Patient remains free of all signs and symptoms of infection.

Documenting interventions

Chart interventions related to:
• temperature readings (including date and times)
• test procedures (including dates, times, and sites of obtained test specimens)
• test results
• skin condition and wound care
• preventive measures (including personal hygiene, oral hygiene, airway suctioning, coughing and deep-breathing measures)
• catheter management procedures (including dates and times of all catheter insertions, removals, and site care)
• equipment and supplies (including particulars of humidification or nebulization of oxygen)
• sanitary measures (for example, providing tissues and disposal bag for expectorated sputum)
• fluid intake
• nutritional intake
• isolation and other precautions
• patient teaching (including toileting and hygiene, hand-washing technique, factors that increase infection risk, and infection signs and symptoms)
• patient's response to nursing interventions
• evaluation of expected outcomes.

Injury, high risk for

related to sensory or motor deficits

Definition

Accentuated risk of physical harm caused by sensory or motor deficits

Documenting assessment findings

Chart assessment findings related to the following:
• Age
• Nature of sensory or motor deficit

• Health history, including cerebral function, mobility, sensory function, use of adaptive devices
• Psychological status, including substance abuse, familiarity with surroundings, mental status, coping skills, self-concept
• Medication use, including understanding of medications, compliance with prescribed regimen, use of over-the-counter medications, interactions
• Knowledge, including understanding of safety precautions
• Medication history
• Pain or fatigue
• Laboratory studies, including complete blood count and differential, coagulation studies
• Diagnostic tests, including chest X-ray, cranial X-ray
• Sensory status, including hearing, vision, touch, taste.

Documenting patient outcomes

Record appropriate expected outcomes on the plan of care. Possible outcomes include:
• Patient identifies factors that increase potential for injury.
• Patient assists in identifying and applying safety measures to prevent injury.
• Patient and responsible caregiver develop strategy to maintain safety.
• Patient performs activities of daily living within sensorimotor limitations.

Documenting interventions

Chart interventions related to:
• observed factors that may cause or contribute to injury
• safety measures (side rails, positioning, and use of call button and bed controls)
• statements by patient and responsible caregiver about potential for injury due to sensory or motor deficits
• observed or reported unsafe practices

• interventions to decrease risk of injury to patient
• patient's responses to nursing interventions
• patient teaching (including safe ways to improve visual discrimination, to decrease risk of burns from sensory loss, to use hearing aids and mobility assistive devices, to ensure household, automobile, and pedestrian safety)
• evaluation of expected outcomes.

Knowledge deficit

related to lack of exposure

Definition

Inadequate understanding of information or inability to perform skills needed to practice health-related behaviors

Documenting assessment findings

Chart the patient's complaints and your physical assessment findings, for example:
• **Chief complaints:** needs information and lacks familiarity with information resources
• Psychosocial status, including age, learning ability (affective domain, cognitive domain, psychomotor domain), decision-making ability, developmental stage, financial resources, health beliefs and attitudes, interest in learning, knowledge and skill regarding current health problem, obstacles to learning, support systems (willingness and capability of others to help patient), usual coping pattern
• Neurologic status, including level of consciousness, memory, mental status, orientation.

Documenting patient outcomes

Record appropriate expected outcomes on the plan of care. Possible outcomes include:
• Patient communicates a need to know.
• Patient states or demonstrates understanding of what has been taught.
• Patient demonstrates ability to perform new health-related behaviors as they are taught,

and lists specific skills and realistic target dates for each.
• Patient sets realistic learning goals.
• Patient states intention to make needed changes in lifestyle, including seeking help from health care professionals when needed.

Documenting interventions
Chart interventions related to:
• patient's statements of information and skills known or unknown, expressions of need to know, motivation to learn
• patient teaching (including learning objectives, teaching methods used, information imparted, skills demonstrated) and patient's responses
• referrals to resource people or organizations who can continue instructional activities after discharge
• evaluation of expected outcomes.

Mobility impairment
related to pain or discomfort

Definition
Limitation of physical movement

Documenting assessment findings
Chart the patient's complaints and your physical assessment findings, for example:
• **Chief complaints:** pain related to movement; decreased muscle strength, control, mass, or endurance; impaired coordination; imposed restriction of movement, including mechanical; inability to move purposefully within the environment, including bed mobility, transfer, and ambulation; limited range of motion (ROM); reluctance to attempt movement
• History of recent surgery, injury, or disorder causing pain or discomfort
• Medication history

• Musculoskeletal status, including coordination, gait, muscle size and strength, muscle tone, ROM, and functional mobility as follows:
   0 = completely independent
   1 = requires use of equipment or device
   2 = requires help, supervision, or teaching from another person
   3 = requires help from another person and equipment or device
   4 = dependent; doesn't take part in activity
• Pain, including environmental and cultural influences, intensity, location, quality, temporal factors
• Psychosocial status, including coping mechanisms, family or significant other, lifestyle, personality, stressors (disease process, finances, job, marital discord).

Documenting patient outcomes
Record appropriate expected outcomes on the plan of care. Possible outcomes include:
• Patient states relief from pain.
• Patient displays increased mobility.
• Patient shows no evidence of such complications as contractures, venous stasis, thrombus formation, or skin breakdown.
• Patient attains highest degree of mobility possible within confines of disease.
• Patient or significant other demonstrates mobility regimen.
• Patient states feelings about limitations.

Documenting interventions
Chart interventions related to:
• patient's observed daily functional ability and changes (use functional mobility scale)
• patient's expressed feelings and concerns about immobility, impact on lifestyle, and willingness to participate in care
• patient's stated level of pain and discomfort and nonverbal cues to pain and discomfort
• observed impairments, pain, and response to treatment

• prescribed treatment regimen for underlying condition and patient's response to treatment and nursing interventions
• medication administration and other supportive measures (including padding extremities to prevent skin breakdown and ensuring correct height of crutches)
• prescribed ROM exercises
• patient repositioning (include times)
• progressive mobilization up to limits of patient's tolerance for pain (bed to chair to ambulation)
• patient teaching (including instructions for using crutches and walkers; practicing techniques to control pain, such as distraction and imaging; understanding need for mobility despite pain; performing ROM exercises, transfers, skin inspection, and mobility regimen) and patient's response
• referrals to counselors or support groups
• evaluation of expected outcomes.

Noncompliance

related to patient's value system

Definition
Unwillingness to practice prescribed health-related behaviors

Documenting assessment findings
Chart the patient's complaints and your physical assessment findings, for example:
• **Chief complaints:** reported or observed challenge to beliefs and value systems, complications, exacerbation of symptoms, failure to keep appointments, failure to progress, inability to set or attain mutual goals
• Age
• Health beliefs
• Patient's perceptions of health problem, treatment regimen, and importance of complying with treatment regimen

• Patient's ability to learn and perform prescribed treatment (activity, diet, medications)
• Financial resources
• Cultural and ethnic influences
• Religious influences
• Educational and language background.

Documenting patient outcomes
Record appropriate expected outcomes on the plan of care. Possible outcomes include:
• Patient identifies factors that influence noncompliance.
• Patient demonstrates a level of compliance that does not interfere with physiologic safety.
• Patient contracts with nurse to perform _____ (specify behavior and frequency).
• Patient uses support systems to modify noncompliant behavior.

Documenting interventions
Chart interventions related to:
• patient's stated reasons for noncompliance
• observed specific noncompliant behaviors
• promoting compliance (including negotiations and terms agreed upon with patient and positive reinforcements provided) and patient's response
• daily progress in complying with treatment regimen
• referrals to counselors or support groups
• evaluation of expected outcomes.

Nutrition alteration: Less than body requirements

related to inability to digest or absorb nutrients because of biological factors

Definition
Change in normal eating pattern that results in changed body weight

Documenting assessment findings

Chart the patient's complaints and your physical assessment findings, for example:

• **Chief complaints:** abdominal pain, diarrhea or steatorrhea, coated tongue, loud bowel sounds, reported weight loss despite adequate caloric intake or reported inadequate caloric intake, digestive problems and, occasionally, pressure ulcers, changes in bowel habits

• GI status related to antibiotic therapy, auscultation of bowel sounds, stool characteristics (color, amount, size, consistency), history of GI disorder or surgery, inspection and palpation of abdomen, pain or discomfort, nausea and vomiting, usual bowel elimination pattern, palpation for masses and tenderness, and percussion for tympany and dullness

• Nutritional status related to change in type of food tolerated, financial resources, height and weight, meal preparation, serum albumin level, sociocultural influences, usual dietary pattern, weight fluctuations over past 10 years

• Intrapersonal or interpersonal factors related to internal or external cues that trigger desire to eat, rate of food consumption, and stated food preference

• Psychosocial status

• Activity level

• Coping behaviors

• Body image as determined by perception of observer and self-perception.

Documenting patient outcomes

Record appropriate expected outcomes on the plan of care. Possible outcomes include:

• Patient shows no further evidence of weight loss.

• Patient tolerates oral, tube, or I.V. feedings without adverse effects.

• Patient takes in _____ calories daily.

• Patient gains _____ lb weekly.

• Patient and family or significant other communicate understanding of preoperative instructions.

• Patient and family or significant other communicate understanding of special dietary needs.

• Patient and family or significant other demonstrate ability to plan diet after discharge.

Documenting interventions

Chart interventions related to:

• daily weight

• daily fluid intake and output measurements (include volume and characteristics of any vomitus and stools—a clue to nutrient absorption)

• parenteral fluid administration

• daily food intake from prescribed diet

• electrolyte levels

• consultations with dietary department or nutritional support team

• any abnormal findings.

If the patient receives tube feedings, document interventions related to:

• concentration and delivery of regular feeding formula or one containing food-coloring additives (especially in patient with altered level of consciousness or diminished gag reflex)

• supportive equipment used, such as an infusion pump

• degree of elevation of head of bed during feeding

• feeding tube placement.

If the patient receives total parenteral nutrition, document interventions related to:

• monitored blood glucose levels and urine specific gravity (at least once each shift)

• monitored bowel sounds (once each shift)

• oral hygiene

• patient teaching (including the reasons for the current treatment regimen, principles of nutrition suited to the patient's specific condition, meal planning, and preoperative instructions if applicable)

• evaluation of expected outcomes.

Pain

related to physical, biological, or chemical agents

Definition

Subjective sensation of discomfort derived from multiple sensory nerve interactions generated by physical, chemical, biological, or psychological stimuli

Documenting assessment findings

Chart the patient's complaints and your physical assessment findings, for example:
• **Chief complaints:** changes in muscle tone (may range from listless to rigid), diaphoresis, increased or decreased breathing effort, stated pain, preoccupation with discomfort (self-focusing)
• Descriptive characteristics of pain, including location, quality, intensity on a scale of 1 to 10, temporal factors, sources of relief
• Physiologic variables, such as age and pain tolerance
• Psychological variables, such as body image, personality, previous experience with pain, anxiety, and secondary gain
• Sociocultural variables, including culture or ethnicity, attitude, and values
• Environmental variables, such as the setting and time.

Documenting patient outcomes

Record appropriate expected outcomes on the plan of care. Possible outcomes include:
• Patient identifies pain characteristics.
• Patient articulates factors that intensify pain and modifies behavior accordingly.
• Patient expresses a feeling of comfort and relief from pain.
• Patient states and carries out appropriate interventions for pain relief.

Documenting interventions

Chart interventions related to:
• patient's description of physical pain, pain relief, and feelings about pain
• observed physical, psychological, and sociocultural responses to pain
• prescribed medication administration (include times, dates, dosages, routes, adverse effects) and comfort measures (such as massage, relaxation techniques, heat and cold applications, repositioning, distraction)
• patient's response to nursing interventions
• patient teaching (about pain and pain-relief strategies) and patient's response
• evaluation of expected outcomes.

Sexuality pattern alteration

related to illness or medical treatment

Definition

State in which an individual expresses concern about personal sexuality

Documenting assessment findings

Chart the patient's complaints and your physical assessment findings, for example:
• **Chief complaints:** reported difficulties, limitations, or changes in sexual activity and expressed behaviors or reactions, such as anger, depressed mood, noncompliance with prescribed therapies, or withdrawal from social interactions
• History of present illness
• Current treatment regimen (medications, therapies)
• Marital status, significant other
• Patient's perception of sexual identity and role
• Usual sexual activity pattern
• Patient's perception of changes in sexual activity resulting from illness or treatment

• Significance of sexual relationship to patient and spouse or significant other
• Emotional reactions (affect, mood)
• Behavioral reactions (specify).

Documenting patient outcomes
Record appropriate expected outcomes on the plan of care. Possible outcomes include:
• Patient voices feelings about potential or actual changes in sexual activity.
• Patient expresses concern about self-concept, self-esteem, or body image.
• Patient states at least one effect of illness or treatment on sexual behavior.
• Patient and spouse or significant other resume effective communication patterns.
• Patient and spouse or significant other use available counseling referrals or support groups.

Documenting interventions
Chart interventions related to:
• patient teaching (about illness and treatment)
• patient's perception of changed sexual patterns
• patient's ability to interact with others
• patient's response to treatment regimen
• referrals to counselors or support persons, such as mental health professionals, sex counselors, or illness-related support groups (I Can Cope, Reach to Recovery, Ostomy Association)
• evaluation of expected outcomes.

Skin integrity impairment, high risk for

Definition
Presence of risk factors for interruption or destruction of skin surface

Documenting assessment findings
Charted assessment findings typically relate to the following:
• History of skin problems, trauma, chronic debilitating disease, immobility
• Age
• Integumentary status, including color, elasticity, hygiene, lesions, moisture, sensation, quantity and distribution of hair, temperature and blood pressure, texture, turgor
• Musculoskeletal status, including numbness, muscle strength and mass, joint mobility, paralysis, range of motion (ROM)
• Nutritional status, including appetite, dietary intake, hydration, present weight and change from normal weight
• Hemoglobin and hematocrit values
• Serum albumin levels
• Psychosocial status, including activities of daily living, mental status, occupation (involving sun exposure), recreational activities.

Documenting patient outcomes
Record appropriate expected outcomes on the plan of care. Possible outcomes include:
• Patient experiences no skin breakdown.
• Patient maintains muscle strength and joint ROM.
• Patient sustains adequate food and fluid intake.
• Patient maintains adequate skin circulation.
• Patient communicates understanding of preventive skin care measures.
• Patient and responsible caregiver demonstrate preventive skin care measures.
• Patient and responsible caregiver correlate risk factors and preventive measures.

Documenting interventions
Chart interventions related to:
• skin condition and any changes
• repositioning patient as scheduled and ordered (including date and time)

• ambulation or active ROM exercises to improve circulation and mobility (including date and time)
• use of skin care devices and supplies (such as foam mattress, sheepskin, alternating pressure mattress, lotions and powders) and effectiveness of interventions
• nutritional intake
• hydration status
• weekly risk factor potential and score (use the Braden Scale)
• patient teaching (including the need to implement preventive measures to promote skin integrity, good personal hygiene habits, signs of skin breakdown, patient and responsible caregiver's demonstrated skill in carrying out preventive skin care measures) and patient's response
• evaluation of expected outcomes.

Sleep pattern disturbance

related to internal factors, such as illness, psychological stress, drug therapy, biorhythm disturbance

Definition
Inability to meet individual need for sleep or rest arising from internal or external factors

Documenting assessment findings
Chart the patient's complaints and your physical assessment findings, for example:
• **Chief complaints:** waking up earlier or later than desired, disorientation, irritability, lethargy, listlessness, restlessness, interrupted sleep, dark circles under eyes, frequent yawning, fleeting nystagmus, droopy eyelids, shaky hands, speech problems, difficulty falling asleep, not feeling well rested
• Age
• Daytime activity and work patterns
• Time the patient usually retires

• Number of hours of sleep patient usually requires in order to feel rested
• Problems associated with sleep, including early-morning awakening, falling asleep, nightmares, sleepwalking, staying asleep
• Quality of sleep
• Sleeping environment
• Activities associated with sleep, including bath, drink, food, medication
• Personal beliefs about sleep.

Documenting patient outcomes
Record appropriate expected outcomes on the plan of care. Possible outcomes include:
• Patient identifies factors that prevent or disrupt sleep.
• Patient sleeps _____ hours a night.
• Patient reports feeling well rested.
• Patient shows no physical signs of sleep deprivation.
• Patient exhibits no sleep-related behavioral symptoms, such as restlessness, irritability, lethargy, or disorientation.
• Patient performs relaxation exercises at bedtime.

Documenting interventions
Chart interventions related to:
• patient's complaints about sleep disturbances
• patient's report of improvement in sleep patterns
• observed physical and behavioral sleep-related disturbances
• alleviating sleep disturbances (such as pillows, bath, food or drink, reading material, TV, soft music) and patient's response
• prescribed medication and patient's response
• patient teaching (including reason for treatment, relationship of regular exercise and sleep, and relaxation techniques, such as imagery, progressive muscle relaxation, meditation)
• evaluation of expected outcomes.

Swallowing impairment

related to neuromuscular impairment

Definition
Inability to move food, fluid, or saliva from the mouth through the esophagus

Documenting assessment findings
Chart the patient's complaints and your physical assessment findings, for example:
• **Chief complaints:** choking (aspiration) spells, difficulty in swallowing, coughing, food stays in mouth and throat
• History of neuromuscular, cerebral, or respiratory disease
• Age
• Sex
• Nutritional status, including appetite, dietary intake, hydration, current weight, and change from normal weight
• Neurologic status, including cognition; gag reflex; level of consciousness; memory; motor ability; orientation; symmetry of face, mouth, and neck; sensory function; tongue movement.

Documenting patient outcomes
Record appropriate expected outcomes on the plan of care. Possible outcomes include:
• Patient shows no evidence of aspiration pneumonia.
• Patient achieves adequate nutritional intake.
• Patient maintains weight.
• Patient maintains oral hygiene.
• Patient and responsible caregiver demonstrate correct eating or feeding techniques to maximize swallowing.

Documenting interventions
Chart interventions related to:
• patient's expressed feelings about current condition
• observed swallowing impairment

• nursing interventions and patient's response (include times of turning and repositioning and degree of elevation of head during mealtimes and for 30 minutes after)
• respiratory assessments and airway suctioning (include dates and times, instances of cyanosis, dyspnea, or choking)
• daily intake and output and weight measurements
• referrals to dietitian and other health services such as speech pathology
• oral hygiene and comfort measures
• patient teaching (including instructions about positioning; dietary requirements; stimuli and feeding techniques to improve mastication, promote swallowing, and decrease aspiration; oral hygiene)
• evaluation of expected outcomes.

Tissue perfusion alteration (cardiopulmonary)

related to decreased cellular exchange

Definition
Decrease in cellular nutrition and respiration because of decreased capillary blood flow

Documenting assessment findings
Chart the patient's complaints and your physical assessment findings, for example:
• **Chief complaints:** chest pain with or without activity, cold and clammy skin, chest congestion, urination difficulties (decreased or absent), fatigue, palpitations, swollen hands or feet, shortness of breath
• Health history, including presence of diabetes mellitus, high cholesterol, hypertension, obesity, smoking, stressful lifestyle, family history of heart disease
• Neurologic status, including level of consciousness, mental status, orientation
• Cardiovascular status, including blood pressure; heart rate and rhythm; heart sounds; pe-

ripheral pulses; skin color, temperature, and turgor; hepatojugular reflux; jugular vein distention; history of congenital heart disease or valvular disorder
• Diagnostic tests, including chest X-ray, electrocardiogram (ECG), exercise ECG, echocardiogram, nuclear isotope studies, cardiac angiography
• Respiratory status, including arterial blood gas (ABG) levels, auscultation of breath sounds, respiratory rate and depth
• Renal status, including intake and output, urine specific gravity, weight
• Integumentary system, including cyanosis, pallor, peripheral edema.

Documenting patient outcomes
Record appropriate expected outcomes on the plan of care. Possible outcomes include:
• Patient attains hemodynamic stability: pulse not less than _____ beats/minute and not greater than _____ beats/minute; blood pressure not less than _____ mm Hg and not greater than _____ mm Hg.
• Patient does not exhibit arrhythmias.
• Skin remains warm and dry.
• Patient's heart rate remains within prescribed limits while he carries out activities of daily living.
• Patient maintains adequate cardiac output.
• Patient modifies lifestyle to minimize risk of decreased tissue perfusion.

Documenting interventions
Chart interventions related to:
• patient's perception of health problems and health needs
• observed physical findings (including heart rate, blood pressure, central venous pressure, pulse rate, temperature, skin coloration, respiratory rate, and breath sounds)
• observed response to activity
• test procedures (including ECG to monitor heart rate and rhythm and results of creatine kinase, lactate dehydrogenase, and ABG analysis)

• prescribed medication administration and oxygen therapy (including dates, times, dosages, routes, adverse effects, equipment, and supplies)
• patient positioning and repositioning to enhance vital capacity and to avoid lung congestion and skin breakdown
• patient teaching (including information about a low-fat, low-cholesterol diet; nitroglycerin or other medications; adverse reactions to medications; activity level; stress management; risk factors for heart and lung disease; the need to avoid straining with bowel movements; and benefits of quitting smoking)
• evaluation of expected outcomes.

Urinary elimination pattern alteration

related to sensory or neuromuscular impairment

Definition
Alteration or impairment of urinary function

Documenting assessment findings
Chart the patient's complaints and your physical assessment findings, for example:
• **Chief complaints:** reported dysuria, frequency, hesitancy, incontinence, nocturia, retention, or urgency
• History of urinary tract disease, trauma, surgery, or infection
• History of sensory or neuromuscular impairment
• Vital signs
• Genitourinary status, including characteristics of urine, cystometry, pain or discomfort, palpation of bladder, postcatheterization problems, presence and amount of residual urine, use of urinary assistive devices, urinalysis, voiding pattern

• Fluid and electrolyte status, including blood urea nitrogen, creatinine, inspection of mucous membranes, intake and output, serum electrolytes, skin turgor, urine specific gravity
• Neuromuscular status, including degree of neuromuscular function present, motor ability to start and stop urinary stream, sensory ability to perceive bladder fullness
• Sexuality status, including capability, concerns, habits, sexual partner
• Psychosocial status, including coping skills, family or significant other, patient's perception of health problem, self-concept, stressors (finances, job).

Documenting patient outcomes
Record appropriate expected outcomes on the plan of care. Possible outcomes include:
• Patient maintains fluid balance; intake equals output.
• Patient voices increased comfort.
• Complications are avoided or minimized.
• Patient and responsible caregiver demonstrate skill in managing urinary elimination problem.
• Patient discusses impact of urologic disorder on self and others.
• Patient and responsible caregiver identify resources to assist with care after discharge.

Documenting interventions
Chart interventions related to:
• observed neuromuscular and urologic status
• patient's expression of concern about the urologic problem and its impact on body image and lifestyle; patient's motivation to participate in self-care
• intake and output, fluid replacement therapy
• medication administration
• bladder training (including times and dates of commode use, Kegel exercises to strengthen sphincter)
• intermittent catheterization (record dates, times, volume eliminated spontaneously, volume eliminated via catheter, bladder balance)

• external catheterization of male patient (include time and date of condom catheter application and changes, supplies used, skin condition of penis)
• indwelling urinary catheterization (include time and date of catheter insertion and changes, condition and care of urinary meatus, kind of drainage system, volume drained)
• suprapubic catheterization (including time and date of catheter insertion and changes, dressing changes, kind of drainage system, supplies used)
• supportive care measures, their effectiveness, and patient's response (including pain control and hydration)
• patient teaching (including teaching about signs and symptoms of full bladder, home catheterization techniques and management, signs and symptoms of autonomic dysreflexia, management of autonomic dysreflexia, emergency measures)
• referrals of patient and responsible caregiver to counselors and support groups
• evaluation of expected outcomes.

Verbal communication impairment
related to decreased circulation to brain

Definition
Decreased ability to speak, understand, or use words appropriately

Documenting assessment findings
Chart the patient's complaints and your physical assessment findings, for example:
• **Chief complaints:** reported or observed disorientation; dyspnea; impaired articulation; reported inability or lack of desire to speak, to identify objects, to modulate speech, to name words, or to speak in sentences; incessant verbalization, phonation difficulties, stuttering or slurring

• Neurologic status, including level of consciousness, orientation, cognition, memory (recent and remote), insight, and judgment
• Speech characteristics, including pattern (garbled, incomprehensible, difficulty forming words), language and vocabulary, level of comprehension and expression, ability to use other forms of communication (eye blinks, gestures, pictures, nods)
• Motor ability
• Circulatory status, including a history of cardiac and circulatory problems, pulse, and blood pressure
• Respiratory status, including dyspnea and use of accessory muscles.

Documenting patient outcomes

Record appropriate expected outcomes on the plan of care. Possible outcomes include:
• Staff consistently meets patient's needs.
• Patient and responsible caregiver communicate at satisfactory level.
• Patient maintains orientation.
• Patient maintains effective level of communication.
• Patient answers direct questions correctly.

Documenting interventions

Chart interventions related to:
• patient's current level of communication, orientation, and satisfaction with communication efforts
• changes in speech pattern or level of orientation
• observed speech deficits, expressiveness and receptiveness, and ability to communicate
• diagnostic test results
• supplies or equipment used to promote orientation (TV, radio, calendars, reality orientation boards)
• promoting effective communication and patient's response
• evaluation of expected outcomes.

Index

A

B

t refers to a table.

C

t refers to a table.

D

t refers to a table.

t refers to a table.

t refers to a table.

I

t refers to a table.

t refers to a table.

J

K

t refers to a table.

L

Lavage, peritoneal, documentation of, 253
Lawsuits against nurses. *See* Malpractice lawsuits.
Lawyers. *See* Attorneys.
Learning needs, patient's
  documenting on initial assessment forms, 198-199
  JCAHO requirements for in initial assessment, 194-195
Learning outcomes
  examples of for chronic renal failure, 223
  how to write concise, 99t
  in outcome documentation system, 97
  writing clear, 223t
Legal process, summary of, 324-325
Legally perilous charting practices. *See* Charting.
Length of hospitalization, effect on documentation, 11
Liability, guarding against, 3
Liability insurance. *See* Insurance, liability.
Licensed practical nurses, code of ethics for, 37
Licensed vocational nurses, code of ethics for, 37
Licensure, role of medical record in, 4
Living wills, 33-35
  filing, 35
  health care facility requirements, 34
  statutory requirements, 33-34
Long-term care settings
  documentation methods in, 160-176
    activities of daily living (ADL) checklists or flow sheets, 162, 175
    effect of regulatory bodies, 161
    guidelines, 175-176
    HCFA requirements, 161
    initial nursing assessment form, 162
    internal documents, 175
    Medicaid requirements, 161
    Medicare requirements, 161
    Minimum Data Set (MDS) form, 162-167
    nursing summaries, 162
    OBRA requirements, 161
    plans of care, 175
    preadmission screening annual resident review (PASARR) form, 162, 169-174
    resident assessment protocol (RAP) form, 162, 168
    standard and required documents, 161-175
  documentation requirements in, 11
LPNs. *See* Licensed practical nurses.
Lumbar puncture, documentation of, 260
LVNs. *See* Licensed vocational nurses.

t refers to a table.

M

Malpractice insurance. *See* Insurance, liability.
Malpractice lawsuits, against nurses, 17-18, 313-330
  attorney's pretrial role, 323-326
  complaint, 29
  courtroom hearings, 30-31
    judge's role, 30-31
    jury's role, 31
    role of documentation, 30
  damage and causation, 18
  defending yourself on the witness stand, 327-330
  discovery, 29-30
    deposition, 29
    interrogatories, 29-30
  duty and breach of duty, 17-18
  not charted, not done, 30-31
  nurse's pretrial role, 314-323
    dealing with insurer, 319, 321-322
    examining the records, 322-323
    finding an attorney, 322
    preserving the medical record, 317, 319
    protecting your property, 323
    settling out of court, 319
    understanding subpoenas, 314-315
  preliminary steps in, 28
  preparations for adjudication, 28-29
  settling out of court, 319
  spotlight on documentation in court, 316-317
  surviving the deposition, 326-327
  understanding the legal process, 324-325
  why nurses are sued, 315
Malpractice lawsuits, examples of actual cases
  breach of duty, 17-18
  care too late, 316
  damage and causation, 18
  deficient policy and procedures manuals, 302
  failing to monitor and review the record, 19
  failure to chart, 302
  failure to use restraints effectively, 290
  inadequate care, 316
  insufficient information, 317
  lax assessment, 316
  missing records, 298
  not charted, not done, 31
  standard of care set by facility's policy, 18-20
  tampering with medical record, 317, 319
Management, nursing, JCAHO standards for, 353
MAR. *See* Medication administration record.

O

t refers to a table.

P

t refers to a table.

t refers to a table.

Index

t refers to a table.

R

t refers to a table.

Index

S

t refers to a table.

t refers to a table.